Experimental Design for Laboratory Biologists

Maximising Information and Improving Reproducibility

Specifically intended for lab-based biomedical researchers, this practical guide shows how to design experiments that are reproducible, with low bias, high precision, and results that are widely applicable. With specific examples from research, using both cell cultures and model organisms, it explores key ideas in experimental design, assesses common designs, and shows how to plan a successful experiment. It demonstrates how to control biological and technical factors that can introduce bias or add noise, and covers rarely discussed topics such as graphical data exploration, choosing outcome variables, data quality control checks, and data preprocessing. It also shows how to use R for analysis, and is designed for those with no prior experience. An accompanying website (https://stanlazic.github.io/EDLB.html) includes all R code, data sets, and the labstats R package.

This is an ideal guide for anyone conducting lab-based biological research, from students to principal investigators working either in academia or industry.

Stanley E. Lazic holds a PhD in neuroscience and a Masters in computational biology from the University of Cambridge and has conducted research at Oxford, Cambridge, and Harvard. He has written several papers on reproducible research and on the design and analysis of biological experiments and has published in *Science* and *Nature*. He is currently a Team Leader in Quantitative Biology (Statistics) at AstraZeneca.

Experimental Design for Laboratory Biologists

Maximising Information and Improving Reproducibility

STANLEY E. LAZIC

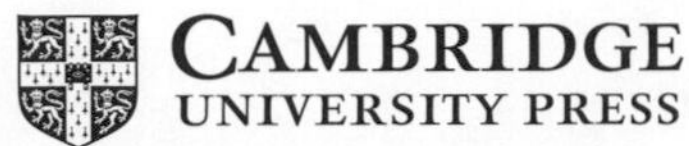
CAMBRIDGE
UNIVERSITY PRESS

CAMBRIDGE
UNIVERSITY PRESS

University Printing House, Cambridge CB2 8BS, United Kingdom

Cambridge University Press is part of the University of Cambridge.

It furthers the University's mission by disseminating knowledge in the pursuit of education, learning and research at the highest international levels of excellence.

www.cambridge.org
Information on this title: www.cambridge.org/9781107074293

First published 2016

Printed in the United Kingdom by TJ International Ltd., Padstow, Cornwall

A catalogue record for this publication is available from the British Library

ISBN 978-1-107-07429-3 Hardback
ISBN 978-1-107-42488-3 Paperback

Additional resources for this publication at https://stanlazic.github.io/EDLB.html

To my teachers and mentors

Contents

Preface

Everything of importance has been said before by somebody who did not discover it.
Alfred North Whitehead

Everything that needs to be said has already been said. But since no one was listening, everything must be said again.
André Gide

True to the above quotes, most of this book's contents have appeared in print before, but often where biologists are unlikely to look – statistics journals and books, and methods papers in other fields. My task is to translate ideas known to statisticians into the language of experimental biology.[1] With a background in both biology (BSc, PhD, postdoc) and data analysis (MPhil in Computational Biology and over seven years working as a preclinical statistician in the pharmaceutical industry), hopefully I am fluent enough in both languages to perform a successful translation.[2]

The contents of this book have little overlap with other statistics-for-biologists books because they mostly focus on statistical analysis. Analysis is but one step of the scientific workflow (Figure 0.1), and before you can analyse data you need to do an experiment. This requires planning, good execution, and quality control checks. These critical topics are rarely taught to biologists, who are expected to learn them on their own. The consequence of this approach is predictable; some biologists obtain the necessary skills, but many do not. This book focuses on the first three steps of the scientific workflow, and data analysis is briefly discussed in Chapter 4.

This book was written to improve the quality of research conducted in academic, government, and industrial labs and institutions. Scientists and funders now recognise that bias and irreproducibility are undermining preclinical biomedical research [2, 5, 28, 30, 42, 80, 83, 84, 123, 172, 240, 251, 305, 316, 342]. There are many reasons why experiments cannot be reproduced (discussed in Chapter 1) and this book focuses on the role that experimental design and data analysis have on making results reproducible.

[1] The term *biology* refers to laboratory-based experimental biology throughout. 'Field biologists' also conduct experiments, and most statistics-for-biologists books target this audience.

[2] There are some novel ideas here, such as the distinction between front-aligned and end-aligned designs (Section 2.11) and the distinction between biological, experimental, and observational units, to replace the biological versus technical replicate distinction (all of Chapter 3).

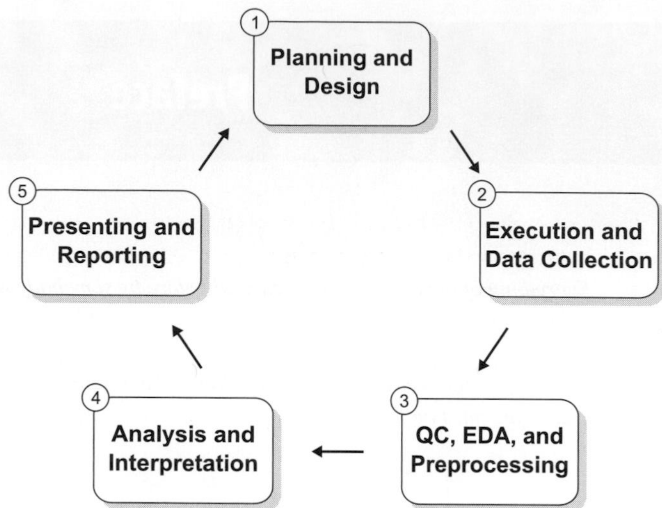

Fig. 0.1 The scientific workflow. This book focuses on steps 1–3. QC = quality control; EDA = exploratory data analysis.

Prerequisites

This book is for experimental biologists, at any level, conducting basic research or with an applied, clinical, or translational focus. Knowledge covered in an introductory statistics-for-biologists course is assumed, and concepts like the standard deviation and common statistical tests such as the t-test, analysis of variance (ANOVA), regression, and correlation should be familiar. It is fine if some time has passed since you formally covered these topics. Mathematical proofs are not included and equations are kept to a minimum, but given the subject, are unavoidable. The emphasis is on the ideas, concepts, and principles, and how to implement them. Hand calculations are unnecessary because statistical software is available.

Quantitative researchers who analyse biological data such as statisticians, bioinformaticians, and computational biologists might also find this book useful. Topics of interest include sources of heterogeneity and confounding in biological experiments (Section 2.12), quality control checks for biological data (Section 6.1), and understanding which types of replication address biologically interesting questions (Chapter 3).

The freely available R statistics language is used for data analysis and graphs.[3] Prior knowledge is useful, but not required. The Appendix gives a brief introduction to R and the examples in the main text assume familiarity with this material. The topics however can be followed without learning or using R. The data sets can be found in the `labstats` package on CRAN[4] and R code can be downloaded from GitHub.[5]

[3] Available at `www.r-project.com`

[4] `https://cran.r-project.org/web/packages/labstats/`

[5] `https://stanlazic.github.io/EDLB.html`

The key prerequisite to derive maximum value from this book is experience conducting biological experiments and analysing the subsequent data – and the more experience the better!

How to read this book

Chapters 1–5 should be read in order as later material depends on earlier ideas, but Chapter 6 on Exploratory Data Analysis can be read at any time. Chapters 1–3 contain no R code, but for Chapters 4–6 sitting in front of a computer and running the code will reinforce the ideas.

Ideas or concepts discussed in detail later in the book will inevitably have to be mentioned earlier. To avoid excessive cross-referencing, the glossary lists the page where the main discussion of the entry is located (if there is one). For example, the term *experimental unit* is mentioned for the first time in this preface, but is discussed extensively in Section 3.2. The glossary entry for this term provides a short definition and indicates that further information can be found on page 96.

Typographical conventions

`Constant width font` is used for R code, R output, and when referring to R functions or objects. Lines of code entered by the user start with '>' or '+'. These symbols do not need to be entered, only the code that follows them. A sign like the one in the margin draws attention to a warning, a key point, a subtlety with R, or a concept that is often misunderstood.

Acknowledgements

This book has benefited greatly from comments by Maarten van Dijk, Irmgard Amrein, and especially Lutz Slomianka. Pierre Farmer and Miguel Camargo also provided constructive feedback on earlier drafts. My wife, Brynn, has read every word in this book, which is beyond the call of duty, and her comments have improved it immensely. I also thank her for her support, well, at least until page 305, at which point she declared, 'You should stop now; no one wants to read that much about statistics.' I didn't always follow everyone's good advice, but I am grateful for their input.

Katrina Halliday and Jade Scard at Cambridge University Press were a pleasure to work with and made the whole process easy and enjoyable. I also thank Judith Shaw for her expert copy-editing. Finally, I would like to thank the developers and contributors of the free software R, Emacs, LaTeX, JabRef, knitr, and Inkscape, which I used to write this book.

S.E. Lazic
Cambridge, 2016

Abbreviations

AIPE	Accuracy in parameter estimation
ALS	Amyotrophic lateral scterosis
ANCOVA	Analysis of covariance
ANOVA	Analysis of variance
AUC	Area under the curve
BMI	Body mass index
BU	Biological unit
CCC	Concordance correlation coefficient
CCLE	Cancer Cell Line Encyclopedia
CI	Confidence (frequentist) or Credible (Bayesian) interval
CRAN	Comprehensive R archive network
CRD	Completely randomised design
CSF	Cerebrospinal fluid
CSR	Complete spatial randomness
CV	Coefficient of variation
DAMP	Damage-associated molecular pattern
df	Degrees of freedom
DoE	Design of experiments
DS	Diallyl sulfide
ED50	Median (half) effective dose
EDA	Exploratory data analysis
ES	Effect size
ESS	Emacs Speaks Statistics
EU	Experimental unit
FORE-SCI	Facilities of Research Excellence – Spinal Cord Injury
FOV	Field of view
GI	Gastrointestinal
GLM	Generalised linear model
GUI	Graphical user interface
Gst	Glutathione-S-transferase
HARKing	Hypothesising after the results are known
HSD	Honestly significant difference
ICC	Intraclass correlation coefficient
i.p.	Intraperitoneally
IQR	Interquartile range

KO	Knock out
LME	Linear mixed-effects model
LOD	Limit of detection
LSD	Least significant difference
MAD	Median absolute deviation
MAR	Missing at random
MCAR	Missing completely at random
MED	Minimum effective dose
MNAR	Missing not a random
NGS	Next generation sequencing
NHST	Null hypothesis significance testing
NIH	National Institutes of Health (USA)
NINDS	American National Institute of Neurological Disorders and Stroke
OU	Observational unit
PCA	Principal components analysis
PI	Principal investigator
PK	Pharmokinetic
QC	Quality control
QRP	Questionable research practice
qPCR	Quantitative polymerase chain reaction
RE	Relative efficiency
RIN	RNA integrity number
RM-ANOVA	Repeated measures analysis of variance
SAP	Statistical analysis plan
SD	Standard deviation
SEM	Standard error of the mean
siRNA	small interfering RNA
SNP	Single nucleotide polymorphism
SOD1	Superoxide dismutase 1 (gene)
SS	Sum of squares
RSS	Residual sum of squares
SUTVA	Stable unit-treatment value assumption
TSS	Total sum of squares
VPA	Valproic acid
WT	Wild type

1 Introduction

To consult the statistician after an experiment is finished is often merely to ask him to conduct a post mortem examination. He can perhaps say what the experiment died of.
Sir Ronald A. Fisher, FRS

Many experiments fail because the data collectors have not been properly trained and many statisticians have their own horror stories to illustrate this.
John A. Nelder, FRS

Modeling is sometimes regarded as primarily a task for subject matter specialists, but in most fields requisite knowledge and understanding of statistics remains thinly spread.
Arthur P. Dempster

This chapter begins by defining reproducibility and discussing non-statistical – mainly psychological – sources of experimental bias. The next section assesses the quality of the published literature and discusses statistical sources of bias. The discussion will be familiar if you have been following the 'reproducibility crisis' over the past several years. The above topics are included to stimulate reflection about your own research practices and to bring together ideas that have been discussed in separate disciplines. The chapter ends with a refresher on statistical inference and a discussion on statistics software.

1.1 What is reproducibility?

An experiment is reproducible when subsequent experiments, by the same or different scientists, confirm the results. The terms *repeatability* and *replicability* are sometimes used interchangeably or with related meanings, but we will use reproducibility as an all-encompassing term. Reproducibility can occur at several levels.[1]

Analytical: Analytical or computational reproducibility refers to obtaining the same results using the original data and a description of the analysis. This is a minimum standard but is impossible to achieve when the data are unavailable. Even if the data are provided in the supplementary material or in public databases, reproducing the results may be hard if the description of the analysis is incomplete [173]. A minimum

[1] Adapted from a report on reproducibiliy by the American Society for Cell Biology: `http://www.ascb.org/reproducibility`

requirement for analytical reproducibility is to provide the data underlying the results and the scripts that produced them. This is simple when using R because the code can be integrated into documents such as reports and publications. For example, large portions of this book have embedded R code, which is evaluated, and then the outputs are inserted into the text document. The `knitr` and `rmarkdown` R packages make this process straightforward [402].

Direct: Direct reproducibility refers to obtaining the same results using the same experimental conditions, materials, and methods as the original experiment. The aim is to make the second experiment as similar as possible to the original, which requires an adequate description of how the original experiment was conducted. Direct replication is the focus of this book, but it may not be immediately clear how better experimental designs can improve direct reproducibility. The brief answer is that a well-designed experiment (1) can isolate the effects of interest from other factors that may influence the outcome, (2) replicates the right aspect of the experiment, and (3) can generalise the results to other times, places, conditions, and samples.

Systematic: Systematic reproducibility refers to obtaining the same results, but under different conditions; for example, using another cell line or mouse strain, or inhibiting a gene pharmacologically instead of genetically. Reasons for a lack of systematic reproducibility are harder to determine because the cell lines might be dissimilar, and what works in one will not work in another. This should not be taken as evidence of poor research practices, and one function of subsequent studies is to find the conditions under which an initial finding holds. Experimental design can help here too, as initial studies can be designed to address the question of generalisability early on.

Conceptual: Conceptual reproducibility refers to obtaining the same general results under diverse conditions, where the aim is to demonstrate the validity of a concept or a finding using another paradigm. The general concept or hypothesis might be 'stress inhibits memory formation', which could be tested in one experiment where people memorise word pairs with loud music playing and in another experiment where rats learn the location of food pellets after a corticosterone injection (a stress hormone). There are many valid reasons why some experiments support the hypothesis and others not – maybe corticosterone, while part of the stress response, is irrelevant for learning. Discrepancies between the results of such experiments do not necessarily indicate poor reproducibility.

A reproducible result was defined above as one that is confirmed by subsequent experiments, but what does *confirmed* mean? One idea is that if the original experiment has a p-value below 0.05, then the experiment is confirmed if the subsequent experiment also has a significant p-value. Although this criterion seems plausible, it has several problems. First, a study with a p-value of 0.03 would be considered irreproducible if the subsequent experiment had a p-value of 0.08. But for all practical purposes the studies may have the same effect sizes and their two confidence intervals (CIs) may overlap substantially. This relationship is shown in Figure 1.1 between the original experiment and the second experiment, New 1. A second problem is that this approach ignores the sample size and power of the experiments. Suppose that a power analysis was conducted based on the results of

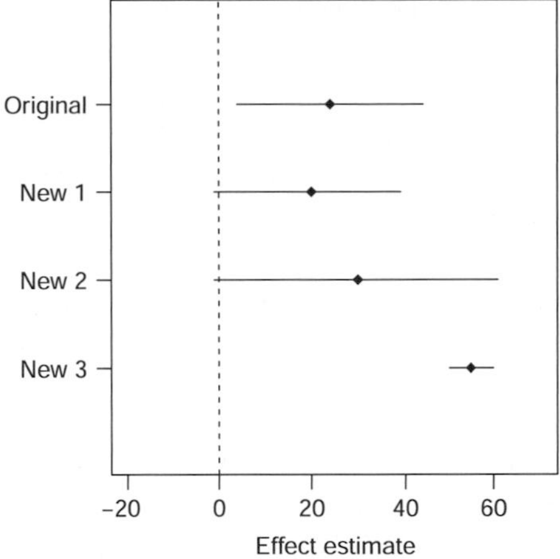

Fig. 1.1 Effect sizes and 95% CI for an original experiment and three follow-up experiments. Using significance as a criterion for reproducibility, only New 3 would be considered to reproduce the original finding, despite the different effect size.

the original experiment and the follow-up experiment uses a slightly smaller sample size and therefore the confidence intervals will be slightly wider, assuming everything else is constant (New 2 in Figure 1.1). Even though the effect size for New 2 is larger than the original, New 2 would not have reproduced the original findings by this criterion. A third problem is that a follow-up study may have a different effect size than the original but would be considered to have successfully reproduced the original if the p-value is significant. This situation is shown for experiment New 3, where the 95% CIs do not overlap with those of the original experiment. There is no agreed criteria for when one experiment can be said to reproduce another, but within a field, scientists 'know it when they see it'.

1.2 The psychology of scientific discovery

It is uncommon for a book on experimental design to discuss psychological aspects of research, but scientific investigations are not conducted in a vacuum; they take place in the context of previous research, are conducted by people who prefer certain outcomes over others, and are constrained by standards and conventions used by research groups and the wider scientific community. Expectations and desires of the researcher and external pressures to publish and to demonstrate creativity and innovation influence how data are analysed, interpreted, and reported. This needs to be acknowledged and discussed because improving reproducibility and 'making more published research true' [172] – one of the aims of this book – cannot be achieved by only improving scientists' maths skills.

Some of the topics discussed below fall within the 'heuristics and biases' field of psychological research. Cognitive biases or cognitive illusions are deviations from true or optimal answers or responses when making estimations, inferences, decisions, conclusions, or judgements [312]. They are cognitive in that they result from perceptual or cognitive

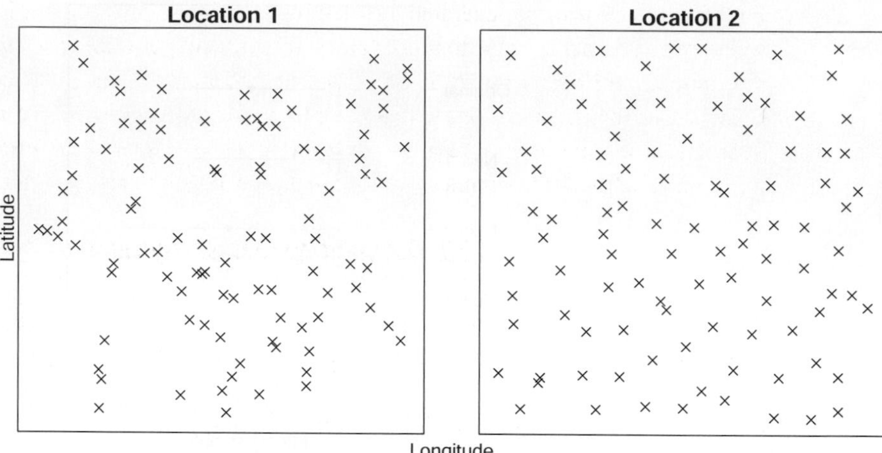

Fig. 1.2 Positions of bombs dropped for two geographic locations. Which location represents the uniform random bombing strategy?

processes instead of, for example, an uncalibrated measuring device. They are also systematic, meaning that the deviations tend to be in a certain direction. They are also hard to avoid. Cognitive biases can influence the design, analysis, interpretation, and reporting of biological experiments and are therefore relevant for scientific investigations. Several such biases are described below, with an emphasis on how they apply to experimentation and statistical inference. Methods for avoiding them are also suggested.

1.2.1 Seeing patterns in randomness

People often see patterns where none exist, including clusters, associations between variables, and sequences of similar values. A fictitious example is given in Figure 1.2. The positions (latitude and longitude) of 100 bombs dropped during a World War II bombing campaign are shown for two different geographic locations. The General wants to know if the enemy is dropping bombs at random, or if they are targeting certain positions more heavily, and he asks you to investigate. Intelligence from the front line indicates that *if* the enemy is using a random strategy, they will randomly sample a pair of latitude and longitude coordinates with equal probability anywhere within the bombing region – known as a uniform random bombing strategy.[2] Was a uniform random bombing strategy used at either of the locations in Figure 1.2? If so, which one? Furthermore, is there evidence at either location for certain positions to be bombed more heavily while others are avoided, possibly reflecting the strategic importance of the positions?

Many would say that the distribution of points at Location 2 represents the strategy of randomly picking a latitude and longitude from a uniform distribution. The positions for

[2] The name arises from sampling latitude and longitude positions from a uniform distribution, where all values between an upper and lower boundary have an equal probability of being chosen.

Location 2 were instead generated by selecting a 10-by-10 grid of equally spaced positions, and then adding some noise to these values. This makes the bomb positions evenly spaced. The random uniform strategy is only used at Location 1. This appears counter-intuitive because there are large regions with no bombs, while other regions have a denser clustering. Such clustering and empty regions are to be expected under a uniform random strategy. Intuition about what randomness looks like does not come easily or naturally.

1.2.2 Not wanting to miss anything

Potentially meaningful patterns like the above example can be formally tested with a statistical analyses, but it is important to avoid using the same data to first find an interesting pattern (such as the lower left empty region of Location 1 in Figure 1.2), and then to statistically test for this pattern. For example, we might try to calculate the probability of seeing no bombs dropped in an area the size of the empty lower left region. Random data – especially if there is a lot of it – will have local regularities and patterns. Picking out one such pattern that catches our attention and then performing a statistical test has implicitly performed many informal tests, in that all of the patterns that *could have been* interesting were examined and discarded without a formal test. For example, it does not appear that more bombs were dropped at higher latitudes compared with lower latitudes (comparing the top versus the bottom half of Location 1). If such a pattern did appear to exist, then we would test that instead. The key principle is: *if a hypothesis is derived from the data, then the ability of the data to support that hypothesis is diminished.* The ability of the data to support a hypothesis can also be compromised by what others do. For example, a PhD student is the first person to analyse a data set and explores it thoroughly. He finds a relationship but is unsure of the appropriate statistical test and so brings it to the principal investigator's (PI) attention. The PI then conducts only one analysis and feels confident that the p-value is valid, because she is unaware of how the data were used to discover this relationship.

Even when a visual-driven inspection of the data is not so pronounced, people want to make the most of the data and to avoid missing anything interesting. This desire is likely greater when the primary result is not significant and then we have to see 'what else we can get out of the data'. One might begin to look for correlations between variables, then again after normalising or correcting for other variables. Then checking for differences between sexes, or the old versus the young, or the less severely affected compared to the most affected, and so on until there are enough interesting findings to report. On the one hand, it seems foolish not to thoroughly examine the data, given all of the work that went into generating it. On the other hand, such a search process can generate many false positives.

There are two approaches to limit the number of false positive results that arise from data-driven discoveries. The first is to divide the analyses into confirmatory and exploratory parts. The confirmatory analysis specifies everything in advance (before seeing the data), including the hypothesis to be tested, the main outcome variable, and the analysis that will be used. The subsequent exploratory analysis allows for greater flexibility to find other relationships of interest, but with the knowledge that the findings carry less weight and are less convincing because they were not predicted in advance, even if attempts have been made to correct for multiple testing. The second approach is to validate the findings, either by conducting a subsequent experiment, or by dividing the data into two parts. Once the experiment is complete, but before any analysis, about 20–30% of the data are removed and locked away. The remaining data are used to find interesting relationships. Once the analysis is complete, the data that were locked away are used to confirm the findings. This is a common approach in the data mining, machine learning, and predictive modelling fields, but it does require enough samples to split into two sets.

People differ in how easily they detect signals in pure noise, find patterns in randomness, or meaning in the coincidental. A sign of 'inferential maturity' is to know where you lie on the spectrum. If you find anything vaguely resembling an association or effect interesting and tend to believe that it is 'real', then pay attention to controlling false positives. If instead you are sceptical and find only large associations or effects convincing, then you risk not further exploring small but true findings.

1.2.3 Psychological cliff at $p = 0.05$

One criticism of p-values is that they encourage dichotomous thinking – the effect or relationship is either significant or it is not – even though evidence is continuous.[3] In the 1960s, Rosenthal and Gaito showed that such a psychological effect exists. They asked psychology researchers and graduate students to rate their degree of belief or confidence in a research hypothesis with p-values ranging from 0.001 to 0.90. They found a 'psychological cliff' at $p = 0.05$ – an abrupt jump in confidence just below 0.05 [331, 332]. A replication experiment by Poitevineau and Lecoutre provided a more nuanced view [313]. They found a strong cliff effect, but only in a subset of subjects; others had a linear or exponentially decreasing confidence as the p-values increased (Figure 1.3).

The cliff effect likely contributes to another misinterpretation of statistical results, which Gelman and Stern have phrased as 'The difference between "significant" and "not significant" is not itself statistically significant' [132]. They are referring to a situation where, for example, Group A is significantly different from the control group, Group B is not significantly different from the control group, and then an incorrect conclusion is made that Group A is significantly different from Group B. If differences between Group A and B are of interest, then they need to be compared directly against each other.

To the extent that a small p-value provides evidence for a research hypothesis, there is no sharp evidential distinction between 0.04 and 0.06. An obvious question is 'What is the correct relationship between a p-value and evidence for a hypothesis?' The short answer is that there is no correct relationship because a p-value says nothing about hypotheses and so the question makes no sense. If you are interested in evidence or the probability that a hypothesis is correct, then likelihood or Bayesian methods are required. These are beyond the scope of this book but good introductions can be found in references [50, 95, 139, 201–204, 269].

[3] Technically, a p-value does *not* provide evidence against a hypothesis. Informally, however, a smaller p-value suggests that an effect is present. The interpretation of a p-value is discussed in Section 1.4.

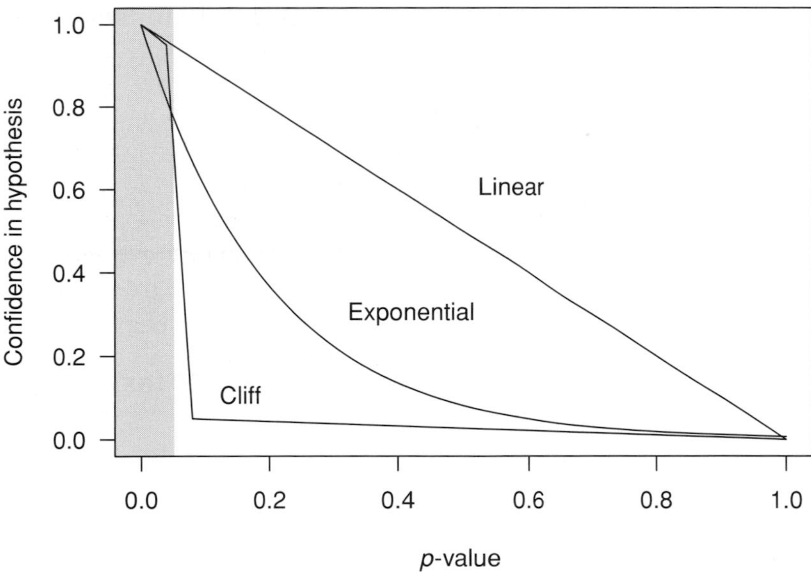

Fig. 1.3 Confidence from p-values. A schematic diagram from Poitevineau and Lecoutre [313]. The confidence in a hypothesis drops rapidly just past $p = 0.05$ for some people. Shaded area is $p < 0.05$.

The key point is that there is nothing special about 0.05, or values on either side, that indicates an abrupt change in what the data have to say about a hypothesis. Gelman and Loken raise two related points about interpreting statistical results [130]. The first is that effects cannot be divided into those that are 'real' and those that are 'not real', based on a p-value. The presence and magnitude of effects and associations are conditional on (1) the sample material used, (2) background variables and conditions (such as laboratory equipment and experimenter), (3) the experimental design (was a blocking factor incorporated), and (4) data preprocessing and the statistical analysis. Since the (true) magnitude of an effect or association is always conditional on so many factors it makes sense to consider how the effect or association varies across diverse situations. Under some conditions the effect may be smaller and the p-value above 0.05, and this does not imply a lack of reproducibility.

Their second point is that the statistical analysis does not determine whether an effect is 'real', just as microscopes do not determine whether bacteria are real, but both microscopes and statistics can help one see things that are not obvious with the naked eye. Effects are determined by the biological process under investigation, the experiment used to probe it, and the data derived from it. Occasionally, effects are so large and clear that no statistical analysis is necessary. When the experiment is more complex and the results less obvious, a statistical analysis only helps one to interpret what is already there. Interpretation of the results may differ depending on the analysis, but so too may a conclusion about a phenomenon depending on the microscope (e.g. light, confocal, or electron). Do not believe a result just because 'the statistics said. . . '.

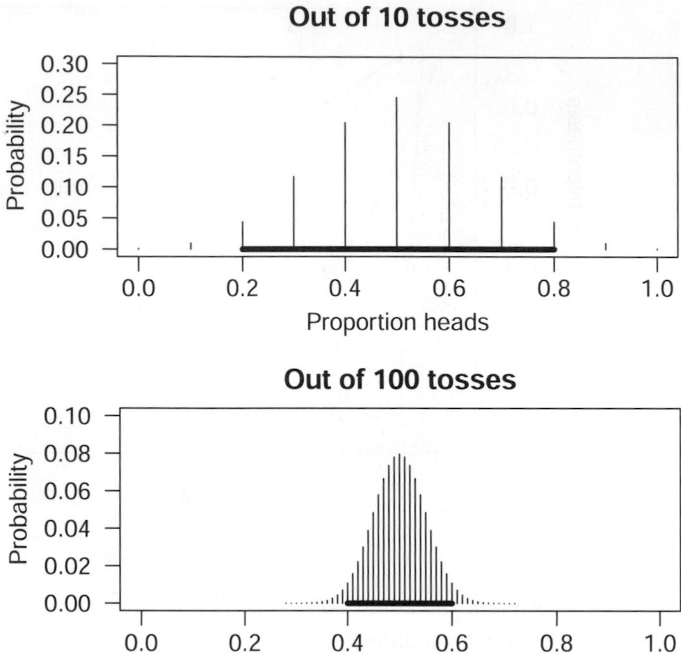

Fig. 1.4 Sampling variability and its dependence on sample size. When tossing a coin 10 times, we expect the proportion of heads to be 0.5, but it would not be unusual to obtain a proportion between 0.2 and 0.8 (thick black line on the *x*-axis). When tossing a coin 100 times (larger sample size), the range of likely values for the proportion is narrower, between 0.4 and 0.6.

1.2.4 Neglect of sampling variability

Sampling variability is the reason that the outcome of a random process differs from run to run. If a fair coin is tossed 10 times, we would expect, on average, five heads and five tails. On any given trial we may get more or less heads, but we would expect most tosses to have between two and eight heads. Rephrasing, the expected proportion of heads is 0.5, with the majority between 0.2 and 0.8. This is sampling variability: we do not always get five heads, and is illustrated in Figure 1.4. Furthermore, as the sample size increases, the variability in the outcome decreases. When the sample size is increased to 100 tosses, we still expect the proportion of heads to be 0.5, but now the majority will lie between 0.4 and 0.6 – a narrower interval. This is the dependence on sample size: the larger the sample size, the narrower the interval of values that we are likely to see. As the sample size increases, we converge to the true proportion of heads when tossing a fair coin. These simple ideas appear often and can lead to incorrect inferences and conclusions if not taken into account. Some examples are discussed below.

Wainer provides two real-world examples [384]. In his first example he shows a map of kidney cancer death rates in the USA, with the top (worst) 10% of counties highlighted.

Counties with high death rates tend to be rural and in the west or midwest, and one might speculate that people in these regions have unhealthy lifestyles or less access to high quality medical care, leading to higher death rates. The interesting twist is that if the counties with the *lowest* 10% of death rates are plotted, they also tend to be in the west or midwest. Counties with the highest and lowest rates are often right beside each other! What is going on? Counties in the west and midwest are sparsely populated, so the addition or subtraction of a few cases will have a larger influence on the cancer rate than in a larger population. Just as in the coin example above, with a small sample size the value of whatever is calculated will fluctuate more widely around the true value. Thus, sparsely populated counties are over-represented at both ends of the death rate distribution.

Wainer's second example discusses the billions of dollars wasted on supporting smaller schools in the USA by educational charities. Smaller schools tend to outperform larger schools on student achievement, and so a logical conclusion is that if larger schools were split into several smaller ones, then student achievement would increase. However, smaller schools are expected to be over-represented in both the top and bottom of the achievement distribution, and that is what Wainer found. Again, with a small sample size (number of students), achievement results will have a wider spread and therefore the tails of the distributions will mostly contain smaller schools.

This phenomenon of larger variances with smaller sample sizes is also relevant for biological experiments. The following situation is often seen in high-throughput screening experiments. The data are simulated, but the example is from a real experiment. Suppose 5000 compounds are tested in a cellular assay and the goal is to find compounds that increase the number of cells expressing a key protein marker. Cells are plated in high-density microtitre plates and images are taken after treatment with the compounds. The total number of cells and the number of cells positive for the marker (which is a subset of the total cell count) are obtained from the images. There are no active compounds in this simulation and so the results are what would be expected from random fluctuations. The distribution of total cell counts across all 5000 wells is shown in Figure 1.5A. The average number of cells per well is 122, but it ranges from 3 to 425. The distribution of positive cell counts across the 5000 wells is shown in 1.5B. The number of positive cells is related to the total number of cells (Figure 1.5C), and the proportion (or percentage) of positive cells is calculated by dividing the number of positive cells by the total number of cells (Figure 1.5D). The proportion was calculated because it supposedly removes the dependence on total cell count. The mean proportion is 0.25 and the range is 0 to 0.8 (the few high values are hard to see in this graph). A cut-off is made based on some criterion such as three standard deviations above the mean of the distribution (dashed line in Figure 1.5D), and all compounds above that are considered 'hits' and will be tested in further experiments. The criterion or threshold used to determine a hit is not important for this example.

Figure 1.5E shows how the *variation* in the proportion of positive cells is dependent on the total cell count, even though the mean no longer is. When cell counts are low, variation is high, and vice versa. The horizontal dashed line is the threshold for hit calling, and all of the hits (high proportion of positive cells) are from wells with few cells. One compound

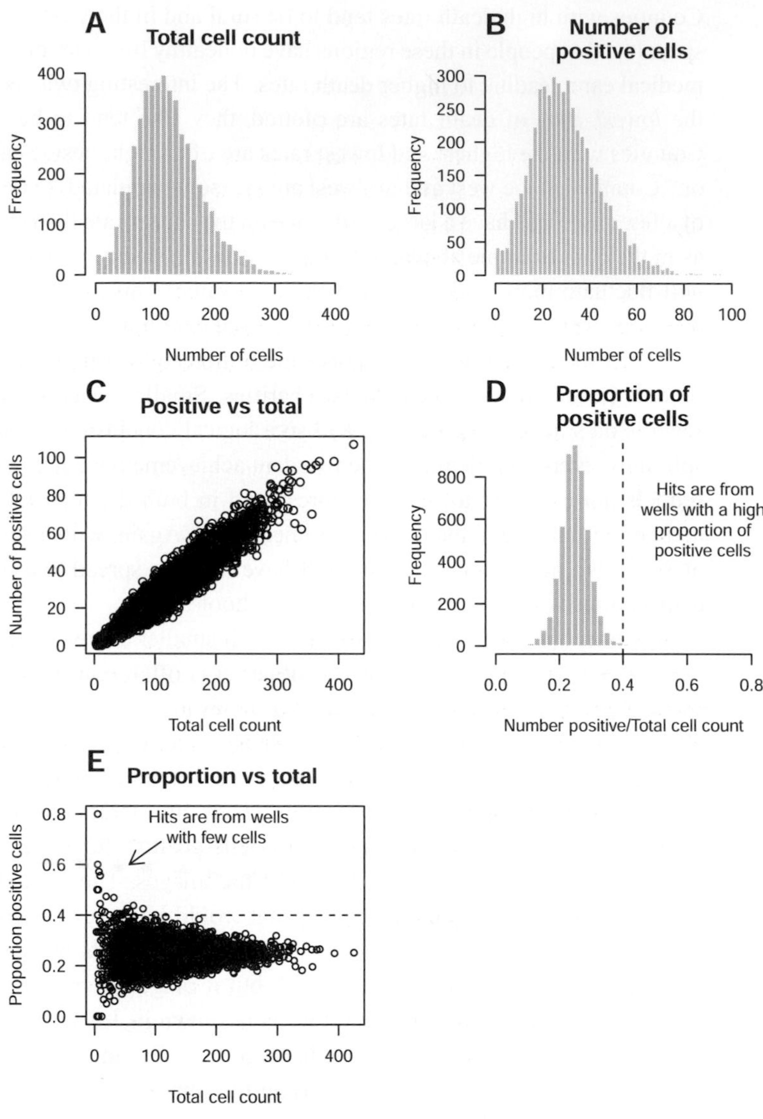

Fig. 1.5 Sensitivity to sample size. The two measured variables are the total cell count and the number of positive cells (A, B). There is a correlation between these variables because the positive cells are a subset of the total number of cells (C). A common strategy to remove the dependence on total count is to take the ratio of positive to total cells, and to look for high ratios (D). However, wells with few cells have the highest ratios (E), which are statistical artefacts.

has a very high proportion of 0.8. This is a statistical artefact but is routinely seen in real experiments and can be mistaken for a true hit. Resources could then be wasted in trying to validate it. But why does this occur? Think of each cell as having a probability of being positive, determined by the flip of an unbalanced coin. Each cell has a 25% chance of being positive (coin lands heads) and a 75% chance of being negative (coin lands tails). If there are only three coins, it is not unusual that all three of them land heads (proportion = 1), especially when 5000 trys are made.[4] If there are 100 coins, it is unlikely that all will land heads.

A subtler example occurs when classifying active compounds according to the reason the compound was selected for inclusion in the assay.[5] For example, some compounds are selected for testing because they bind to proteins in a biochemical pathway believed to be relevant for the disease. Alternatively, epigenetic mechanisms might be important and so any compound that is known to affect DNA methylation or histone acetylation is included. Also, a set of chemically diverse compounds are often used to cover a broad range of the chemical space. At the end of the screen it is usually of interest to see if one of the three compound sets (pathway set, epigenetic set, diverse set) is enriched for hits. For example, if 12% of the epigenetic compounds tested are hits while only 4.5% of the pathway set and 6% of the diverse set are hits, then epigenetic mechanisms might be important and further effort should be focused here. But it would not be surprising for the epigenetic set to have an unusually high or low percentage of hits if it contained only 50 compounds, while the pathway set had 5000 and the diverse set 50 000. Thus, the percentage of hits does not provide enough information to make conclusions about the compound sets. Can you think of examples from your own experiments where sampling variability might provide a different interpretation of the results?

Sampling variability is also important when assessing the reproducibility of results. Some researchers are surprised when they obtain different results after repeating an experiment, especially when great effort was spent to make the replication as similar as possible to the original experiment. 'Different results' are usually defined as one with $p < 0.05$ and the other with $p > 0.05$. Comparing p-values is not a good way of assessing reproducibility, either within or between laboratories (see Figure 1.1). It is impossible to exactly reproduce an experiment, but even if it were possible, the results would not be identical because of sampling variability. Just like tossing a coin 10 times gives a different number of heads every time, estimating the difference between two groups will give a different estimate every time the experiment is conducted. An example is shown in Figure 1.6, where hypothetical data were generated with a mean difference of 0.5 in each of the 10 experiments. The mean differences and 95% CI are shown, along with the p-values. Half of the p-values are significant and the other half are not. This does not indicate lack of reproducibility and reflects the variation that one would expect due to sampling variability alone, as this was a simulated example and so all other sources of variation are under complete control. Compare Experiment 9, which is significant, and 10, which is not. The estimated mean difference is nearly identical in the two experiments, but Experiment 9 just happened to have better precision (narrower 95% CI) and therefore a smaller p-value. The mean differences from the 10 experiments range from 0.25 to 0.95 and the p-values range from 0.008 to 0.256, and are entirely due to sampling variation. *Large differences in significance can be associated with small differences in the underlying effect.*

[4] The probability of obtaining three heads when the probability of each is 0.25 is $0.25 \times 0.25 \times 0.25 = 0.015625$. If you try this 5000 times, then you would expect $5000 \times 0.015625 = 78$ of those times to get all heads.

[5] I thank Pierre Farmer for this example.

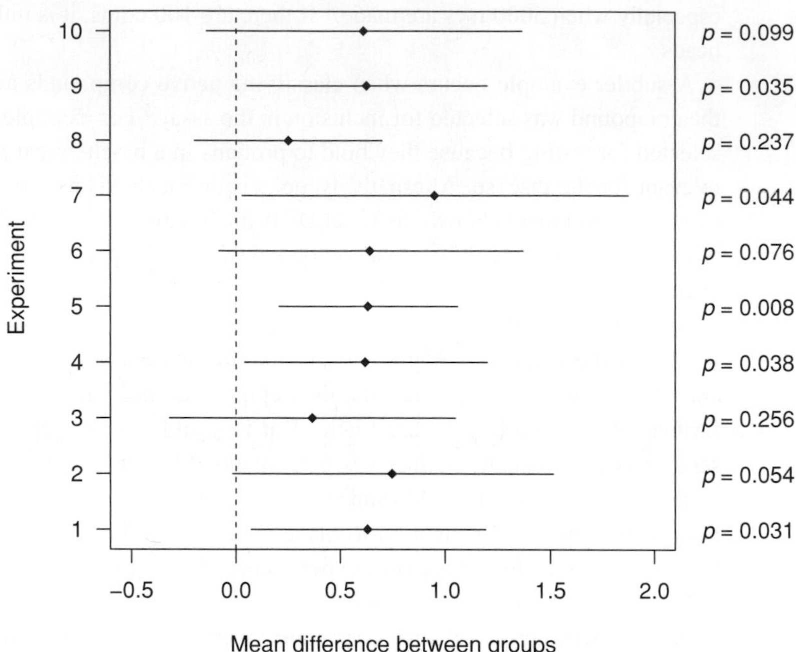

Fig. 1.6 Sampling variability for experimental outcomes. Simulated data from 10 perfectly controlled experiments with a true mean difference of 0.5, and a constant variance and sample size. Variation in the estimated mean difference, 95% CIs, and *p*-values are just a reflection of sampling variability and are within the range of expected values, despite only half of the *p*-values being significant.

1.2.5 Independence bias

Independence bias is the tendency to overestimate the evidential value of new data, especially when the data are correlated with existing data. It leads to the belief that many significant results provide much stronger support for a hypothesis than they actually do. Suppose we are interested in whether a compound increases muscle strength in humans. We randomly assign 20 people to either the compound or placebo control group and assess their strength after 4 weeks of treatment.[6] The subjects' strength is measured on three barbell exercises: bench press, deadlift, and squat. The three strength variables have the following p-values when testing for the effect of the compound: $p = 0.01$, $p = 0.03$, and $p = 0.02$. How convincing are the results? How likely is it that all three p-values would be significant if the compound was inactive? Many people informally reason that although there is a 0.05 chance of a false positive result, three significant results provides convincing evidence for the effect of the compound, even if the p-values are not very small. More formally, if there is a 0.05 chance of a false positive result, the probability of three false positives is $p = 0.05 \times 0.05 \times 0.05 = 0.05^3 = 0.000125$. Since this total probability is

[6] This experiment could be improved by taking the subjects' baseline strength into account, but we ignore this for the sake of simplicity.

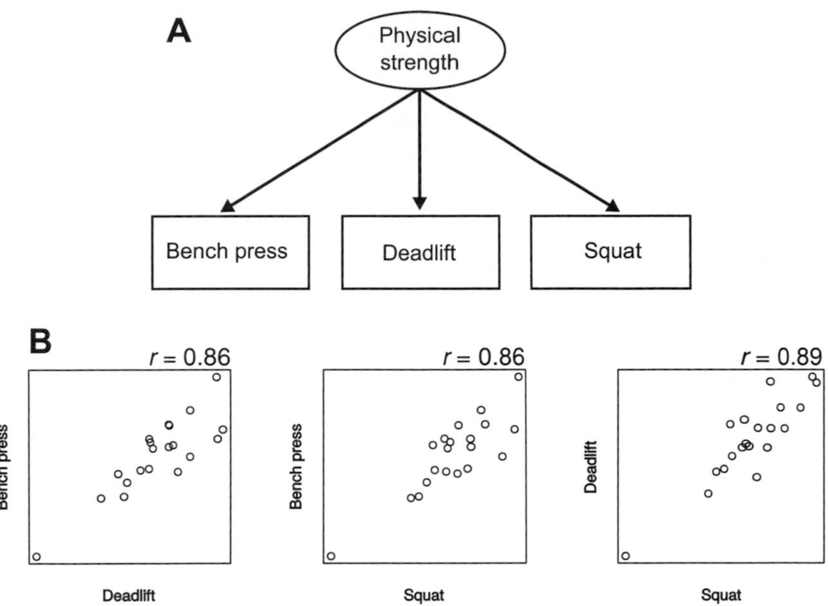

Fig. 1.7 Latent and measured variables. Three measured variables are measuring different aspects of physical strength – the underlying latent variable – and are therefore highly correlated (A). The scatterplots (B) show the relationships between the measured variables along with the Pearson correlation (*r*).

small, it is unlikely that all three tests would be significant if the compound is inactive. The mental bias arises because the three measured outcomes do not provide *independent* pieces of information about the effect of the compound. The total probability calculated is only valid if the three *p*-values are independent, which would occur, for example, if the values were from three different experiments using different people. At the other extreme, if the three measured outcomes are perfectly correlated, then they would all be significant or none of them would, the second and third *p*-value provide no new information once we known the first. The higher the correlation between the variables the greater the redundancy in the information they provide.

The three variables in this example are highly correlated because they are all measuring the same thing – the people's strength. The three exercises are all capturing different aspects of physical strength, but the high correlations are expected. Strength, like many aspects of biology, is hard to define and often cannot be measured directly. Other examples include inflammation, disease severity or stage, cognitive functioning, psychological and emotional states, and even gene expression. These are not directly observed or measured like a person's weight. Variables that cannot be directly measured are called *latent variables.*[7] Figure 1.7A shows the relationship between latent and observed variables for the physical strength example. Figure 1.7B shows scatterplots of 20 simulated values for the three measured variables, with an average correlation of 0.87 between them. Assume

[7] The observed variables are called *manifest* or *indicator* variables, but these terms tend to be discipline specific. We use the terms *observed* or *measured* variables.

that 10 of these values are the controls and the other 10 are the treated people, and that the compound has no effect. What is the probability *all three* statistical tests will have a p-value of less than 0.05? Based on a simulation (not shown) it is about 0.02, just below the usual 0.05 cut-off, but much higher than 0.000125 if independence is assumed. The three significant p-values provide some evidence for an effect of the compound, but it is almost as likely as obtaining one significant p-value.

Highly correlated variables do not provide independent evidence for an effect because they are often different measures of a single underlying effect. The above example used physical strength, but the same problem arises with gene, protein, or metabolite levels as these tend to be co-regulated.

There are several ways to avoid over-interpreting the degree of evidence provided by many correlated variables. First, one variable can be defined beforehand as the primary outcome, and then only this variable is used for testing hypotheses or making a decision. A primary outcome can be chosen based on the literature, after pilot experiments, or during assay development. For example, the outcome with the greatest sensitivity to discriminate between negative control and positive control samples could be chosen, or the variable with the smallest coefficient of variation (CV). The primary outcome is then used for all subsequent experiments because it has been validated as the best variable. Criteria to consider when choosing a primary outcome are discussed in Section 5.1. This approach works well in theory, but often not in practice, because if the result for the primary variable is not significant, but one of the other variables is, many researchers would find it hard to stick with the original plan and base their conclusions on the primary outcome, especially if a significant result is desired. A drawback of the primary outcome approach is that the other variables have some additional information that remains unused. It seems wasteful and inefficient that data are collected but not put to use. One way the additional data could be used is to reduce measurement error. For the strength example, one person may have a stiff shoulder on the day of testing, another may have a sore knee, and another a bad back. Depending on how much an exercise involves an injured body part, a single measurement can underestimate the true strength of a person. If the three measurements could be combined, then a better estimate of overall strength could be obtained.

This brings us to the second method of dealing with many correlated variables: combine them into a set of fewer variables that still relate to the latent variable of interest. We could for example add the amount lifted in the three exercises to obtain a new variable called 'total weight':

$$\text{Total weight} = \text{Bench press} + \text{Deadlift} + \text{Squat}$$

Total weight is a linear combination of the original three variables and can be used as the primary outcome in an analysis. The measured variables are all of the same kind and have the same units (e.g. kilograms) so a simple summation is meaningful. When the observed variables have different units, summing them creates a variable that is hard to interpret. Another problem with adding variables is that variables with larger values will have a larger influence on the total than variables with smaller values. Exercises where a lot of weight can be lifted will contribute more to the total than exercises where less can be lifted. This is undesirable and we would like all variables to contribute equally to the total. Ideally, we would like a general method to combine variables of different types, where each variable makes the same contribution. Fortunately, many methods are available and the two most common are *principal components analysis* (PCA) and *factor analysis*. The popularity of each method varies widely by scientific discipline. Shipley [354] and Grace [140] discuss the use of such latent variable models in biology to reduce measurement error.

Related to this are *composite measures*, which are a combination of several measured variables, but they may be on different scales. For example, an overall assessment of disease severity or disease burden is composed of several subscales such as the degree of cognitive and motor impairment, which are assessed on a zero (no impairment) to five (complete impairment) scale. The sum of the subscales gives the overall disease severity score. Although composite scores have the advantage of reducing the number of outcome variables, different patterns on the subscales will be obscured. For example, one patient has mostly cognitive impairments, another mostly motor impairments, and a third is mildly impaired on both. Their composite score can be the same, despite differences in their disease manifestation. For this reason, composite scores are especially problematic when looking for associations between clinical outcomes and gene expression or imaging biomarkers.

1.2.6 Confirmation bias

Confirmation bias is the tendency to search for, interpret, focus on, and recall information that confirms a research hypothesis and can manifest itself in many ways. For example, suppose a microarray study is conducted and a list of differentially expressed genes between diseased patients and healthy controls is derived. It is common to provide support for a gene in this list by citing previous studies that found an association between the gene and the disease in question. A PubMed search[8] is conducted using the disease name plus a gene of interest as search terms. The papers found will tend to be those that show a link or association with the gene and the disease, and this may seem to provide support for the findings of the microarray study. But how convincing is this approach (ignoring for the moment that the papers found will be of varying quality and provide various degrees of support for the gene of interest)? What about the studies that examined the gene (or protein) in this disease but *did not* find it to be relevant? There could be many papers that addressed the same research question, but only those that mention the disease and gene in the title or abstract will be found with a PubMed search, and they will tend to be ones with statistically significant results (Figure 1.8). The studies returned from a literature search could be mostly those with false positive results. This is especially true with -omics experiments, where all genes are examined but only a few will be mentioned in the title or abstract, and will therefore be found with a PubMed search. In the above example, there has been no attempt to find negative results, for example, by searching for the disease and gene using the Gene Expression Omnibus (GEO) database.[9] A GEO search will find the

[8] `www.ncbi.nlm.nih.gov/pubmed`.

[9] The GEO homepage is `http://www.ncbi.nlm.nih.gov/geo/`, and GEO Profiles can be used to find the expression profiles for a gene in a disease or other experimental condition by using 'gene AND disease' as search terms (`http://www.ncbi.nlm.nih.gov/geoprofiles/`).

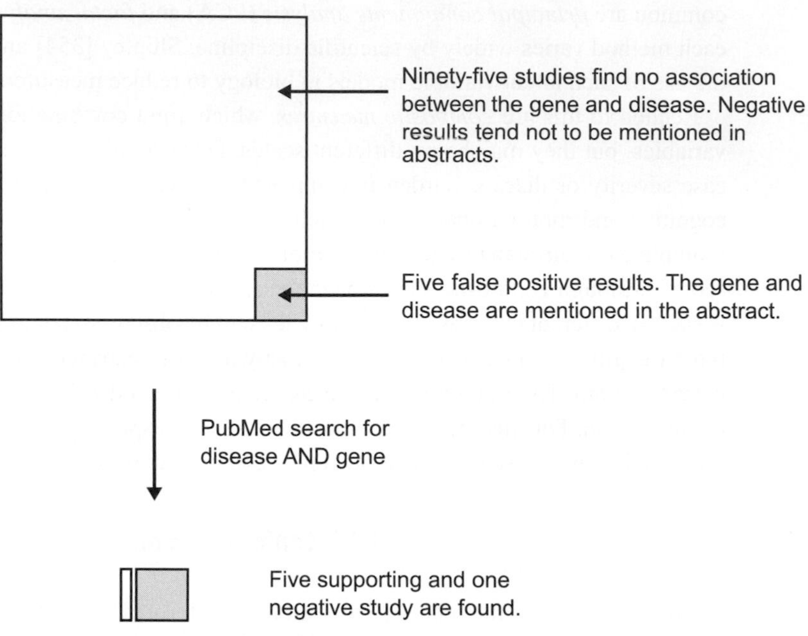
100 relevant studies
Ninety-five studies find no association between the gene and disease. Negative results tend not to be mentioned in abstracts.
Five false positive results. The gene and disease are mentioned in the abstract.
PubMed search for disease AND gene
Five supporting and one negative study are found.

Fig. 1.8 Confirmation bias in literature searches. The tendency to only search for papers that support findings instead of all papers that potentially disconfirm findings. PubMed searches will tend to return positive results because they are more likely to be mentioned in the title or abstract.

gene of interest across all of the microarray and NGS studies it contains that mention the disease. One can then see how many relevant studies were conducted and the number that did not find the gene to be differentially expressed between patients and healthy controls.

Confirmation bias can also occur during the analysis and interpretation of data. Suppose that the data are slightly skewed, and a decision is made to log-transform it. An analysis is conducted on both the raw and transformed data, and if only one of these analyses provides a significant result for the main comparison of interest, then it is the result that is reported. It is as if *by definition* the correct analysis is the one that gives the significant result; the other analyses that were conducted are disregarded because they do not support the research hypothesis.

Another source of confirmation bias occurs when deciding which data to include in a publication to 'tell a story', and which references to cite when supporting a claim. Data that do not fit with the overall story may be excluded. There is also the tendency to minimise the importance of negative results and to cite them less – especially in the biological sciences [108]. Confirmation bias is hard to avoid, but efforts can be made to find negative results and ensure that they are not discounted and are appropriately cited. Tetlock suggests that confirmation bias can be mitigated by simply rewording the question [367]. For example, in addition to asking 'is there an association between this gene and disease?', which biases one to find supporting evidence, also ask 'why is there no association between this gene and disease?', which focuses the search on finding negative evidence.

1.2.7 Expectancy effects

Expectancy effects occur when a scientist's expectations influence measurements or assessments. For example, if transgenic mice are expected to exhibit more of one behaviour compared with wild-type controls, then subjective ratings of behaviour can overestimate their prevalence in the transgenic mice. Or, if no differences are expected between litters of animals or batches of samples processed separately, then subtle clustering of data points may be ignored or attributed to random noise.

A classic example of expectancy effects is the story of N-rays – a story rooted in poor experimental design [194, 296]. In 1903, French physicist Rene Prosper Blondlot claimed to have discovered a new type of radiation, which he called N-rays, and many respected scientists reproduced his results. It was an important finding and received a lot of attention from the scientific community. N-rays were supposedly emitted from organic objects and biologists and medical doctors became interested.

N-rays were detected by subjectively assessing the brightness of a spark or the darkness of photographic plates. The researchers were not blinded during these assessments and they saw what they expected and wanted to see: when we do X, the spark gets brighter. The effects however disappeared in later experiments when researchers were unaware of the experimental condition when assessing the brightness of the spark, that is, when they were *blinded* [194].

Between 1903 and 1906, some 300 papers on N-rays were published by 100 scientists [296]. A couple of years after their discovery, few believed in the existence of N-rays, and science appears to be working as it should: a claim was made, scientists investigated, and eventually the truth was found. On the other hand, if expectancy effects had been controlled from the start, 100 scientists need not have wasted their time. Blinding (Section 2.5) and randomisation (Section 2.3) could have prevented the expectancy effects.

1.2.8 Hindsight bias

Hindsight bias is the tendency to find explanations for results that were not predicted – often consistent with one's hypothesis or the prevailing paradigm. It is mainly a problem for exploratory experiments (as opposed to confirmatory experiments, see Section 2.1) and occurs whenever an unplanned or unanticipated effect or association is statistically significant, and we conclude 'that makes sense' or 'I knew it all along' [390]. Sometimes the explanation is not obvious, but after some thought and a PubMed search, one can appeal to some theory or find a couple of papers that can be marshalled in support of an explanation. With almost 25 million entries in PubMed, something useful can be found. Furthermore, given the number of false positive results in the literature, it is not hard to find at least one paper that supports any given finding. The only way to validate such results is to admit that they were not predicted, make a prediction about what will be found in a *new* experiment, and then conduct the new experiment [135]. When an explanation comes after the result, it is extremely weak and unconvincing. Researchers may develop different explanations for the same results depending on their background knowledge and the papers they stumbled across in their internet search. The proposed explanation may be true, but the only way to know for sure is to test it in a subsequent experiment.

Hindsight bias can be avoided by making a prediction before the experiment is conducted. It helps to write down the expected results of the experiment; for example, that the treated group will express Gene X at a higher level. One could go a step further and predict the size of the effect and its uncertainty, such as a 2-fold increase with a 95% CI between 1.5- and 2.5-fold. The estimate can be based on effect sizes commonly seen in the literature for related experiments or a pilot study. Maybe write down a value for an unbelievably large effect. This helps to calibrate predictions and intuitions. If the result is a 10-fold increase, then the usual reaction of excitement might be tempered with concern of why the prediction was so different and why the effect is so large. Is there another source of variation that is influencing the results? Furthermore, if Gene X is the same between groups but Gene Y and Gene Z are differentially expressed, then one cannot claim these results were expected.

1.2.9 Herding effect

Herding behaviour is the tendency to follow the scientific crowd when it comes to theories believed and methods used (either experimental or statistical) – science is not immune to fashionable trends. For example, a protein or biological process is believed to be critically important for a disease. Then, everyone moves on to study another protein or process that is now thought to be of greater importance. In drug discovery, many companies chase after the same targets at about the same time. Such herding behaviour makes it hard to publish findings that go against the prevailing view. And when such results are published, they may be ignored by the research community. Olson argues that findings are ignored when they do not contribute to the overarching narrative that scientists use to understand and interpret results,[10] and cites his own work in marine biology as an example [300, p. 211].

The herding effect can also occur at the level of a research group, where all members have the same beliefs, are trained in the same methods, and conduct experiments to support a single point of view. This can lead to *scientific inbreeding*, where replications are not truly independent because they have the same biases and errors as the original experiment [170].

Herding behaviour is a problem because there may be few people that take a critical view of a research area, demand that assumptions are checked, and seriously consider alternative explanations.[11] A risk is that contradictory or negative results are suppressed and experiments are run again until the 'right' answer is obtained. Such behaviour is hard to overcome because we often take basic premises as given, and then try to extend scientific knowledge

[10] A similar idea to Kuhn's concept of a *paradigm* [206].

[11] Not fully appreciating how alternative explanations can account for observed results is a problem in the field of adult neurogenesis [217, 218, 223], where I spent my PhD and postdoc years.

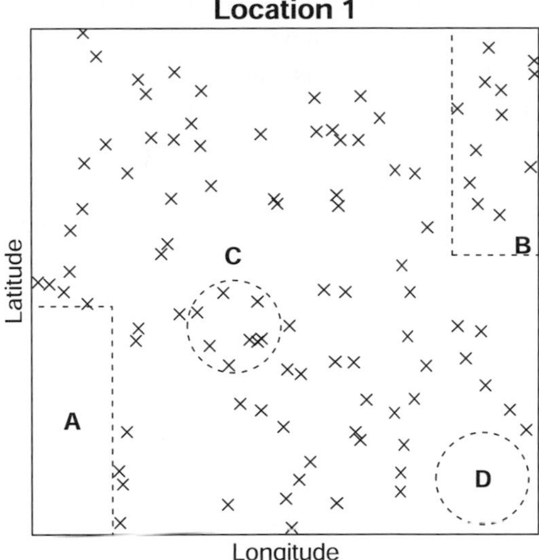

Fig. 1.9 Positions of dropped bombs. Regions (A) and (B) are fields, Region (C) is a power plant, and Region (D) is a munitions factory.

in a certain direction. The admonishment to be an independent thinker is unlikely to be helpful, as most people – scientist or otherwise – already believe that they are.

1.2.10 How the biases combine

The above biases and mental misrepresentations often work together to distort scientific results. As an illustration, we return to the example of whether bombs are dropped at random at Location 1 from Figure 1.2. The graph is reproduced in Figure 1.9 and further information is added. Recall that the General asked you to determine if the bombs are dropped at random, or if some positions are targeted more heavily while others are avoided. Also recall that these positions were generated by randomly selecting latitude and longitude pairs from a uniform distribution.

After discussing with colleagues, reading the literature on bombing strategies, and looking at what others have concluded about previous bombings, the consensus is that the enemy is unlikely to randomly drop bombs (herding effect). So when you start to analyse the data there is an expectation that you will find further evidence, and this is what you set out to do (confirmation bias). A first look at the bomb positions suggests that there may be some areas that are more heavily bombed while others have few bombs (seeing patterns in randomness). For example, you notice that Region A in Figure 1.9 has no bombs in it. After some further investigation you find that this region is mostly an empty field, which makes perfect sense because a field is not of strategic interest (hindsight bias). Furthermore, you notice that Region C has a denser clustering of bombs. This region is close to – but not exactly encompassing – a power plant, which is of definite strategic importance (hindsight bias). You know the importance of a formal statistical analysis and develop the idea that by calculating the area of a region relative to the total area, and then given the total number of bombs dropped, you can work out if the region has significantly greater or fewer bombs than expected. Your analysis confirms your intuitions that Region A has significantly fewer bombs than expected and Region C has significantly more! You examine other areas that might suggest an over- or under-representation of bombs (not wanting to miss anything), but nothing else is significant, and so you conclude that the power station was the only specific position targeted (psychological cliff at 0.05).

It is clear how several biases combined to produce the incorrect conclusion. There are additional issues. First, the absence of bombs in Region A is taken as evidence for avoiding locations with no strategic importance, such as an empty field. But Region B is also an empty field, and the bombs here are not taken as evidence *against* this hypothesis, either because the number of bombs in this field was not checked, or if it was checked, the results were downplayed because they were inconsistent with expectations. In either case, it is another example of confirmation bias.

Second, Region A was defined as not of strategic interest because it was mostly an empty field. But what if it contains a dairy farm, and the field is for the cows to graze? Is it now of strategic importance? What if the dairy farm produces high protein rations from milk products for the army? If there were more bombs than expected in Region A, then we could have made the story that the enemy is targeting the food supply (hindsight bias). What is considered strategically important is not defined beforehand. There was nothing *a priori* interesting about the patch of land contained in Region A until it was observed that there were fewer bombs there. Third, the clustering of bombs in Region C is taken as evidence for targeting important positions (the power plant), but the lack of bombs in Region D is not taken as evidence against this hypothesis. Suppose Region D is a munitions factory. Again, what is of strategic importance is not defined beforehand, and how close do the bombs have to be to a strategic location to be included in the count? Recall that Region C was *close to* a power plant. How close is close? Furthermore, why is Region A defined as a rectangle and Region C a circle?

A fourth, much subtler point, is that the analyses are not independent, and so the two significant p-values are correlated (independence bias). If there is an unusually high number of bombs in one region, then by definition, there must be fewer in the remaining region. It is similar to testing if eight heads out of 10 coin tosses is significant, and then testing if two tails out of 10 tosses is also significant. Since the number of tails is equal to the number of tosses minus the number of heads, the two p-values are redundant. Since the regions are not defined beforehand, the dependence is not as strong as in the coin example.

Pleased with your analysis you decide to share the results with the General, who is happy to see that his belief in a non-random bombing strategy has been vindicated. He will recommend you for a promotion and also suggests that you distribute the findings more widely. You decide to deposit them in either the repository of **NAT**ional **U**seful **RE**ports or the **C**entral **EL**aborated **L**ists, making sure to support your conclusions by citing earlier reports that came to the same conclusion (but not those that found the opposite results; confirmation bias). There is now one more piece of evidence to add to the collection that argues in favour of targeted non-random bombing by the enemy. And the cycle continues. . .

This was a fictitious example, but the parallels with experimental biology are clear. There was no fraudulent activity, the analysis was technically correct and, superficially, many of the steps seem sensible. But taken together, the approach led us astray. The question remains about how we should have proceeded. Certainly, more could have been defined before the analysis was started, including what is a strategic target (there can be several priority levels), how close do bombs have to be to the target to be included in the count (information on the accuracy of the enemy bombers can be used). This narrows the options available for finding patterns in pure noise. In addition, fake data generated by random uniform sampling of positions could have been included, and the analyst not told which data are real and which are fake [64]. This introduces blinding at the analysis stage. One could even withhold information that fake data are included. If the analyst can make a convincing argument that the fake data show signs of non-random bombing, then their conclusions about the real data become suspect.

A key mistake was trying to prove non-randomness from the start instead of trying to disprove randomness. This is, again, an example of confirmation bias, where we are trying to confirm our hypothesis of targeted bombing instead of trying to disprove the opposite hypothesis of random bombing. The problem with trying to confirm non-randomness is that we have to specify what particular type of non-randomness we want to test, and this led to the data-driven selection of whatever looked interesting. To disprove the hypothesis of random bombing, we only have to reject the hypothesis of *complete spatial randomness* (CSR) without specifying how exactly non-randomness will manifest itself. Methods exist for testing CSR but are not discussed here (see [96]). If the data are consistent with CSR, then there is no need to investigate further.

1.3 Are most published results wrong?

The heading for this section is inspired by Ioannidis' conclusion that most published results are false [168] (and in a subsequent paper he argued that the effect size is often overestimated in those studies that reached the correct conclusion [169]). The short answer is that many papers provide insufficient information to assess whether the experimental design and statistical analysis are appropriate or whether the investigators engaged in any questionable research practices, such as reporting only favourable results. There has been a good deal of introspection by the biomedical research community lately regarding bias and the lack of reproducibility [2, 5, 28, 30, 42, 80, 83, 84, 123, 172, 240, 251, 305, 316, 342], which suggests that there are serious problems with current biomedical research. These discussions have led top journals (e.g. *Science*, *Science Translational Medicine*, *Nature*, and the *Nature* series of journals) to implement stricter reporting standards [3, 183, 271], and the National Institutes of Health (NIH) to pilot various methods for improving the reproducibility of research – including training in experimental design for NIH intramural postdoctoral fellows [80]. In addition, *Science* has recently introduced a Statistical Board of Reviewing Editors, who will check manuscripts and recommend those that should receive a more thorough review [270]. Below we discuss several lines of evidence suggesting that much of the literature is of questionable value, including anecdotal comments from statisticians and scientists, empirical studies examining the quality of published reports, large-scale attempts at replication, and anonymous questionnaires given to scientists asking about questionable research practices that they have observed or engaged in.

1.3.1 What statisticians say

This chapter opened with quotes from eminent statisticians on the quality of experiments and analyses conducted by scientists. Statisticians are in a unique position because they see the raw data and interact with scientists before papers are published. They are often exposed to 'the real story' instead of the sanitised version that gets published. They are also less invested in the outcome – it's not their hypothesis being tested – which enables them to be more impartial. Applied biostatisticians also work with many research groups and have a broad exposure to how biologists conduct experiments. Given statisticians' knowledge on designing experiments and making inferences from data, such comments should cause one to pause and reflect on the quality of experiments in the biological sciences. Nelder's comment opening this chapter 'and many statisticians have their own horror stories' alludes to statisticians' widespread concern. It is noteworthy that Fisher's comment was made in 1938 and Nelder's and Dempster's over 60 years later, suggesting that the quality of experiments has not improved over time. Fisher made his statement at a statistical congress and Nelder and Dempster commented in statistics journals [93, 290]. In all cases the comments were directed at fellow statisticians – who perhaps nodded their heads knowingly – but their concerns were not communicated to biologists. Further comments from statisticians on experimental quality and statistical inference are below and most were published in journals or books that biologists are unlikely to read.

> *In practical situations many scientific or industrial investigations are doomed to fail. There are many and varied reasons for this, but the most often encountered reason is simply that the investigation was not properly planned. Many investigators fail to understand that careful pre-planning is essential for a successful experiment.* ([153, p. 30])

> *. . . the statistician should request a detailed description of the experiment and its objectives. It may then become evident that no inferences can be made or that those which can be made do not answer the questions to which the experimenter had hoped to find answers. In these unhappy circumstances, about all that can be done is to indicate, if possible, how to avoid this outcome in future experiments.* ([373, p. 559])

> *. . . how many investigators are fully aware of all of the potential sources of bias in their experimental protocol and understand how to incorporate them into the design and allow for them in the analysis to avoid any negative impact on the conclusions?* ([305, p. 734])

> *There is a disturbing tendency for techniques to be used by people who do not fully understand them and the standard of statistical argument in scientific journals can best be described as variable.* ([70, p. 214])

> *One of us worked for many years across multiple research groups at a large medical school and was occasionally asked to evaluate the work of other research groups, with*

access to all data and staff. It was alarming how often mistakes occurred and went undetected. ([131, p. 4])

Today's medical journals are full of factual errors and false conclusions arising from lack of statistical common sense. ([59, p. 335])

Statistical thinking is the statistical incarnation of 'common sense'. 'We know it when we see it', or perhaps more truthfully, its absence *is often glaringly obvious.* ([397, p. 223])

We think that the problem is that often researchers do not admit uncertainty or variation; they think they've already made their discovery, and they think of various data-collection and data-analysis rules as technicalities that should not get in the way of science. After all, if you've published a paper with nine statistically significant results, it would seem like you've discovered a pattern that could only occur once in $(1/20)^9$ *by chance, a probability that would seem too extreme to be seriously whittled away by minor methodological issues.* ([130, p. 54])

It is often the case (e.g., in biology) that the experimental worker shows a certain, indeed a strong, prejudice against statistical work. ([411, p. 3])

One thing has become painfully clear to me in twenty years of extensive teaching, statistical consulting, reviewing, and interacting in ecology: ecologists' understanding of statistics is abysmally poor. Statistics should naturally be a source of strength and confidence... Unfortunately, it is all too frequently a source of weakness, insecurity, and embarrassment. ([94, p. 332])

There was little interest for the principles of sound statistical design and analysis of experiments. (From a workshop on statistical thinking for scientists in the pharmaceutical industry.) ([375, p. 65])

Some biologists may be offended by these comments, but consider what biologists might say if statisticians started conducting experiments in the lab without regard for good practices such as using experimental controls and validating reagents. The point remains, designing experiments and analysing data are core activities in experimental biology, and many who are expert in these areas of scientific discovery think that the general level of knowledge among biologists is insufficient. Biologists are not at fault – formal education and training in these areas are minimal and biologists have to go out of their way to learn more about topics that many find intrinsically boring and disconnected from their scientific activities. That many biologists do not see how statistics and experimental design are critical for their research is a failing of the statistics community. Biologists want to do good science and will readily learn something if it will improve their research. The rigid formality of setting up a null hypothesis (that is known to be false), comparing it with an alternative hypothesis (that is uninteresting), calculating p-values that do not say anything about hypotheses and confidence intervals that do not provide confidence, is enough to convince many biologists that statistics has nothing useful to offer.

It is not obvious how statistics and experimental design can improve scientific discovery and it is the responsibility of statisticians (or those writing about statistics) to make this connection for scientists.[12] Focusing on experimental design is one way of making statistics more relevant for biologists – the approach taken in this book – because it is closely related to scientists' day-to-day activities. A second approach is to use Bayesian methods for statistical inference instead of frequentist methods. Introducing an unfamiliar method of inference in a book primarily about experimental design would take us too far afield and that is why frequentist methods have been used in Chapter 4. McElreath [269] and Kruschke [203] provide excellent introductions to Bayesian analysis.

1.3.2 What scientists say

Biologists may be dismissive of what statisticians think, maybe because statisticians are perceived as lacking biological knowledge or are pedantically obsessed with trivial matters and miss the bigger picture.[13] Concerns that scientists have about their own areas of research are often not captured in the literature but traded over a beer at conferences, although a few reports are now appearing. One example is from Glenn Begley; he relates how he was unable to replicate results published in *Cancer Cell*, and when discussing this with the (respected) senior author of the paper, Begley was told that the experiment was conducted many times, and only the one positive experiment was published [83]. Professor Ulrich Dirnagl discusses a paper he reviewed that excluded three animals in the treated group without mentioning it [83]. The methods stated that 10 animals were used in the treated group, but only seven animals were shown in a figure. The study was testing a new compound to see if it would protect the brain after a stroke. As it turns out, the missing three animals in the treated group had died of a massive stroke, and their exclusion made the treatment appear effective.

A detailed account of science gone wrong is by John Maddox (editor of *Nature* at the time) and colleagues, who had visited the lab of Dr Jacques Benveniste to scientifically audit a remarkable yet unlikely finding [255]. Benveniste had published a paper in *Nature* demonstrating that highly diluted solutions of anti-IgE showed biological activity, which could be interpreted as evidence in support of homeopathic medicine [91]. The paper came with an editorial reservation at the end and an accompanying opinion piece on when to believe the unbelievable [1]. During their week-long stay in Benveniste's lab, Maddox and colleagues described a remarkable list of poor experimental practices, including measuring control samples a second time if the results were higher than the treated samples – because the first reading 'must have been incorrect' – or excluding results that failed to 'work', defined as not in line with expectations. Experimenters were not blinded and thus observer bias could have been introduced. In addition, there was an undeclared conflict of interest as a company that produced homeopathic medicines funded two of the authors on the paper. Perhaps the most interesting feature is the psychology of the scientists and how

[12] Many statisticians have successfully made this connection – George Box and J. Stuart Hunter are personal favourites. Google 'Stu Hunter Teaches Statistics' and watch the first YouTube video on *What is Design of Experiments – Part 1* (`https://www.youtube.com/playlist?list=PL335F9F2DE78A358B`) as an example.

[13] Fisher was just as much a biologist as a statistician, his appointment at Cambridge University was the Balfour Chair of Genetics; he was not based in a mathematics or statistics department.

they were able to explain away results that were evidence against their hypothesis, accept uncritically results that supported their views, and how this justified recounting until the 'correct' answer was obtained or excluding data altogether.[14] The most troubling aspect of such research practices is just how common they are.

Lack of reproducibility is not a recent phenomenon, but it is interesting to speculate why attention has increased recently. In 1673 Robert Boyle wrote:

> *You will find* [. . .] *many of the experiments published by authors, or related to you by the persons you converse with, false and unsuccessful* [. . .] *you will meet with several observations and experiments which, though communicated for true by candid authors or undistrusted eye-witnesses, or perhaps recommended by our own experience, may, upon further trial, disappoint your expectation, either not at all succeeding constantly, or at least varying much from what you expected.* (Quoted in Fisher [121, p. xv])

1.3.3 Empirical evidence I: questionable research practices

Martinson and colleagues anonymously asked 3247 NIH-funded scientists if they had engaged in a list of questionable research practices (QRPs) during the previous 3 years [260]. Overall, they found that 33% of scientists reported engaging in at least one of their top 10 most serious behaviours, 0.3% of respondents admitted to falsifying data, the most serious item on Martinson's list; 6% admitted to not presenting data that contradicted their previous results, 12.5% said that they overlooked others' flawed or questionable interpretation of data, 15.5% said that they changed the design, methods, or results in response to pressure from a funding source, 13.5% admitted using inadequate or inappropriate research designs, and 15.3% dropped observations from analyses based on a gut feeling that they were inaccurate. A meta-analysis of 18 studies by Fanelli found that 2% of scientists admitted to fabricating, falsifying, or modifying data or results at least once, and 34% admitted to other QRPs [106]. When asked about colleagues, admission rates were 14% for falsification and up to 72% for other QRPs.

More recently, John and colleagues anonymously asked 2155 psychologists if they had engaged in a list of 10 QRPs [177]. Unlike Martinson's study there was no time limit, and so scientists responded if they had *ever* engaged in a behaviour. This led to much higher estimates, and the results are grim. Overall, 0.6% admitted to falsifying data, but 63.4% failed to report all dependent measures (i.e. selective reporting), 15.6% stopped collecting data earlier than planned because the desired results were obtained, 45.8% reported 'rounding off' p-values (e.g. reporting 0.054 as <0.05), 45.8% admitted to selectively reporting studies that 'worked', 38.2% said that they excluded data after looking at the impact of doing so on the results, and 27% admitted to reporting an unexpected finding as having been predicted from the start. Lest you think that psychologists are an exceptionally unethical group, when the results were broken down by discipline, neuroscience (the closest group

[14] Dr Benveniste's rebuttal can be found in *Nature* and *Science* [34, 35]. The Wikipedia page for Jacques Benveniste contains more information about the story (`http://en.wikipedia.org/wiki/Jacques_Benveniste`). His findings have not been substantiated during the subsequent 25 years.

to experimental biologists) had one of the highest rates of QRPs (clinical was the lowest). In addition, when broken down by research type, laboratory and experimental research had the highest rates (clinical was again the lowest). Also of note, Bakker and Wicherts found that 41% of manuscripts in the psychology literature had discrepancies between the reported sample size and the data used in the statistical analyses (which can be determined from the reported degrees of freedom), indicating that some data had been dropped without mention [19]. This is similar to the 38.2% self-report estimate by John and colleagues [177].

These estimates are likely conservative because those who engage in QRPs may be less likely to respond to questionnaires, and even if they did respond, the questions may not have been answered honestly. Engaging in *some* of the above behaviours does not imply misconduct, dishonesty, or an attempt to deceive. There may be ethically justified reasons for stopping a study early if a definitive answer has been reached, especially with human or animal subjects. In addition, there may have been legitimate reasons for not including all data, such as instrument failure. Scientists are provided with little guidance on acceptable and unacceptable research practices. Even so, such practices, especially when they are not mentioned in a paper, can distort the research record.

1.3.4 Empirical evidence II: quality of studies

A separate issue to that of questionable research practices is the quality of studies. A goal of all experiments is to obtain unbiased estimates of effect sizes and an appropriate precision of those estimates.[15] These results are then used to support or refute a theory or hypothesis, plan further experiments, make treatment decisions for patients, or approve a new drug – none of which can be done well with biased estimates or faulty precision. There are two main areas where experiments fail. The first is in the design and execution of the experiment, and the second is in the analysis and interpretation. Several studies have examined the quality of published reports in biology, and the results are not encouraging.

Two main problems identified with the design and execution are a lack of randomisation and a lack of blinding [20, 25, 31, 87, 154, 158, 189, 253, 254, 279, 308, 327, 329, 341, 348, 378], which is determined from the description in the methods section of manuscripts. Some studies may have been randomised and blinded but the authors failed to report this. However, studies that do not mention using randomisation or blinding have larger effect sizes compared with studies that report using these techniques (reviewed in reference [97]), which is consistent with poor experimental practices leading to inflated outcomes. Hooijmans and colleagues have developed a risk of bias questionnaire for animal studies based on a similar questionnaire used to assess clinical trials [160]. Few preclinical studies would receive an acceptable score based on these criteria. Studies occasionally examine a particular aspect of the published literature such as the correct use of statistical tests, whether data

[15] There is the concept of a bias-variance trade-off in statistical modelling, where a model that is slightly biased can predict future observations better than an unbiased model because of a reduction in variance. This is much less of a consideration when analysing data from designed experiments with only a few parameters.

have been removed without mention, or a mismatch between test statistics and *p*-values, and the conclusions are never good [37, 125, 222, 294, 299].

Another major issue is pseudoreplication, an artificial inflation of the sample size [216], that usually occurs when the biological unit of interest differs from the experimental unit or observational unit. For example, many studies apply an experimental intervention to pregnant female rodents (experimental unit) but then observe the effects in the offspring (biological unit of interest and the observational unit). The sample size is the number of pregnant females and not the number of offspring when testing the effects of the intervention (discussed in Chapter 3). The valproic acid rodent model of autism uses such an approach and only 9% (3/34) of studies correctly identified the experimental unit and thus made valid inferences from the data [222]. Such errors are also common in the polyriboinosinic:polyribocytidilic (Poly I:C) acid model of schizophrenia [219].

An important issue for *in vivo* experiments are litter effects, or the litter-to-litter variation in the outcome variables [148, 159, 164, 222, 263, 386, 415]. This is a large and under-appreciated source of variability which can increase both false positives and false negatives. Manuscripts rarely discuss how litter effects were taken into account. This topic is discussed further in Section 2.12.5.

Once again it is instructive to turn to a case study, this time involving the superoxide dismutase (SOD1) transgenic mouse model of amyotrophic lateral sclerosis. Preclinical studies using this animal model showed enough efficacy for several different drugs to proceed to clinical trials, where none proved to be effective [344]. A meta-analysis of the preclinical literature showed that only 31% of studies reported randomly assigning animals to treatment conditions and even fewer reported blind assessment of outcomes [32]. It also appears that there were unpublished studies that failed to confirm the initial findings [344]. A large scale and properly conducted study by Scott *et al.* did not support previous findings and also uncovered sources of variability that could explain the false positives in the literature, such as litter effects [346].

When it comes to analysis and reporting, an incongruity between test statistics and *p*-values occurred in 11% of papers published in 2001 in *Nature* and the *British Medical Journal* [125], with similar results in two psychiatry journals [37]. These may be due to rounding, typographic, or copy-and-paste errors, or perhaps errors in analysis. Another study by Bakker and Wicherts found comparable results in the psychology literature [18]. The Bakker paper was particularly thorough in that they contacted the authors of the original publications and so were able to reanalyse some of the data. They found that 15% of papers had at least one error which led to a change in conclusion, defined as a *p*-value changing sides of 0.05 after the recalculation. Furthermore, they noted that these errors tended to be in one direction, making non-significant results significant. Bakker and Wicherts make the point that one cannot conclude that these are attempts to deceive, as a non-significant *p*-value may be double-checked and scrutinised more and thus corrected, whereas a significant *p*-value goes unquestioned. Another interesting finding was that authors of the original publications that responded to Bakker's first email request for data had fewer errors than those that responded after a second email request one week later. Perhaps the second group are less conscientious, explaining both the increased number of statistical errors and the delay in replying, or perhaps they are aware that the proper way to round

0.04938 to two decimal places is 0.05 and not 0.04. Such 'errors' might account for the 'peculiar prevalence of p values just below 0.05' [92, 198, 228, 261, 325]. Another study by the same group found that the reluctance to share data was associated with a higher prevalence of reporting errors and that the unwillingness to share data was greater when the errors had a bearing on statistical significance [394].

Many of the above errors are likely clerical and attributed to carelessness, and although they decrease the overall quality of published results they are hard to eliminate completely. More troubling is when incorrect inferential procedures are used. For example, suppose a scientist wants to show that a compound has an effect only in normal mice, but not in mice that have the gene for a putative target knocked out. The proper method of addressing this question is testing the drug × genotype interaction effect (discussed in detail in Section 2.8), but *half* of the neuroscience papers in *Science* and *Nature* and other top neuroscience journals do not analyse such data correctly [294]. Instead, many researchers try to support their hypothesis by demonstrating that the difference between the drug and control group is significant in the wild-type mice ($p < 0.05$) but not in the knock-out mice ($p > 0.05$). Although there is a certain logic to this, it is an incorrect analysis because, as Gelman puts it, 'the difference between "significant" and "not significant" is not itself statistically significant' [132]. Not a single study in their sample of cellular and molecular neuroscience articles published in *Nature Neuroscience* used the correct procedure [294]. Some effects were large and the conclusions unlikely to change if reanalysed with appropriate methods. For others, the conclusions might need to be revised.

1.3.5 Empirical evidence III: reproducibility of studies

The previous two subsections discussed questionable research practices and the quality of studies, and further issues are discussed below. The big question is whether these affect the overall conclusions and therefore the body of scientific knowledge. Perhaps not all of the outcomes examined are reported in papers, unusual data points are routinely dropped, and incorrect analytical methods are common, but is it likely that the correct conclusion is still reached most of the time? It would appear that the answer is no. Scientists at Amgen were able to confirm the results in only 6 out of 53 (11%) landmark papers [29], and at Bayer only about one third of studies (14 out of 67) could be reproduced [287, 318]. These reports were from target validation efforts at the two companies. When a new molecular target for a disease has been identified and published, pharmaceutical and biotechnology companies invest a large amount of effort to reproduce the results and to gather further evidence to validate the connection, otherwise any further investment in pursuing this target would be a waste of time and money. These replication efforts by industry are a serious attempt at establishing real effects.

Another large scale replication effort was the FORE–SCI programme (Facilities of Research Excellence – Spinal Cord Injury) organised and funded by the American National Institute of Neurological Disorders and Stroke (NINDS) [361]. Twelve published spinal cord injury/repair studies were selected based on their quality, size of the beneficial effect, whether clinically relevant endpoints were used, and how easily the methods could be translated into the clinic (reported in Steward *et al.* [361]). These studies were then independently conducted, and the results were not encouraging. Six of the twelve studies failed to replicate the original findings and four studies had inconclusive, mixed, or a partially replicated result. Only two studies fully replicated the original reports.

Mobley and colleagues conducted a survey at the MD Anderson Cancer Center asking scientists if they had tried to reproduce a finding from a published paper and if they were successful [278]. More than half of the 434 respondents said that they were unable to reproduce the original finding; 78% of respondents tried to contact the authors to obtain more information, with 18% receiving no response, and 43% receiving a negative or indifferent response. In only 33% of the cases were differences resolved. Furthermore, 44% of all respondents and 60% of junior faculty and trainees reported having difficulty publishing the contradictory results.

The American Society for Cell Biology conducted a survey of their 8000 members and found that over 70% of the 869 respondents were unable to reproduce at least one study, and that 33% of respondents said they were told that another group had tried and failed to reproduce their findings.[16] The response rate was low and the numbers are hard to interpret because the number of studies that the scientists tried to replicate is unknown. Nevertheless, the results suggest that there is room for improvement.

Finally, the Open Science Collaboration conducted a large scale replication of 100 psychology studies, which included 270 contributing authors and took 4 years to complete [301]. Of the original studies, 97% reported significant results, but only 36% of the replication studies did, despite having power greater than 90%. In addition, the replication effect sizes were about half of the original estimates, and in only half the cases were the original effect size estimates within the 95% confidence interval of the replication estimate. The results are not encouraging and there is no reason to think that preclinical biomedical research is any different. A similar large scale replication effort is underway in oncology research.[17]

1.3.6 Empirical evidence IV: publication bias

Publication bias occurs when certain types of results have a greater probability of being reported than others. Reported results tend to be those that are statistically significant ($p < 0.05$) and support a research hypothesis. Thus the existence and magnitude of effects will be biased if positive results are more likely to be published than negative results. Publication bias can arise if entire experiments are not submitted, or if only certain results from an experiment are included in the final publication while others have been omitted. It could also arise if editors tend to reject papers with non-significant results. How do we know that publication bias exists? It is often estimated in systematic reviews and meta-analyses. Systematic reviews are less common in preclinical compared with clinical research [341], and the data are mainly based on animal models. Nevertheless, publication bias is detected in many preclinical studies [32, 254]. Another method of assessing publication bias is to

[16] `http://www.ascb.org/reproducibility/`
[17] `https://osf.io/e81xl/`

compare the number of reported significant results to the number of expected significant results, given the power of the studies and assuming various plausible effect sizes. Tsilidis and colleagues found excess significant results in animal studies of neurological conditions using this approach [368]. Another method to assess the extent of publication bias is to ask researchers what percentage of experiments that they have been involved in were eventually published. A survey of Dutch scientists reported a median value of 80%, or that 20% of their studies went unpublished [366]. Another finding which suggests widespread publication bias is that almost all cancer biomarker studies report significant results [209], yet few make it into the clinic.

Occasionally, the number of studies conducted is known, making it possible to check whether results were reported for all, and to determine the reasons for non-reported results. Such a case was recently reported in the social sciences and found that significant results were more likely to be published [122]. The findings likely apply to preclinical biomedical research, as well as the reasons researchers gave for not publishing the results. These include (1) the belief that it would be hard to get the results published or that others would not be interested, and (2) publication was deprioritised as efforts were shifted to other projects. Researchers may reason that it is better to focus on experiments that are going well instead of preparing 'unsuccessful' experiments for publication, which likely end up in a low-impact journal.

1.3.7 Scientific culture not conducive to 'truth-finding'

Academic science has been described as a tournament market, much like professional sports or the music and movie industries [124]. It is characterised by intense competition for big rewards, where small differences in ability or productivity are amplified into large differences in recognition and pay-offs. While this may encourage high levels of productivity, it can have perverse consequences. Publications – the number, the journal, the position in the author list, and the number of citations – are the primary outcomes by which biologists are judged and from which the rewards follow (a faculty position, tenure, scientific prizes, and so on). Biologists are incentivised to publish in journals with high impact factors, preferably as first or last author; but this is hard because of the limited number of papers accepted by top journals (which has been termed *artificial scarcity* [408]). Publications are required not only to obtain rewards, but often just to survive in science [66]. It is unsurprising that scientists try to maximise publication output, which may require trade-offs with the quality of research, and on occasion, the truth – fraud in extreme cases, but much more common are the questionable research practices discussed above.

The November 2012 issue of *Perspectives on Psychological Science* was devoted to the topic of reproducibility and several articles touched on cultural issues faced by researchers and how they can distort science. The titles are informative: 'Science or art? How aesthetic standards grease the way through the publication bottleneck but undermine science' [134], and 'The rules of the game called psychological science' [17]. These points apply equally well to experimental biology, including how the fetish for novelty reduces incentives for replication studies and how the desire for 'a good story' influences how the results are written and reported, such that the data appear to support a hypothesis perfectly. Both papers raise the point about competition and Giner-Sorolla summarises the issue well: '[S]ympathy and collective self-interest among psychologists may very well overcome principled research practices. Anyone who stands on principle, unless very lucky in results, will fail to compete effectively' [134].

Fiedler takes the argument further and suggests that because strong, impressive findings – that is, a good story – are what the scientific community and others want, researchers select the experimental factors, treatment levels, sample material, background variables, boundary conditions, time points, and outcome variables to maximise the size and consistency of the effects that are obtained [116]. On the one hand, someone is considered a good scientist if they can choose from a wide variety of options just those that maximally show an effect or phenomenon. On the other hand, it is misleading when large and consistent effects do not apply more broadly under different and perhaps more realistic conditions. Scientists may be reluctant to explore the rest of the 'experimental space' if it means finding smaller or non-existent effects under some conditions and thus producing a more complicated or nuanced story (or such results might just be omitted from a publication). This is a real concern for translational research because animal experiments may have been unintentionally optimised to show large effects instead of typical effects, or at least the variability of effects and how they depend on the animal model, background conditions, or outcome variable. What appears to be impressive preclinical findings then fails to translate to human studies.[18] A similar problem also arises in clinical trials, which typically use a homogeneous patient group (e.g. non-smoking males, between 18 and 65 years of age, with no comorbidities), a narrow subset of the disease spectrum (e.g. only mild disease severity), and outcomes that may be easy and objectively measured, but not necessarily relevant to patients [161].

The Mobley study mentioned earlier asked trainees (1) if they experienced pressure from a mentor to prove the mentor's hypothesis, even though the data fail to support it (Yes = 31%), (2) if they were pressured to publish findings of which they had doubt (Yes = 19%), and (3) if they were aware of mentors that required high impact publications before a trainee could successfully leave the lab (Yes = 49%) [278]. Although people may reasonably differ in the amount of evidence they require to convince themselves that a hypothesis is true or that a phenomenon is real, these findings suggest that there is pressure on junior scientists to obtain the 'right' answers and then publish them in selective journals. This study was restricted to one institution, but the experience of these trainees is likely similar elsewhere.

Incentive structures and pressures to publish differ between preclinical industrial research and academia. There has been little research into how these differences relate to bias or reproducibility but one study looking at statins found that non-industry sponsored

[18] There are many reasons why preclinical results may not translate, but if much of the research was based on the maximal effects possible in animal models, and if these only occur under a narrow set of conditions, then it is less likely that the translation to humans will be successful.

preclinical studies had effects that were almost three times larger compared with industry sponsored studies [197, 252]. Another study by the same group showed that publication bias was more evident in the non-industry sponsored studies [10]. The reasons for these findings are unclear, and their consistency across other research areas is unknown, but it deserves further investigation.

1.3.8 Low prior probability of true effects

The probability that a result is true partly depends on the probability that it is true before the experiment is conducted – known as the *prior probability* [168, 169, 295]. For example, suppose an investigator wants to test if mobile phone radiation affects gene expression in the brains of mice. He randomly assigns a group of mice to be exposed to radiation and has a control group that is not exposed. He then analyses the expression of five genes that he believes – based on previous research and biological knowledge – to be relevant for mobile phone electromagnetic radiation. If an effect is found in one or more of the genes, the results will have a relatively high probability of being true because the genes were selected specifically because they were believed to be relevant or sensitive to this experimental intervention. Compare this with an alternative approach where the investigator uses a microarray to analyse the changes in expression of 20 000 genes. Most genes will be unaffected by the radiation and thus the prior probability for most genes will be low, yet one would expect 1000 genes to have an (unadjusted) p-value of less than 0.05 ($0.05 \times 20\,000 = 1000$). Even with a correction for multiple testing (discussed in Section 4.1.3) there will still be many false positives that get reported, and even though they are statistically significant, they are unlikely affected by mobile phone radiation. Let us perform a few calculations to fix ideas. Assume that only 5 of the 20 000 genes will be truly affected by the radiation ($5/20\,000 \times 100 = 0.025\%$). We would expect 1005 p-values less than 0.05: 5 differentially expressed genes (assuming that there were no false negatives, that is, all 5 were detected as significant) and 1000 false positives. This means that more than 99% ($1000/1005 \times 100$) of the genes that we would call differentially expressed are actually false positives.

A trend in the biological sciences is the ability to measure more and more outcomes quickly and inexpensively. This includes all of the '-omics' technologies, high content image analysis, and automated recording of many behavioural parameters in animal studies. In earlier times only a few outcomes could be measured and they were likely carefully chosen and had a higher prior probability of being affected by an experimental intervention, compared with more recent studies. But as it becomes easier to measure a greater number of outcomes, the prior probability of any particular outcome decreased. The number of false positives is likely increasing over time, and there is evidence that the number of significant results is increasing [107]. Unless we think that scientists are getting better at predicting or verifying their hypotheses, the other explanation is more false positives. We know there is a problem when highly uncertain preclinical research is often significant but Phase III clinical trials are successful just over half of the time [98]. Such trials have a much higher probability of success because they are based on previous Phase I and II trials plus years of preclinical research. They also have enough power and have statisticians to deal with the design and analysis.

Why it's good (and bad) to be a biologist

Biologists have it easy when doing science compared with other disciplines – which is a good thing – and this is manifested in many ways. First, biologists can often create large effects. The expression of a gene can be reduced over 90% using small interfering RNAs (siRNA), or increased several fold by other means. These are enormous effects compared with what other disciplines can achieve. For example, imagine a social intervention that decreases crime by 90% or some new teaching method that improves student test scores several fold. Many disciplines deal with effects of small or modest size and require much more careful experimentation and sophisticated analyses to separate signal from noise. Second, experimental biologists have relatively homogeneous samples, such as cell lines or genetically similar mice, which are also reared and housed under identical conditions. Thus, the variability between experimental units can be extremely small, making it possible to detect small effects with few samples. Compare this with conducting a study on animals in the wild, patient populations, or first year undergraduates, as psychologists often do. Third, it is often possible to experimentally control many relevant variables, such as temperature, pH, concentration, humidity, duration, housing conditions, diet, and so on. It is usually possible to hold steady important factors that may influence and thus add noise to the outcome. In field studies, it is impossible to control the weather, and in clinical trials researchers usually have little control over patients' lifestyle or environment. Fourth, it is often easy to reproduce the treatment across subjects. For example, if 10 rats are to be given 5 mg/kg of a compound before a meal by gavage once a day for 10 days, the experimenter can be certain that this has occurred, and can make note of any deviations from the protocol. An experimenter can be less certain that 10 people will take a pill under a prescribed dosing regimen. Some people will forget to take the pill, they may take it at different times of the day, they may take it *after* a meal, they may decide to stop taking it if they feel better, and they may not record all of these deviations, which can introduce noise and possibly bias in the data, making it harder to detect true effects. Fifth, it is much easier to infer causality in highly controlled experiments, making statistical adjustments to equate groups on relevant variables unnecessary. Compare this with an economist who is interested in whether inflation affects (i.e. has a causal influence on) unemployment. They can only measure the relevant variables and require complex analytical methods to try to establish causality. Sixth, biologists often deal with directly observable phenomena such as number of cells, death (yes/no), or degree of pathology. Contrast this with a psychologist measuring well-being, a clinician measuring quality of life, or an ecologist measuring biodiversity. These nebulous concepts are hard to define and measure, requiring greater consideration by the experimenter, a greater number of outcome variables, and more complex analyses. Seventh, biology experiments usually have only a few explanatory variables; there are usually few experimental treatments and perhaps a variable related to a biological factor such as sex, age, or genotype. This makes the analysis straightforward compared with epidemiological studies which can have many variables related to diet, lifestyle, education, occupation, environmental exposures, medical history, and perhaps genetic information. Knowing which variables to include in the analysis is not a trivial exercise. Eighth, biologists usually generate their own data to directly address a research question and are less likely to use a secondary data source that was collected for one purpose but is then used for another one. An example is a Phase I clinical trial designed as a dose-ranging study, but is later used to look for biomarkers of efficacy. Finally, there are few negative consequences for biologists or journals of being wrong [28, 130]. It is unlikely that any single laboratory experiment or publication using animal models or cell cultures will influence public policy, alter the treatment of patients, influence large financial decisions (at least in academia), or lead to a lawsuit – there is little pressure to ensure that the results are correct.

To summarise, experimental biologists have it easy compared with other disciplines. But this comes at a cost. Because biologists can often get by with minimal knowledge about experimental design and statistical inference, there is little incentive to develop these skills. The correct qualitative answer (e.g. compound X increased phosphorylation of protein Y) can often be obtained even with a poor design and a meaningless p-value. But it is not always so easy. Sometimes the effects are small; using highly homogeneous samples means that the results may not be applicable more widely (e.g. in a different strain of animal), there may be environmental, technical, or extraneous factors affecting the outcome that cannot be held constant, and it may be hard to reproduce the treatment exactly (e.g. transfection efficiency may differ between wells). At best, this will lead to more noise in the data, making it harder to detect treatment effects. At worst, it will lead to biased results which can (1) indicate that an effect is present when none exists, (2) mask a true effect, or (3) provide an incorrect estimate of the size of an effect, depending on whether the bias is in the same or opposite direction of the true effect.

Another reason why experimental biologists have not more fully developed their statistical skills is the division of labour between those who generate data – wet lab biologists – and those who analyse it, such as computational biologists, bioinformaticians, or biostatisticians. No one can be an expert in all fields and there is a need for specialist skills in data analysis, especially for high-dimensional -omics experiments. But if analyses can be handed off to others, there is little pressure to expand one's own analytical skills. The data generator/analyst division is a dangerous cleavage of two skill sets that all experimental scientists should have. Science suffers when researchers cannot analyse their own data and understand and critique the methods commonly used in their field. Contrast this situation with physics; there are no 'computational physicists' that analyse data generated by the 'experimental physicists'. All physicists have good quantitative and computational skills, and they also know a lot about about physics. Biology should head in the same direction.

1.3.9 Main statistical sources of bias in experimental biology

As discussed above, bias can be introduced many ways. Some are especially important in biology and are related to the design and analysis of experiments. The first (in no particular order) is treating exploratory or learning studies as confirmatory studies. This distinction is discussed in Section 2.1, but here we just mention that the purpose of a confirmatory study is to test a few specific hypotheses under a narrow set of conditions. The classic example is a Phase III clinical trial, which has a predefined main outcome variable, one or very few comparisons of interest (e.g. treatment versus placebo), a specified population of patients, and a narrowly defined set of conditions under which the experiment will be conducted. A learning or exploratory study, on the other hand, trys to gain as much information as possible about the experimental and biological system – the conditions under which effects are present, how individuals differ in their response, which outcome variable is the most sensitive, and so on. There is no defined hypothesis and investigators are interested in discovering any type of effect. A learning study can be prone to false positives because of the many effects examined and they should be followed by a confirmatory study to verify and validate the findings. The problem is that many biological experiments tend to be learning experiments, but are then presented as confirmatory experiments. Significant effects are written as if they were predicted in advance and investigators can easily convince themselves that 'we knew it all along' that these results would be obtained. Whatever the results, they can be made to fit into a theory or to support some hypothesis. This has been called Hypothesising After the Results are Known (HARKing; [185]).

A second source of bias relevant to biologists is 'researcher degrees of freedom' which is the flexibility that scientists have in selecting outcome variables to present, removing troublesome data, transforming variables, adjusting/normalising/correcting variables (e.g. dividing by body weight), the choice of model or statistical test, whether a one- or two-tailed test will be used, and whether to collect more data [282, 355]. This can lead to trying many options until the 'right' answer is obtained and then presented as the only analysis of an *a priori* hypothesis. For example, Chan and colleagues compared the outcomes of clinical trials that were published in journal articles with the outcomes as specified in the study protocol – in other words, comparing what the authors defined as the primary outcome before conducting the study with what they actually reported. They found that 62% of trials had at least one primary outcome that was added, removed, or changed [68]. Follow-up studies by the same group found similar results between 40 and 62% [69, 104, 105]. Preclinical studies rarely define primary and secondary outcomes, which means that any result that supports a hypothesis of interest can be reported.

A third problem that affects the analysis of many biological experiments is the confusion between experimental units and observational units. This distinction is discussed in Chapter 3 and is important because it relates to how the sample size is defined. The experimental unit (EU) is the smallest entity, unit, or piece of experimental material that can be randomly and independently assigned to different treatment conditions [67, 114, 153, 274] and to increase the sample size or 'N' it is necessary to increase the number of experimental units. Observational units (OU) on the other hand are the entities on which measurements are made, and they may or may not correspond to the EUs. To understand the difference, consider an experiment in which 10 people are randomly assigned to receive either a pill that is hypothesised to lower blood pressure or a placebo control pill. After taking the pill, blood pressure measurements are taken from the left and right arms of all people. There are 10 people, but 20 measurements. Since people were randomly assigned to the treatment conditions, the people are the EUs, and the sample size is the number of people ($N = 10$). Arms are the OUs, and an analysis using all 20 measurements (e.g. a t-test) would have an inflated sample size and p-values that are too small. This is called pseudoreplication [165]

Box 1.1 Main statistical problems affecting the validity of studies

Design
- Treatment effects confounded with biological and technical effects
- Incorrect experimental unit defined → replicating the wrong thing
- Lack of randomisation
- Low power

Execution
- Lack of blinding
- Lack of randomisation
- Optional stopping

Analysis
- Incorrect experimental unit → inflated sample size/wrong error term
- Poor or inappropriate model
- Multiple analyses (researcher degrees of freedom)
- Incorrect interpretation of results
- Selective reporting (dropping observations, outcomes, or whole experiments)

and has been discussed in the literature repeatedly [89, 216, 222, 376, 377], but remains a persistent problem.

A fourth issue is when the effect of interest is difficult or impossible to estimate because it is mixed up, or confounded, with other biological or technical effects. As an example, consider the above blood pressure experiment, but the five people in the treatment condition are male and the five in the placebo condition are female. The effect of treatment is said to be completely confounded with the effect of sex and cannot be estimated. Unless one assumes that there are no differences between sexes, the experiment is a failure. Partial confounding would occur if there is an imbalance in the sex ratio between the treatment groups (e.g. the treatment group has a 4:1 ratio of males to females while the placebo group has a 1:4 ratio), which can also pose inferential problems. Confounding can also occur between treatment effects and technical factors and is nearly impossible to diagnose from reading a manuscript. It is therefore an underappreciated source of bias. Such confounding is the root of many horror stories that Nelder was referring to in his quote opening this chapter and what Fisher was referring to when he said that a statistician may be able to say what an experiment died of. It is usually possible to avoid or minimise confounding by an appropriately designed experiment and is discussed in Chapter 2.

A final common source of bias is inappropriate or inadequate statistical models. These include inappropriately treating the data as normally distributed (e.g. the data may be bounded below by zero if the data are counts, or they may be bounded below and above if the data are proportions or percentages), ignoring censoring (e.g. in experiments where latencies are measured, the experiment may finish before the event occurred for some subjects), not including important explanatory variables in the model (e.g. relevant subject characteristics or technical factors), and not taking dependencies in the data into account (e.g. the dependencies between the two observations per person in the above blood pressure example).

Taken together, methodological concerns, cultural factors, and publication practices distort the scientific record such that much of the published literature is of questionable value [58, 143, 408]. And doing more experiments will not necessarily allow us to weed out false claims or converge to the truth [171]. To this we can add citation bias, which occurs when results that support the hypothesis of the author are more likely to be cited [141, 142], or citations to papers that do not provide support of the stated claim [176]. Scientists differ in how much they believe published results; some are sceptical until further papers support initial findings while others assume the correctness of results until contradictory evidence arises – especially if the first result was published in a prestigious journal. The purpose of the preceding discussion was not to disparage science or scientists, but to raise awareness of issues that temper the credibility of the public record. It was also to draw attention to the central role that experimental design and statistical inference have in the generation of scientific knowledge.

1.4 Frequentist statistical inference

There are several paradigms or schools of statistical inference and biologists mostly use *frequentist* methods – the methods you were taught as an undergraduate in the biological sciences.[19] Educators find frequentist concepts hard to communicate, students find them hard to comprehend, and scientists often misunderstand and misapply them in practice. Nevertheless, another try is made below.

Frequentist methods were largely developed by Sir Ronald Fisher (who introduced the concept of a null hypothesis and *p*-values as evidence against the null) as well as Jerzy Neyman and Egon Pearson (who introduced Type I and II errors,[20] power, alternative hypotheses, and deciding to reject or not reject a null hypothesis based on a pre-specified significance level). Fisher had different views on statistical inference to Neyman and Pearson and some have argued that the combination of their ideas in statistics-for-scientists books and courses has made statistics confusing [72, 163]. Two different versions of frequentist methods are discussed below, and the only difference is where the emphasis is placed; the mathematics is identical.

[19] Frequentist methods are also called classical, orthodox, or 'error statistics' by some authors, but the term frequentist will be used.

[20] Type I errors are false positives (declaring that an effect exists when there is no effect) and the false positive rate is traditionally denoted as α. Type II errors are false negatives (declaring that an effect is absent when it exists) and are denoted as β. The more informative terms 'false positive' and 'false negative' will be used.

Box 1.2 **Stats quiz: A *p*-value of 0.05 tells you . . .**

(a) The probability that the null hypothesis (H_0) is true (that is, the probability of 'no effect' is 5%).
(b) There is a 95% chance that the alternative hypothesis (H_1) is true (there is a high probability that the effect is real).
(c) The chance of replication exceeds 95%.
(d) The chance that the result is a false positive is 5%.
(e) Something about the magnitude of an effect; a low *p*-value indicates a large effect.
(f) The probability of obtaining the same or even more extreme results, given that the null hypothesis is true.
(g) Some combination of the above (please specify).

Null hypothesis significance testing (NHST)

The most common variant of frequentist inference is called null hypothesis significance testing (NHST), which you were likely taught in an introductory statistics class. The focus is on calculating a *p*-value and then deciding whether to reject the null hypothesis, which we will denote as H_0, based on a pre-specified cut-off, such as a *p*-value below 0.05. Given the central role that *p*-values have in this method of inference and the (sometimes pathological) importance placed on them by many scientists, one would expect that scientists know the definition of a *p*-value and the information they provide. Unfortunately, when asked, many scientists cannot define a *p*-value. Please take a moment to choose an answer to the quiz in Box 1.2 before continuing.

Goodman writes

> Writing about *P*-values seems barely to make a dent in the mountain of misconceptions; articles have appeared in the biomedical literature for at least 70 years warning researchers of the interpretive *P*-value minefield, yet these lessons appear to be either unread, ignored, not believed, or forgotten as each new wave of researchers is introduced to [. . .] medical research.

How did you do? Only one option is correct, and it is (f). Goodman discusses *p*-value misconceptions in detail and it would be a good paper to read if you selected an incorrect option [136]. A simple way of doing well on this type of quiz is to remember two things. First, a *p*-value is the probability of the *data*. If an option suggests that a *p*-value is the probability of a hypothesis (a and b), an error rate (d), or an effect size (e), then it is incorrect. Second, a *p*-value is a conditional probability, meaning that it is the probability of something, given that something else is true. Specifically, the *null hypothesis is given or assumed to be true*. While option (c) refers to the probability of (future) data, it does not state that the null hypothesis is true, given, or assumed. Hence, (f) is the only remaining option.

⚠ To reiterate, a *p*-value is *the probability of the data, or more extreme data, given that the null hypothesis is true.* It can be written *P*(Data observed or more extreme data $|H_0 = \text{TRUE})$. The '|' is read as 'given', and the above is usually abbreviated as $P(\text{Data}|H_0)$. To clarify this definition let us use a coin tossing example. Suppose we have a coin and we are interested in making an inference about the bias of the coin. We are interested in testing if it is a fair coin, defined as having an equal chance of landing heads or tails. We will define the bias of the coin as the propensity to land heads up and we will denote this quantity with the Greek letter theta (θ).[21] If the coin is fair then $\theta = 0.5$; it will land heads up 50% of the time, on average. How can we test if a coin is fair? We could flip it many times and count the tosses that land heads. Suppose we toss the coin 20 times and it lands heads on 15 of these tosses. We were expecting 10 heads out of 20 tosses if it was a fair coin but observed 15. The question before us is: 'Are the observed 15 heads far enough away from the expected 10 heads to conclude that the coin is not fair?' Alternatively, we could ask if the observed bias of the coin $15/20 = 0.75$ is far away from the expected value of $10/20 = 0.5$. But how do we define 'far enough away' between what we expect and what we observed? The frequentist solution is to use a reference distribution based on all possible outcomes of tossing a *fair coin* 20 times, along with the probabilities of those outcomes.[22] Then, we compare our observed result against this distribution to see if it is unusual. Where does this reference distribution come from? It is a theoretical distribution, but suppose for the moment that we know nothing about theoretical statistical distributions. We could generate a reference distribution by taking a coin that is known to be fair ($\theta = 0.5$), toss it 20 times, and count the number of heads. If this procedure is repeated 1 million times we would obtain the reference distribution and it would tell us how a *fair coin* is likely to behave (Figure 1.10).

The height of the bars in Figure 1.10 is the probability of obtaining that number of heads and the sum of the heights of all the bars equals one. We would see that obtaining 10 heads out of 20 tosses is the most common outcome and obtaining 15 heads is much less common. The observed data is not used to generate the reference distribution. It would take a long time to generate such a distribution by repeatedly tossing a fair coin, and this is where theoretical distributions make life easier.

A fair coin will land with 15 heads 1.48% of the time (this is hard to estimate from the graph but can be easily calculated; it is the height of the bar at $x = 15$, and then multiplied by 100 to convert the probability into a percentage). Since this value is small, we might infer that our coin is unfair because 15 heads is unusual for a fair coin. The problem with this approach is that the probability of getting *any* specific outcome is low. For example, 10 heads out of 20 tosses will occur 17.61% of the time with a fair coin (the height of the tallest bar in the graph, when $x = 10$). In other words, the expected or most likely outcome does not happen all that frequently. This occurs because there are 21 possible outcomes (0, 1, 2,..., 20 heads) and the total probability is spread out over these possibilities. The situation gets worse if there are a greater number of possible outcomes (say if we flipped the coin 50 times instead of 20). The solution used by frequentist statisticians is to calculate

[21] We could have defined the bias as the propensity to land tails up. This is arbitrary and makes no difference. We assume that the coin is tossed fairly, meaning that it is not tossed in such a way to favour one outcome or the other.

[22] Technically, the reference distribution is called a sampling distribution.

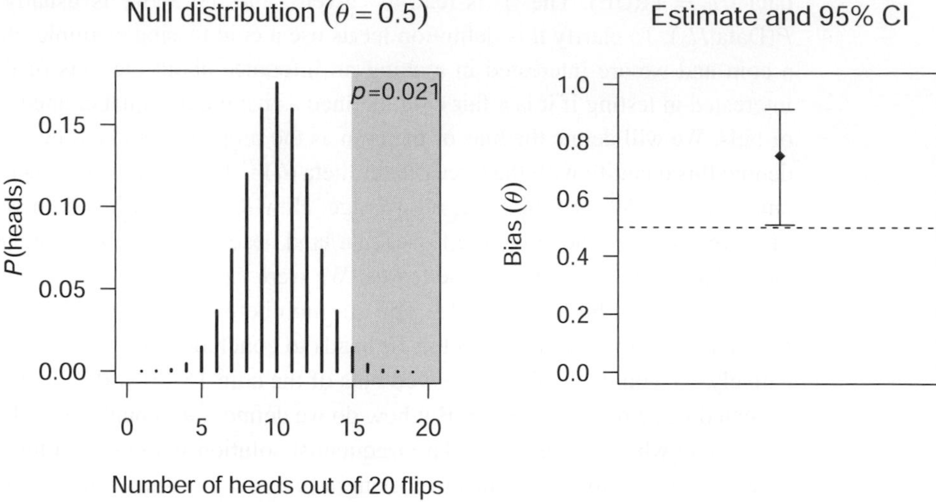

Fig. 1.10 Frequentist inference for the bias of a coin. The left graph is the theoretical reference distribution of coin flips for a fair coin ($\theta = 0.5$). The grey region is the region of the distribution that is greater than or equal to the observed data ($\geq$15 heads). The *p*-value is equal to the sum of the heights of the bars in the grey region. The right graph plots the best estimate of the bias and 95% CI.

the probability of not just the observed outcome, but also more extreme outcomes (16, 17, 18, 19, and 20 heads), which brings us back to the definition of a *p*-value: it is the probability of the observed data, *or more extreme data*, given that the null hypothesis is true. In our example the data are 15 heads out of 20 tosses, and the more extreme data are 16–20 heads, which deals with the first part of the definition (and equals $p = 0.021$; grey region in Figure 1.10). The 'given that the null hypothesis is true' part refers to how we generated the reference distribution. Recall that we are interested in testing if the coin is fair, so the null hypothesis is that the coin is fair ($H_0 : \theta = 0.5$) and therefore we generated the reference distribution by tossing a coin that is known to be fair ($\theta = 0.5$) a million times.

The logic of frequentist inference is to first enumerate all of the possible outcomes, along with their probabilities, to generate a reference distribution based on a null hypothesis fixed by the researcher. This distribution is then used to calculate the probability of the observed results or anything more extreme, which we mentioned previously can be written as $P(\text{Data}|H_0)$. If this probability is low then one can conclude either that H_0 is true and an unlikely outcome has occurred, or that H_0 is false, but we do not know which option is correct. Because unlikely outcomes are unlikely, we favour the second option. The logic can be broken down as follows:

1. If the coin is fair, then 15 heads or more is unlikely.
2. We observed 15 heads.
3. Therefore the coin is not fair (or the coin is fair and an unlikely event occurred).

This procedure has struck many as backwards because a hypothesis is treated as fixed and the probability of the data is calculated $P(\text{Data}|\text{Hypothesis})$. However, once an experiment is conducted, the data are fixed, and a scientist wants to make a probabilistic statement about a hypothesis $P(\text{Hypothesis}|\text{Data})$. The two probabilities can be very different. Consider the probability that a person with lupus (taken as given) has a rash $P(\text{Rash}|\text{Lupus})$ versus the probability that a person with a rash (taken as given) has lupus $P(\text{Lupus}|\text{Rash})$. The first probability is very high because a rash is a symptom of lupus and the second probability is low because there are many reasons why someone might have a rash other than lupus. This inversion between what a p-value tells you and what you want to know is the main reason for the misinterpretation of p-values, and also likely why frequentist methods are hard to teach and understand.

It also follows from this approach that using a relevant and appropriate reference distribution is critical for making correct inferences. In our example we tossed the coin 20 times and counted the number of heads. Thus, the reference distribution was based on many hypothetical tosses of $N = 20$. Suppose that we used another tossing procedure where we kept tossing the coin until we obtained 15 heads, and it happened to take 20 tosses. The data are the same, 15 heads out of 20 tosses, but the method of generating the data differs. In the first case the number of tosses is fixed while in the second case the number of heads is fixed. The data are identical, but the reference distributions and therefore the p-values differ, depending on which method is used. If we use one method for tossing and the other method's reference distribution, the p-values will be incorrect. Frequentist inference is dependent on the *sample space*, which is the space of all possible outcomes. If the total number of tosses is fixed, the possible outcomes are 0 to 20 heads. If the number of heads is fixed, then the minimum number of tosses is 15, with no upper limit. Thus, the calculation of a p-value is dependent on the space of possibilities.

Frequentist methods and the null hypothesis significance testing approach have many critics [79, 133, 136, 139, 178, 193, 245, 360]. A brief list includes:

- p-values do not tell scientists what they want; they provide the probability of the data given H_0, and scientists would like the probability of H_0 or H_1 given the data. Indeed, it is not even meaningful to talk about the probability of a hypothesis in frequentist inference.
- The calculation of a p-value is based on unobserved data, in other words, on data that might have occurred but did not. This seems odd, and there is evidence that this is not a natural way of thinking [306].
- The null hypothesis of exactly 'no effect', 'no difference', or 'no association' (sometimes called the *nil* hypothesis) is often false. For example, many biological processes will have some non-zero association, and differences between sexes or litters on many variables are rarely exactly zero. What does a p-value tell us when calculated from a reference distribution that is based on a false premise?
- It is hard to support a null hypothesis. One either rejects or does not reject H_0; much like a criminal case, a person is declared guilty or not guilty, but not innocent. Often the interest is in concluding that two groups are the same, or at least 'similar enough' for practical purposes, and the application of frequentist methods is not straightforward.
- p-values are widely misunderstood – even by statisticians [224].

- Encourages dichotomous thinking – a result is either significant or it is not – and thus automates reasoning and can lead to a psychological cliff at $p = 0.05$ [313, 331].
- A small p-value could reflect a large sample size or precise data instead of a meaningful difference between groups.
- Leads to publication bias because significant results ($p < 0.05$) are more likely to be published.
- The probability of false positives is constant (usually set at 0.05) regardless of the sample size. This is also counter-intuitive; as the sample size increases, surely one should be able to come to the correct conclusion.
- p-values depend on the (often unstated) intentions of the scientist. For example, when to stop collecting data (after 20 tosses, after 15 heads, or after 1 minute of tossing), or whether one is interested in detecting departures from the null in one or two directions.

Criticism of frequentist methods has increased in recent years, with few arguing that they are well suited for scientific discovery [267], or at least acknowledging that the approach has some positive characteristics [349, 391]. Nevertheless, this has become the dominant paradigm used by scientists for analysing data.

Parameter estimation

A second approach to frequentist inference is parameter estimation. Here, the focus is not on testing a hypothesis and obtaining a p-value, but rather obtaining an estimate of the size of an effect (the parameter) and uncertainty in that estimate. In a comparative experiment the estimate is called an *effect size* and it could be the difference between the means of the control and treated group, along with a 95% confidence interval. In many experiments estimating the effect size is more important than testing a hypothesis. Often it is known beforehand that there will be some effect and rejecting a null hypothesis is uninteresting and uninformative. Some have suggested that focusing on parameter estimates can overcome some of the problems with NHST, especially the focus on p-values and the dichotomous thinking that follows [88]. But inference is still based on a reference distribution and confidence intervals have a frequency interpretation as well. Similar to p-values, confidence intervals are often misinterpreted by researchers [155]. Box 1.3 is a quiz on the interpretation of confidence intervals adapted from Hoekstra *et al.* [155]. Assume the 95% CI is from an experiment comparing the difference between two means, which of the statements in Box 1.3 are true?

Options (a)–(d) refer to the probability of the true mean difference, that is, the effect size or parameter. Since frequentist methods cannot make probabilistic statements about parameters or hypotheses, these options are incorrect. Just like a p-value, a confidence interval does not tell us the probability of a hypothesis or parameter value, but is often misinterpreted in such a way. Option (e) refers to our belief about the true mean difference, and since frequentist methods rule out subjective probabilities, this option is incorrect. Since *confidence* is a mental state, a *confidence interval* suggests that we can be 95% certain that the true value of the estimate is between the upper and lower bound. Much like the term

Box 1.3 **Stats quiz: A 95% CI of 2.1–3.5 tells you ...**

(a) The probability that the true mean does not equal zero is at least 95%.
(b) The probability that the true mean equals zero is smaller than 5%.
(c) The null hypothesis (mean difference of zero) is likely incorrect.
(d) There is a 95% probability that the true mean difference lies between 2.1 and 3.5.
(e) We can be 95% confident that the true mean difference is between 2.1 and 3.5.
(f) If we repeat the experiment many times, the true mean difference will be between 2.1 and 3.5 95% of the time.
(g) If we repeat the experiment many times, the true mean difference will be between the upper and lower interval.

significance, the common meaning of *confidence* interferes with the statistical definition. Options (f) and (g) are similar, the only difference is that option (f) includes the specific interval values, whereas option (g) refers to unspecified upper and lower values. Option (f) is incorrect precisely because it gives a numeric interval from this experiment.  *'Confidence' refers to the long-run properties of the procedure and not the value of estimate.* For any given experiment, the true value is either in or out of the 95% CI, and so the probability is either zero or one. In this hypothetical experiment, the 95% CI was from 2.1–3.5. The true mean difference either is or is not between these values. If the experiment is conducted a second time, the upper and lower CI values will be different (say, 1.9–3.3), and again, the true value either is or is not contained within this CI. A 95% CI tells you that if the experiment is repeated many times, we expect that 95% of the time the intervals will contain the true value of the parameter. This, again, is not what is desired for scientific inference, but it is hard to *not* think and talk about CIs as representing a range of intervals that are somehow more credible than values outside of the interval. The only consolation is that a Bayesian analysis (which can make statements about the confidence of certain values over others) will often correspond to frequentist CIs, and so an incorrect interpretation may coincide with the correct one. Morey and colleagues provide an excellent discussion on the interpretation of confidence intervals and how they relate to Bayesian credible intervals [280].

Plotting estimates and confidence intervals is a good way to summarise the results of an experiment. The results for the coin tossing example are in the right graph of Figure 1.10. The horizontal reference line is at $\theta = 0.5$; which was the null hypothesis that the coin is fair. Since the lower 95% CI does not cross $\theta = 0.5$ (although it is close) the null hypothesis is rejected, but the true bias of the coin is uncertain because the 95% CIs are wide. The graph tells us what we already know, that $\theta = 0.5$ is not a plausible value for the bias of this coin, but we also get an impression of the precision of the estimate. These graphs are even more useful when comparing many effects from a single experiment or the same effect across multiple experiments. It is easy to notice trivially small effects that have small p-values (because of a large sample size for example) and effects that may not be statistically significant, but are large and biologically or clinically meaningful. In the latter case this could prompt one to collect more data to reduce the uncertainty in the estimate.

This section emphasised the limitations of the frequentist approach to inference, partly because the limitations are why many scientists misinterpret p-values and confidence intervals. Bayesian methods are conceptually simpler but are not discussed because both frequentist and Bayesian methods will lead to similar conclusions in experiments with few parameters, little prior information, and a reasonable sample size [175, p. 550], which describe the examples used in Chapter 4.

1.5 Which statistics software to use?

There are many statistical software packages available, each with advantages and disadvantages. R is a powerful open-source statistical package used by many statisticians and is becoming popular in other fields. The main drawback of R is that it takes more time to learn compared with point-and-click software. This may discourage some people, but if you are a younger scientist, then it is worth investing time to learn how to use professional statistics software – you'll be using it for the rest of your career. Some of R's advantages are listed below.

Free. R can be downloaded for free from the R-Project website (`www.r-project.org`). R runs on all major operating systems (Windows, Mac, Linux), and there are many free manuals, reference sheets, mailing lists, blogs, and wikis for beginners.

Excellent graphics. R can produce an enormous variety of production-quality graphical output in all of the standard formats (e.g. PDF, EPS, JPEG, PNG, TIFF, SVG). It is also possible to create specialised graphs from scratch.

Can import files from other statistical software. Data files from Minitab, SAS, SPSS, Stata, and others can be imported into R, allowing for an easy transition from your current favourite software. In addition, R can easily read plain text and Microsoft Excel files.

Large user community. R has a respected group of core developers who maintain and upgrade the basic R installation, but anyone can contribute add-on packages that provide additional functionality, such as specialised statistical tests or graphical functions. There are thousands of such packages available. In addition, there are online user groups where you can post questions and others will answer them (listed in the Appendix).

GUIs available. The basic R installation has a command line interface, which may be new for those used to a point-and-click graphical user interface (GUI). To ease the transition to R, the RCommander package provides an interface resembling other statistical programs (`http://socserv.socsci.mcmaster.ca/jfox/Misc/Rcmdr/`). After an analysis is selected from the menu, the commands are printed to the screen so that you can see and learn how to use them. The `Rcmdr` package is installed and loaded as any other R package.

Learn to program. R is not just a statistical package, but a programming environment, allowing users complete control over all aspects of data analysis. Learning R means you learn the basics of computer programming, a skill that every scientist should know. Writing programs or scripts enables you to automate repetitive tasks, which will reduce errors and free time for more important things.

Speak the language of your bioinformatics/statistics colleagues. Modern biomedical research often involves collaboration among people with different scientific backgrounds and expertise. Knowing the basics of a tool used by bioinformaticians, computational biologists, and statisticians enables you to communicate better with your collaborators and to share information and data more easily.

Make maths easier. R is a fancy calculator and can easily replace spreadsheet software. Also, R enables you to dissociate knowing what to do from how to do it, that is, the computation. For example, suppose you want to conduct a sample size calculation based on results from a recent publication and the paper reports the mean difference between two groups ($M = 3.1$), the total sample size ($N = 10$), the t-statistic ($t = 3.92$), and the p-value ($p = 0.004$). The paper does not report the standard deviation (SD), which is required for the sample size calculation. You do need to know that a t-statistic is calculated from the other variables (Eq. (1.1)) and that the p-value is not needed.

$$t = \frac{M}{\mathrm{SD}/\sqrt{N}}. \tag{1.1}$$

If you are confident with algebra you can rearrange Eq. (1.1) and substitute the numbers to give

$$\begin{aligned} \mathrm{SD} &= \frac{M\sqrt{N}}{t} \\ &= \frac{3.1\sqrt{10}}{3.92} \\ &= 2.50078. \end{aligned} \tag{1.2}$$

If your algebra is a bit rusty you can perform a simpler rearrangement by subtracting t from both sides of Eq. (1.1) to give

$$0 = \left(\frac{M}{\mathrm{SD}/\sqrt{N}}\right) - t. \tag{1.3}$$

Now we let R find the value of SD that makes Eq. (1.3) equal zero. First, we create a function for Eq. (1.3) and call it `f`. The function allows us to enter values for the mean, sample size, and t-statistic, which are indicated in the parentheses after the word `function` in the code below. The second line of code is the right hand side of Eq. (1.3). R's `uniroot()` function is then used to solve `f` for the unknown SD. The `lower` and `upper` arguments give the range of values for the SD between which R will search for the solution. The answer is the same as we calculated above to four decimal places.

```
> f <- function(M, N, t, SD){
+     (M / (SD / sqrt(N))) - t    # Equation 1.3
+ }
>
> uniroot(f, M=3.1, N=10, t=3.92, lower=0, upper=100)$root
[1] 2.50079
```

The point is that you need some high-level knowledge of what is required (the unknown SD can be calculated from the *t*-statistic equation), but then let R deal with the low-level computation and algebra. Indeed, most of your homework problems from first year calculus can be answered with R's `deriv()` and `integrate()` functions.

Structures how you think about data analysis. Data analysis is mostly fitting models to data, and software should allow you to think and analyse data in that framework. If the software requires you to point and click in one sub-menu to do a *t*-test and then in another to do a two-way ANOVA because you want to include another categorical variable in the analysis, you are left with the impression that *t*-tests and ANOVAs are different beasts (an idea reinforced by statistics cookbooks that discuss these as separate topics). They are both examples of linear models, the same R function (`lm()` or `aov()`) can be used for both analyses and the assumptions of both are checked in the same way. This point is probably hard to appreciate until you start using R to model data.

Further reading

Problems with frequentist methods: Cohen [79] is a classic paper and Goodman [136] and Stang [360] focus on biomedical research.

Bayesian inference: An article by Dienes [95] and several by Kruschke [201, 202, 204] and a book [203] provide excellent introductions to Bayesian methods, although with examples in psychology. McElreath's recent book is also great [269] and Lee and Wagenmakers very nice book requires little mathematical background (although all examples relate to cognitive modelling) [225].

Catalogue of biases: Lindner lists several biases in preclinical experiments [240], Sackett lists 56 biases in medical research [338], and Barber discusses 10 in psychological research [21]. Another list by Strasak and colleagues contains 47 common statistical errors in medical research [362].

Miscellaneous: The scientific audit that took place to verify the results published in *Nature* on the 'High-dilution' experiments is described by Maddox *et al.* [255]. The issues discussed in a paper entitled 'False-positive psychology: undisclosed flexibility in data collection and analysis allows presenting anything as significant' are highly relevant for biologists as well [355]. *Nature's* News Feature on the SOD1 mouse model of amyotrophic lateral sclerosis is an account of how easy it is for poor quality studies coupled with publication bias to lead a whole field astray [344]. A paper entitled 'Statistical thinking and statistical practice: themes gleaned from professional statisticians' provides many quotes from anonymous statisticians about their interactions with scientists and clients [307]. Finally, if you are interested in the philosophical, sociological, psychological, and methodological issues of reproducibility in biomedical science, a recent book by Maiväli provides an excellent discussion [256].

2 Key Ideas in Experimental Design

The development of the design of experiments is one of the greatest contributions of statistical science to science and technology. Yet, almost nobody knows anything about it!

John A. Nelder, FRS

. . . if all our engineers and scientists had some understanding of even the simplest principles of efficient experimental design a quantum leap could occur in the rate of development of our knowledge and of our ability to solve our problems.

George Box, FRS

This chapter introduces concepts and principles from the branch of statistics known as the design of experiments (DoE). A well-designed experiment has the following characteristics:

1. Effects can be estimated unambiguously and without bias.
2. Estimates are precise.
3. Estimates are protected from possible one-off events that might compromise the results.
4. The experiment is easy to conduct.
5. The data are easy to analyse and interpret.
6. Maximum information is obtained for fixed time, resources, and samples.
7. The findings are applicable to a wide variety of subjects, conditions, and situations.

These aims can only be achieved by *planning* the design, data collection, and analysis, and not by making decisions after the experiment is underway or completed. We begin this chapter by making a distinction between learning versus confirming experiments. The goals of these two types of experiments differ and influence the design and subsequent analyses [353]. We then discuss an equation that relates four types of effects to the variability in the outcome variable. This equation lies at the heart of experimental design and much of the book is devoted to working out its implications. The rest of the chapter introduces concepts such as randomisation, sampling, blocking, and factor arrangement. How to combine these aspects to meet experimental objectives is deferred to Chapter 5. Finally, we discuss sources of heterogeneity and confounding and how they can ruin experiments if uncontrolled.

Table 2.1 Examples of questions for learning (left) and corresponding confirming (right) experiments.

Learning experiment questions	Confirming experiment questions
• Does the drug have toxic side effects (at what dose, given for how long, in which tissue)?	• Does 5 mg/kg of the drug given once a day for 5 days increase blood creatinine[a] concentration?
• Does stress affect rodent behaviour (what kind of stress, for how long, on what behavioural tasks)?	• Does fox urine odour (a stressor) affect the amount of food Wistar rats consume during the first 24 hours after exposure?
• How does exercise affect cognitive functioning of older people (what type of exercise, how much, which aspect of cognition)?	• Does 30 min of aerobic activity (treadmill running) at 60% VO_2 max[b], 3 days a week for 6 weeks, in males between 55–70 years of age, improve performance on a mental rotation task?

[a] Increased creatinine indicates kidney damage.
[b] VO_2 max is the maximal oxygen uptake and is a measure of a person's aerobic fitness.

2.1 Learning versus confirming experiments

Experiments can have two general goals: to learn something new, or to confirm a previous finding or test a specific hypothesis [54, 56]. Sheiner discusses the differences between learning and confirming experiments in his classic paper [353], and the distinction is important because it affects the decisions made about the design. The aim of a learning or exploratory experiment is to discover as much as possible about the sample material or the phenomenon under investigation, given time and resource constraints. The aim of a confirming experiment on the other hand is to verify, confirm, or validate a result, which was often derived from an earlier learning experiment. Examples of learning experiments and corresponding confirming experiments are listed in Table 2.1.

The examples on the left in Table 2.1 do not test hypotheses but ask more general questions such as 'what happens if I do this?' (uncertainty in where or how the effect will be observed) or 'under what conditions might I observe X' (uncertainty in what will cause the effect to occur). The examples on the right not only supply further experimental details but ask more specific questions.

Suppose we are interested in testing the effect of a compound on rodent behaviour. When little is known about the compound it would be foolish to select a single hypothesis to test under a narrow set of conditions in the first experiment. At what dose do the effects appear? A dose that is too low will appear ineffective. Is the dose–response relationship monotonic? If not, overdosing may not have an effect either. At what time after injection does the behavioural effect occur, when is this maximal? Test too early or too late and the effect may be missed. Is the effect the same across species and strains? Choose the wrong species and the effect may be missed. Which behaviours are affected and which outcome is the most sensitive? Does the route of administration matter, sex, age, and so on?

How can an experiment be designed with so many unknowns? An aim of early experiments should be to address as many of the above questions as possible by using a wide variety of factors and measuring many outcomes. It would make sense to test several doses covering a wide range, at multiple time points, in multiple species, and examine the effects on many behavioural outcomes. It is impossible to examine every factor or outcome that might be of interest and decisions and compromises will have to made. No hypothesis is tested here, we are only exploring potential effects of the compound. The trade-off is that for fixed time and resources many things can be learnt, but the estimates will be less precise than if fewer factors were used. If the purpose is to learn from the experiment, then this is a good compromise because chances of finding effects across many factors and outcomes are maximised, and how the size or even existence of effects depends on these factors.

If a friend asks you to fetch their keys from the kitchen, a sensible search strategy would be to first cast your glance over the room, check under the newspaper on the table, and peer into a drawer or two. Without any other information it would not make sense to spend 5 minutes investigating the back half of the top drawer in one cupboard. A breadth-first search can narrow down the possibilities, allowing for more focused follow-up searches. Statistical significance is not the major concern in learning experiments, there may be large and biologically meaningful effects observed that do not reach the standard criteria for significance – this is not a failed experiment, but indicates areas where further investigations are likely to lead to important results.

Once exploratory experiments are complete, one is in a much better position to design subsequent experiments to test specific hypotheses. A problem with much of the published literature is that no distinction is made between learning and confirming experiments, resulting in two negative consequences. First, experiments are narrowly focused and do not explore enough of the design space,[1] much like beginning a search for keys by intensively examining a single drawer instead of exploring more widely. If multiple research groups conduct similar experiments but all have small design spaces, it may be hard to get a broad view of the field when experiments differ so much. What may at first appear to be conflicting results could be the result of experiments conducted in different regions of the design space where the existence or the size of the effects differ.

The second problem is that learning experiments tend to be reported as confirming experiments, where significant results are reported as if they were hypothesised before the experiment was conducted. The species in which no effect was present may be excluded, along with some non-significant behavioural tests, and much is made about the single significant result with the large effect, and the other outcomes that were 'trending towards significance', citing the relevant theory and literature to make the results plausible. This contributes to false positive reports in the literature.

An argument can be made to designate experiments as either exploratory or confirmatory, or at least indicate which results in a manuscript are exploratory and which are confirmatory [190, 383]. The same data cannot be used to both learn and confirm, although

[1] The design space or design region is the set of all possible values that the predictor variables can take.

Table 2.2 Design options for learning and confirming experiments. Adapted from Sheiner [353].

Design feature	Learning	Confirming
Subjects	Heterogeneous	Homogeneous
Environment	Varied	Standardised
Treatments	Many	Few
Factor levels	Many	Few
Design space	Large	Small
Randomisation	Yes	Yes
Blinding	Possibly	Yes
Blocking	Yes	Yes
Outcomes	Many	Few
Time points	Many	Few
Controls	Few	Many
Analysis	Bayesian	Hypothesis testing

experiments can have both a learning and confirming component.[2] Independent data are required for confirmation. High-dimensional -omics experiments are learning experiments and ideally they should be followed by a confirmatory experiment. There is still value in publishing only a microarray study for example, because others can use it to design confirmatory experiments, but it needs to be presented accurately and completely.[3]

The distinction between learning and confirming experiments is not absolute as one can learn something new in a confirmatory experiment, but it is useful to consider the main purpose of the experiment. Table 2.2 displays the main differences between learning and confirming experiments. Learning experiments tend to use heterogeneous subjects or samples (both sexes, different ages, multiple species or strains, multiple cell lines, and so on), under several environmental conditions (standard housing and enriched), test multiple treatments (multiple compounds with the same mechanism of action, multiple positive and negative controls), many factor levels (not just present or absent but low, medium, and high), and multiple time points.

For both types of experiments the basic principles of randomising, blocking, and blinding are still necessary. There may, however, be some advantages to knowing the treatment conditions in a learning experiment, may allow you to detect unusual patterns or interesting observations that are not a part of the formal data collection process. For example, animals in the treated group may appear more docile or there may be fewer cells in one experimental condition. A blinded researcher might notice variation in behaviour or cell count, but

2 Cross-validation is an exception but usually requires larger sample sizes than that found in many biology experiments.

3 Microarray studies are often followed by qPCR measurements for selected top genes, but the same samples are used. This is not an independent confirmation of the results; qPCR measures the same thing using another technology, and might be useful if the quality of microarrays is questioned, either as a general technology or the arrays used in a study. Also, beware of looking to the literature for confirmation of -omics results as it is almost always possible to find at least one paper that supports any interesting finding.

may not realise that they correspond to treatment groups. Toxicologists have been debating the pros and cons of knowing the treatment groups when making pathological assessments. An argument in favour of knowing the groups is that results from one outcome (e.g. kidney histology) can influence the assessment of the others (e.g. levels of serum creatinine, which are related to kidney function) [157]. Although collecting data unblinded can introduce bias, this may be less of a concern in exploratory experiments because there are no hypotheses to test that the researcher is psychologically or emotionally invested in demonstrating. With a 'let's see what happens' mindset, knowing the treatment groups allows both planned and unplanned observations to inform future confirmatory experiments.

Experiments typically have negative and positive control conditions (discussed in Section 2.10) that are used as reference groups to compare treatment effects against and to verify that experimental assumptions hold. Controls are always beneficial, but some may be less important in learning experiments because with fewer control groups, more treatment groups can be included. This is a trade-off, and suitable options will vary from experiment to experiment. Having multiple control conditions is useful for confirming experiments because they enable stronger conclusions to be drawn when experimental assumptions can be verified.

The analyses from exploratory and confirmatory experiments also have a different emphasis. Sheiner suggests that Bayesian methods are more appropriate for learning experiments while frequentist methods are better suited for confirming experiments. Since exploratory experiments have no defined hypothesis, hypothesis testing at fixed significance levels makes little sense [54]. The aim is to generate hypotheses that can be tested in subsequent confirmatory experiments by finding effects that look interesting, however defined.

2.2 The fundamental experimental design equation

Before discussing the fundamental experimental design equation three terms discussed extensively in Chapter 3 need to be defined. *Biological units (BUs)* are the entities that we would like to make an inference about. Humans, animals, and cells are common biological units used in experiments, and the purpose of a study is to learn about biological units. Many experiments replicate the BU, but a valid experiment can be conducted with only one. *Experimental units (EUs)* are the smallest entities, units, or piece of experimental material that are randomly and independently assigned to a treatment condition [67, 114, 153, 274]. Examples include a person, animal, litter, cage or holding pen, fish tank, culture dish, well, or a plot of land. *Only replication of the experimental unit is genuine replication* – that is, only increasing the number of EUs increases the sample size (N). The EU may or may not correspond to the BU. *Observational units (OUs)* are the entities on which measurements are made, and they may differ from the EU and BU. This tripartite distinction is meant to replace the terms *biological replicate* and *technical replicate*, which do not define the key aspects of samples.

Equation (2.1) is the most important one in this book, and variations of it have been described elsewhere [153, 375]. It matters because it shows how four types of effects can influence the outcome, and forces one to think about factors that might need to be controlled, manipulated, or held constant in an experiment. It is also a generic statistical model that shows how you can divide the data into independent pieces that correspond to the influences you care about (treatment effects), and other pieces that correspond to influences that would otherwise get in the way (technical and biological effects). Examples of each type of effect are given below the four terms.

$$\text{Outcome} = \underbrace{\text{Treatment effects}}_{\substack{\text{Environment}\\ \text{Compound}\\ \text{Inhibitor}\\ \text{siRNA}\\ \text{Dose}\\ \text{Time}}} + \underbrace{\text{Biological effects}}_{\substack{\text{Sex}\\ \text{Age}\\ \text{Weight}\\ \text{Litter}\\ \text{Genotype}\\ \text{Species}\\ \text{Cell line}}} + \underbrace{\text{Technical effects}}_{\substack{\text{Technician}\\ \text{Batch}\\ \text{Plate}\\ \text{Cage}\\ \text{Array}\\ \text{Day}\\ \text{Order}\\ \text{Source}}} + \underbrace{\text{Error}}_{\substack{\text{Experimental}\\ \text{Treatment}\\ \text{Sampling}\\ \text{Measurement}}} \tag{2.1}$$

The *outcome* is the measured variable that you want to make an inference about. It is also called the *response*, *criterion*, or *dependent* variable. Examples include the expression of a gene or protein, performance on a behavioural test, or the number of apoptotic cells in a histological sample. Most experiments will have multiple outcomes and the discussion below applies to both univariate and multivariate outcomes.

Treatment effects are the effects caused by the manipulations and interventions of the experimenter. Drawing a conclusion about the treatment effects on the outcome is the main reason for conducting the experiment. Treatment effects usually receive the most attention when designing an experiment and examples include the effect of knocking down a gene with a small interfering RNA (siRNA), the effect of different environmental conditions that animals are reared in, or the effect of inhibiting an enzyme. Treatment effects (as well as biological and technical effects) are also called *factors* and the values that a factor can take are called *factor levels* or just *levels*. For example, 'compound' is a factor that could have levels 'absent' and 'present'; environment is a factor that could have levels 'standard' and 'enriched'.

Biological effects are differences that arise from intrinsic properties of the samples or sample material and are not actively manipulated by the experimenter. An example is differences between sexes. Males of many species are larger than females, and if the outcome is body weight, some variation in the outcome will be due to the sex of the animal. An important decision in the planning stage is whether to include only one sex, thereby holding this variable constant, or to include both sexes. The advantage of including both is that the conclusions about treatment effects will apply to both sexes. It is also possible to detect if the treatment effect is larger in one sex (called an *interaction effect* and discussed in Section 2.8). If only males are used, we would have to make an assumption, which may or may not be reasonable, that males and females are similar enough to argue that the results found in one sex can be extrapolated to the other. This is an argument by analogy and is not a statistical conclusion. A disadvantage of using both sexes is that the design, analysis, and interpretation of the results can be more complex. Another disadvantage is that more parameters are estimated with a fixed sample size and thus the power to detect treatment effects is reduced.

Technical effects are the properties of the experimental system that can influence the outcome. Whereas biological effects are due to the intrinsic properties of the samples, the technical effects are due to all of the other properties of the experiment. For example, extracting RNA in separate batches may introduce differences between samples in different batches. Or, samples for a microarray study might be hybridised and scanned over several days, which might introduce differences between days. Microtitre plates – especially the higher density 384 and 1536 well plates – often have edge effects, where wells along the edge differ from wells in the centre of the plate. Variables that are of little interest but may affect the outcome are called *nuisance variables*.

There are many potential technical effects that can influence the results. Researchers need to know which are the most important and then either hold them constant (e.g. process all samples in one batch) or ensure that the treatment effects are not mixed up with the technical effects; for example, if control samples are in the first batch and treated samples are in the second. Two appropriate aphorisms when thinking about technical effects are 'know thy experimental system' and 'hope for the best but plan for the worst'.

Error is the variation in the outcome that cannot be explained or attributed to the treatment, biological, or technical effects, or any combination of interactions. It is the background noise that remains after all of the signal has been removed and, despite the name, has nothing to do with an experimental mistake. Casella defines error as 'the inability of the experiment to replicate itself' [67, p. 45].

There are several sources of error and it may not be possible to distinguish all of them in an experiment (Figure 2.1). *Treatment error* is the inability to exactly replicate the treatment across experimental units. For example, animals injected with a compound do not receive exactly the same amount because of variations in the injection procedure. Also, injections may be given in the wrong location (e.g. an intraperitoneal injection ends up elsewhere) thus altering the compound's pharmacokinetics. Or, when lesioning a brain region, the exact location and size of the lesion may vary from animal to animal. In clinical studies, patients are given a drug to take, but some patients may not comply with the instructions. Treatment error can often be reduced by refining and standardising procedures and is likely why results become more stable as researchers become more experienced.

Treatment error usually cannot be estimated because it is inseparable from *experimental error*, which reflects the natural biological variation from experimental unit to experimental unit, even after taking into account the relevant biological effects such as differences between sexes, ages, genotypes, and so on. Experimental error will be large when humans are the experimental units, smaller when animals are, and smaller still with *in vitro* studies. Even if treatment error can be reduced to zero, the measured response will differ because of unknown and unmeasured properties of the experimental units.

A third source of error is *sampling error*, which occurs because a sample is rarely identical to the population from which it was derived. Whatever is measured on the sample will be higher or lower than the true population value. And different samples will have different estimates. Sampling error is important in much of statistics, but is less relevant in experimental research because the experimental material (rodents, cell lines, patients) are usually not sampled from a population. In experimental biology, subsampling is more common, which involves taking multiple (sub)samples from experimental units. For example, it is

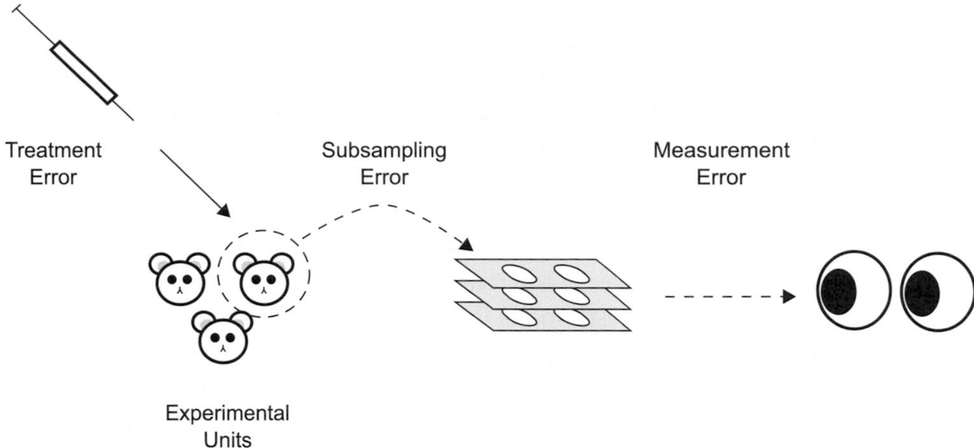

Fig. 2.1 Sources of error. The inability to replicate the treatment exactly for each EU leads to treatment error, which usually cannot be estimated. Variability amongst EUs plus treatment error leads to experimental error – the relevant error for testing hypotheses about treatment effects. Multiple subsamples (e.g. histological sections) can be taken from each EU, but subsamples will not be identical, leading to subsampling error (these are not true replicates and do not contribute to *N*). The inability to perfectly measure the outcome leads to measurement error, which can be estimated by measuring the same (sub)samples multiple times.

often unfeasible to count all cells in a brain region (the population consists of all cells in the brain region), so several histological slices through the brain region are taken, the number of cells on each slice are counted, and then used to estimate the total number of cells in the brain region.[4] In this example each animal is a sample (experimental unit) and each slice is a subsample. Uncertainty due to subsampling error can be reduced by taking more subsamples. This distinction is critical for making appropriate inferences and is discussed in Chapter 3.

There is the potential for confusion between how samples and subsamples are defined here and how they are defined in other statistics books, especially books in the social sciences. Here, *sample* always refers to experimental units and so sampling error results from some experimental units being included in the experiment, but others could have been. Imagine in Figure 2.1 a large population of mice from which the three mice in the diagram were sampled. The arrow pointing from the population to the three mice would be the sampling error.

A final source of error is *measurement error*, which occurs because measurements are never perfect. Measurement errors can arise in several ways. First, measuring devices can be imprecise; for example, if weight can only be recorded to the nearest gram. Second, the sample material can be of poor quality. It may be hard to measure a structure of interest in a histological section when there is high background staining. Third, there can be error in the definition of what is being measured. For example, measuring 'depression' in rats by

[4] Stereology is the field that deals with counting cells in 3D structures efficiently and without bias [13, 283].

using total immobility time on the forced swim test. Also, there may be nonlinear relationships between what is measured (e.g. fluorescence) and what the measurement represents (e.g. gene or protein expression, concentration of a substance). Fourth, there is error due to the experimenter. For example, the definition of an apoptotic cell will differ between researchers, and for the same researcher on different occasions. Finally, there is error due to the experimental procedure. Rats do not sit still when they are weighed, and the reading on the scale fluctuates.

Measurement error can be quantified if measurements are repeated on the same sample material; for example, if two measurements of body weight are made on all of the rats. Differences in the measurements for the same rat represent measurement error. Experimental error is usually greater than subsampling error, which is usually greater than measurement error. This is not surprising because we expect differences between animals to be greater than differences between two measurements made on the same animal.

There are two reasons why these distinctions between sources of error are important. First, if you want to reduce error, then you need to know where to look and what methods to use. If the values of the outcome are noisy, then one can systematically go through potential sources of error and see if there is scope for reducing it. For example, if treatment error is large then including more experimental units will improve the precision, but taking more subsamples (e.g. more tissue sections on each animal) will not help. Alternatively, if subsampling error is large one can take a greater number of subsamples. Including more experimental units will always improve precision, but it is often easier and less expensive to take more subsamples (e.g. more tissue sections per animal than more animals). If the measurement error is high, one can take duplicate or triplicate measurements; for example, measuring the weight of rats twice. Once again, it is often easier and less expensive to take more measurements than to include more experimental units or subsamples.

The second reason for distinguishing between sources of error is that only some sources are relevant for testing hypotheses, and using the wrong source will give meaningless results. We return to this idea often, but here we just note that experimental error (differences between experimental units plus treatment error) is the appropriate error for testing hypotheses; it is the noise from which the signal must stand out. This means that if more tissue sections (subsamples) are used, or more measurements taken, we do not increase the sample size, even though we have more values. Only by increasing the number of animals (experimental units) can the sample size be increased.

Several comments are in order. First, the categorisation of effects into treatment, biological, and technical is not absolute; one person's biological or technical effect is another person's treatment effect. For example, age could be a biological effect because it is a property of the subjects that might be related to the outcome, but is not scientifically interesting. Alternatively, age could be considered a treatment effect if the experimenter wants to test a hypothesis about age differences. These categories can help structure one's thinking about sources of variability, but they should not be made overly rigid.

Second, not shown in Eq. (2.1) are the interactions between treatment, biological, and technical factors. An interaction occurs when the existence, magnitude, or direction of a treatment effect depends on the levels of one or more biological or technical factors, or even another treatment factor; for example, there would be an interaction between treatment (e.g. compound versus control) and sex if the treatment had an effect in males but not in females. Interactions between treatment and biological factors are more likely (and of greater interest) than between treatment and technical factors. Interactions are discussed in Section 2.8.

Third, it is necessary to avoid confounding treatment effects with biological or technical effects. The influence of technical effects is often not considered when planning experiments and this occurs for several reasons. First, treatment and biological effects are inherently more interesting and are the focus of the experiment. Second, the potential for technical effects to influence the outcome is underappreciated and the magnitude of these effects is often underestimated. Some scientists may acknowledge that collecting data over 2 days instead of 1 may introduce more noise, but believe that it is likely to be negligible, and that running the controls on the first day and the treated group on the second should not be a problem. This view is often an untested assumption and not based on previous experiments that were designed to detect such effects, or based on the literature. If large treatment effects are expected, then technical effects will have little influence on the overall interpretation of the data, but hoping that technical effects are small relative to treatment effects and are therefore ignorable is a gamble with little upside (administratively easier) and a large downside (a useless experiment).

Fourth, the person planning the experiment may not be the same as the person conducting it. In an academic lab, the principal investigator may decide on which treatments and levels should be included and the execution is left for a PhD student to determine. In an industrial setting, the lab head may plan the experiment with the project team and the details are left for a technician to work out. Thus, not all relevant factors are considered in the design phase, and often the easiest or most straightforward approach is taken, instead of one that has statistically desirable properties. For example, control samples may all be processed together followed by the treated samples, instead of in a random order, or all of the treated animals may be housed in one cage and all of the controls in another, instead of having mixed cages.[5] Although experiments are easier to conduct, the potential for technical factors to bias the results is introduced.

Fifth, when technical effects are seen, it forces one to think about what other underlying factors are responsible for the observed effects. For example, if differences between cages are observed, it is usually not the cage itself that is causing the differences – they are all similar plastic and metal boxes. Considering how the cages differ suggests new variables to explore. The important underlying factor could be the location of the cage in a room or rack (e.g. temperature, light, or noise gradients) or maybe cages are a proxy for the order of data collection if animals are brought on a cage-by-cage basis into the testing room. Some of the main sources of technical effects are discussed in Section 2.12.

Sixth, an important distinction is between *common cause* variation and *special cause* variation. Common cause variation is the variation that is usually present and attributable

[5] There may be good reasons for not having mixed cages, the point made here is that this can introduce a source of bias that was not considered in the design stage.

to a known source. For example, there may be consistent differences between litters or between the edges and centre wells of a microtitre plate. Since common cause variation is known before the experiment is conducted, the experiment can be designed to take it into account. Special cause variation is the result of a one-off event that is not usually seen but affected the results in one experiment. For example, suppose that there are, in general, no differences between litters, but in this particular experiment one or two pregnant dams suffered from an infection during pregnancy that introduced differences between the offspring. Such effects could greatly reduce the value of the experiment if whole treatment arms are lost, or they could masquerade as treatment effects if only one litter was used in each of the control and treated groups. Special cause variation is harder to guard against, but precautions can still be taken. For example, if samples need to be processed in batches, it would be a good idea to avoid having all the controls in one batch and treated samples in another, as a one-off event that affects a batch can make the experiment worthless. More likely, it would be impossible to distinguish a batch effect from a treatment effect and a spurious 'discovery' will have been made. Another example is the order of data collection or sample processing; even if there is usually no time trend, randomising the order will protect against the rare time that it does occur.

Seventh, when studies have multiple patients or human samples, inferences can be made about patients or people in general. In animal studies, there are usually multiple animals, and inferences can be made about other animals, as well as a qualitative (non-statistical) inference about humans – to the extent that the biology is similar or the disease model reflects the human condition. What can a cell line tell us about a disease, biological process, or people in general? This is a problem for much of preclinical research because replication does not occur at the ideal level (biological replication), greatly reducing the scope of inference. *Generalising* refers to making broad inferences from the observation of many particular instances. It is necessary to replicate the units that one wishes to generalise to, and which may differ from the units that need to be replicated for a valid statistical test. Most biomedical research consists of doing X to Y under conditions Z and observing the outcome. Here, X is the experimental intervention, Y is the sample material, and Z is the background conditions (temperature, pH, concentration, plating density, incubator, and so on). Generalisability increases as X, Y, and Z are diverse or vary over a wide range. For example, varying X is often of experimental interest such as examining multiple concentrations of a drug instead of only one, or making observations across time instead of at only one time point. When using a heterogeneous population or sample material (Y varies) then the results will be applicable more broadly. Similarly, when the background conditions vary, then the results are not specific to a narrowly defined set of conditions. For many cell culture studies variation in Y is nearly zero, and a convincing demonstration of a phenomenon will usually require it to be robust under many background conditions Z, by conducting the same experiment on separate days.

Finally, the above points show why it is hard to teach statistics and experimental design to undergraduates. The analysis follows the design, and well-designed experiments require biological and technical knowledge that undergraduates do not yet have. How would they know that atmospheric ozone affects the fluorescent signal intensity from microarrays and that this could be a potential confounding variable [57, 110]? Healy puts it nicely: 'Indeed, it is not easy to inculcate a properly quantitative approach to affairs until some experience of affairs has been acquired' [149].

2.3 Randomisation

When doing an experiment we need to decide which experimental units will be assigned to which treatments. This is called *treatment assignment* or *treatment allocation* and we can think of it as either assigning treatments to EUs or EUs to treatments. The gold-standard method is to make the assignments randomly for each EU.

What are the benefits of randomisation? First, it ensures that groups are, on average, comparable on both observed and unobserved variables. It is unlikely that two groups will be identical, especially when the sample size is small. For example, with a total sample size of six rats, it is impossible to divide them into two groups of three such that the exprcssion of all genes is similar (at least one gene will be higher in all three rats in one group). This does not diminish the usefulness of randomisation because it ensures that, *on average*, the groups will be similar, even when we do not know which variables should be similar between groups.

For any given randomisation, there might be a large imbalance on the observed variables; for example, more females in the control group. Scientists often wonder if another randomisation to get a 'better' arrangement is legitimate or if this is cheating. If the first randomisation is unsuitable then it is fine to randomise again. But we have to be careful how 'suitable' is defined. Ensuring that the number of males and females are balanced between the treated and control conditions is fine, but re-randomising to have fewer animals with a severe disease phenotype in the treated condition is unacceptable. If there are covariates that should be balanced between experimental conditions, then forming blocks is one way to ensure a good balance on the first randomisation (see Section 2.4 below).

If it is permissible to use multiple randomisations until a suitable arrangement is achieved, then what is the advantage of randomising compared with selecting experimental units to achieve a nice balance? This brings us to the second advantage of randomisation: it removes the effect of conscious and unconscious experimenter biases. If researchers are allowed to haphazardly allocate experimental units to the treatment conditions, then subtle differences between the EUs might influence their allocation. Furthermore (third advantage), randomisation is a useful device to *convince others* that no systematic biases are present and that the EUs were assigned so as not to bias the results. This is important when convincing the scientific community about the validity of the results. Randomisation can also help maintain blinding by making it hard to guess the treatment groups of EUs.

Finally, randomised designs are easier to conduct, analyse, and interpret. Complex blocking or matching strategies to balance many covariates make the design and analysis harder, perhaps for only a small increase in precision. There may be non-random ways which are better by some criterion but random assignment ensures that the assignment mechanism is ignorable so that a simpler analysis can be conducted and the results are less sensitive to prior assumptions.

2.4 Blocking

Treatment effects can be hard to detect when the experimental error is large; that is, when variation between experimental units is large. This variation could occur due to any of following:

1. EUs are heterogeneous.
2. EUs form recognisable subgroups (e.g. male and female).
3. EUs are grouped into batches to simplify the conduct of the experiment and this may introduce differences between EUs in different batches.

A solution to the first problem is to select EUs that are as homogeneous as possible, but if they are all the same, the results cannot be generalised to more diverse EUs. Also, it may not be possible to find enough homogeneous experimental units. Fortunately, blocking can be used to efficiently estimate treatment effects when variation between the EUs is large. The idea is to divide the experimental units into subgroups of similar units at the beginning of the experiment. Similarity is based on variables that either affect the outcome or that we would like to have balanced between treatment groups. Then, randomisation to the treatment conditions occurs *within* each of the subgroups (Figure 2.2).

The homogeneous subgroups are called blocks and the test for treatment effects uses multiple homogeneous subgroups instead of one large heterogeneous group. For example, suppose that we are interested in testing if a 2-week high-protein diet increases body weight in rats. Suppose that before the start of the experiment a baseline measure of food consumption is recorded for 1 week. Some rats will eat more than others and it is expected that they will be heavier regardless of diet. Treatment effects will be harder to detect with a completely randomised design because the amount that rats eat is an uncontrolled variable. Some variation in final body weight will be due to the amount of food consumed and this will add noise to the data. A more efficient design would be to first group the rats into homogeneous subsets based on baseline food consumption. This could be done by ranking the rats from heaviest to lightest eaters and then grouping them into pairs by taking the first two rats (the two that ate the most during baseline), then the next two in the list, and so on. The difference from a completely randomised design is that one rat within each pair is randomised to one of the treatment groups, and the other rat is then assigned to the remaining treatment group. Each rat in a pair is expected to eat a similar amount of food during the experiment because they have been matched on their baseline food consumption. By removing this source of variation, the comparison between rats in a pair will be mostly unaffected by the amount of food they eat, allowing treatment effects to be more easily detected. The test for a treatment effect is made between each pair of rats, and then averaged over all pairs. Complete randomisation ensures that on average – meaning across many such experiments – baseline food consumption will be balanced across the two groups. Blocking ensures that *in this experiment* the two groups will be balanced.

In the above example, baseline food consumption was a continuous variable that was used to create matched pairs (blocks). A second reason for heterogeneity between

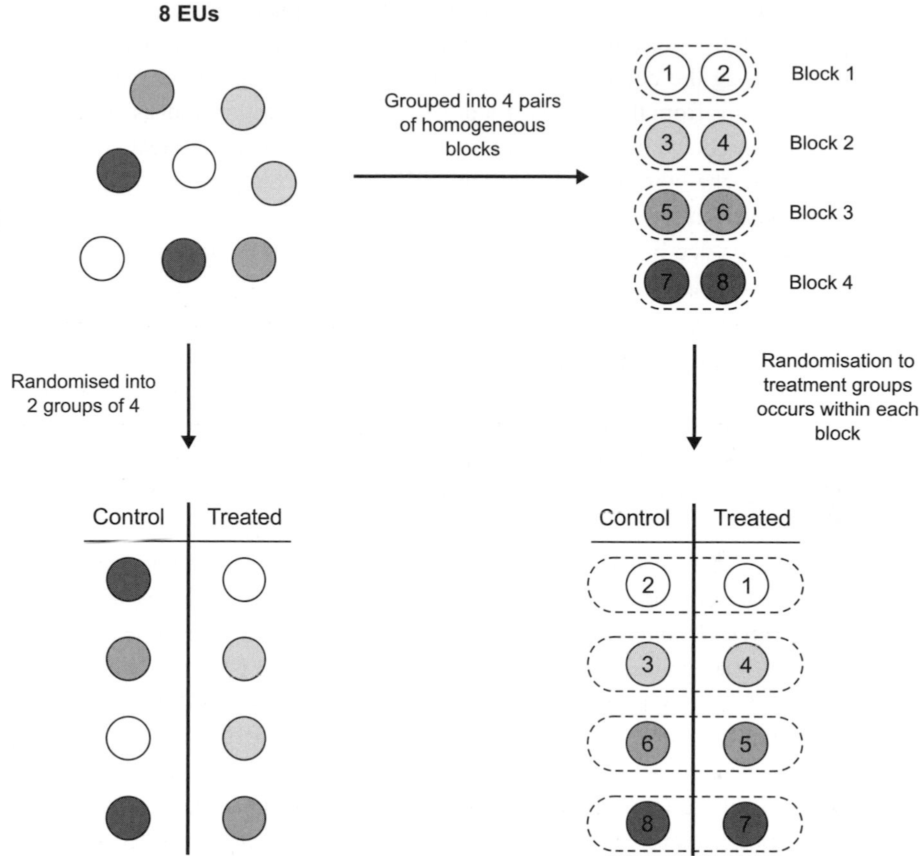

Fig. 2.2 Blocking can increase the precision of treatment effect estimates with heterogeneous experimental units (indicated by the degree of shading). Eight EUs can be randomised directly into two groups, or they can first be paired into four homogeneous subgroups (blocks) and then randomised to treatment conditions within pairs, such that one EU from each pair is in each treatment condition. Adapted from Bolstad [51].

experimental units is because they form recognisable subsets or subgroups, and the EUs within a subgroup are more alike than EUs between subgroups. The subgroups are typically defined by biological factors such as sex, litter, age, and so on. For example, male rats tend to be heavier than females, and part of the variation in the outcome will be due to sex differences. One could first divide the rats into males and females, then randomly assign members of each sex to the treated or control groups. This ensures that an equal number of males and females are in each treatment condition (assuming that the total number of rats is evenly divisible by the number of treatment conditions).

The third reason for heterogeneity between experimental units is that technical artefacts influence the outcome. Large experiments often need to be divided into smaller batches and run as a series of mini experiments. Even if the EUs are homogeneous at first, the process of batching may introduce differences. Cell culture experiments are often repeated multiple times over several days and the results combined for a single analysis. The values of the outcome variables often vary considerably from day to day and this variation is usually dealt with by 'normalising' the results relative to the control group for each day. For example, setting the control group to 100% and calculating a percentage or fold change of other groups from the control group. Although this mostly removes the day (block) effects, it is a poor choice for several reasons. First, it can make the variance of the control group smaller than the other groups (see Figure 6.7 for an example). Second, it hides the magnitude of block effects, which others can use to plan their experiments. It is useful to know if the difference between days is large compared with the treatment effects. Third, aspects of a poorly designed experiment can be easily hidden; for example, severe imbalance between experimental conditions and blocks, or that some experimental conditions were not tested in some blocks. Finally, if this type of *ad hoc* adjustment for block effects is done, then it would be better to subtract the mean of the whole block instead of the mean of the control group only, although this is not recommended (see the discussion associated with Figure 6.7 for more information).

Blocking variables are usually biological or technical factors that are known to influence the outcome but are not scientifically interesting. Blocking variables are used to reduce the experimental error and to obtain more precise estimates of treatment effects but there is usually no interest in testing a hypothesis or calculating a p-value for block effects. However, one scientist's block (e.g. sex) may be another scientist's experimental variable of interest.

Blocking is only beneficial if the blocking factor accounts for variance in the outcome, and the more variation that the blocks account for, the greater the efficiency of the design compared with a completely randomised design. Blocking can also reduce the efficiency of a design if the blocks account for little or no variation in the outcome because additional parameters are being estimated. The general rule is often stated as 'block what you can and randomise the rest'. These concepts and the benefits of blocking will become clearer when we go through numerical examples (Section 4.4).

Blocked designs are classified into *complete block* designs, where each treatment appears in each block and *incomplete block* designs, where blocks do not contain all treatments. Incomplete block designs usually occur when there are not enough experimental units within a block for all of the treatments to be tested. For example, suppose litter is used as a blocking variable and the litter size varies between 8–12, but there are 15 treatments to be tested and thus all treatments cannot be tested in all litters. Incomplete block designs will not be considered as they are rare in experimental biology and they are covered in almost all books on experimental design (Mead *et al.* is the most relevant for biologists [274]).

2.5 Blinding

Blinding refers to concealing information about treatment groups or other aspects of the experiment from subjects, researchers, and others involved with the experiment. Blinding is used to reduce bias that can arise when this information is known (Box 2.1). Human

Box 2.1 **Blinding**

Who should be blinded?

- Human subjects or patients.
- Researchers conducting the experiment.
- Caregivers, animal facilities staff, and others who interact with the subjects.

What information should be concealed?

- The experimental group when assessing the outcome.
- The future treatment group of subjects during pre-treatment interventions such as inducing a lesion.
- Previous values when multiple observations are made on the same experimental or observational units over time.
- The values of other outcomes from the same experimental or observational units.
- Information that provides clues about treatment groups.
- Information indicating which experimental units are in the same treatment condition, even if the experimental condition of the groups remains unknown.

subjects might respond differently when they know the treatment group that they are in. For example, subjects in the treated group might report that they feel better compared with subjects in the control group because of their expectation that the treatment will have a positive effect (placebo effect), or because they wish to please the experimenter. Blinding human subjects removes these potential biases as alternative explanations for the observed results. Blinding may, however, be difficult or unethical; for example, when comparing a surgical intervention with a pharmaceutical treatment, blinding might require that some patients receive a sham surgery. Subjects may use clues to guess their treatment group. When subjects provide informed consent they are told of potential side effects of the experimental interventions. Subjects may deduce the group they are in by the side effects they experience, and this knowledge can then influence the results.

In addition to concealing information about treatment groups from the subjects, it is also desirable to conceal this information from the experimenter. This prevents the experimenter from intentionally or unintentionally influencing the results, especially for outcomes that involve subjective judgements or assessments, such as determining disease severity or degree of pathology; for example, by assigning scores of 0, +, ++, or + + +. The primary purpose of blinding experimenters is not to prevent unscrupulous researchers from manipulating the results but to protect against unconscious biases.

When only subjects are blind, the experiment is *single blind*, and is irrelevant for rodent and *in vitro* experiments. When both subjects and experimenters are blind, the experiment is *double blind*. These terms are taken from the clinical trial literature, where it is usually easier and more important to blind subjects. Hence, either studies blind subjects only (single blind), or both subjects and experimenters (double blind), but never experimenters only. In preclinical experiments, it is only the experimenters that are blind, as rats and cells do not have expectations about treatment outcomes. One does occasionally see preclinical experiments described as double blind, and the authors usually mean the experimenter was blind. Unless active steps were taken to conceal the treatment groups from subjects, preclinical experiments should not be described as double blind.

The third group of people that should be unaware of the treatment conditions are those who interact with subjects. For animal experiments, this includes the animal facilities staff, since they might give some groups 'special treatment'; for example, by handling some animals more gently or interacting with them more, which could influence the results. For human experiments, caregivers, nurses, and family members are included in this third category.

What information should be concealed? For subjects, they should remain unaware of their treatment condition for the duration of the experiment. For experimenters, there are six pieces of information that can be withheld. The first and most important is the treatment group to which the experimental or observational units belong when assessing outcomes, as this is the most likely place where bias can arise. In addition, experimenters should be blind when interacting with the biological or experimental units before assessing outcomes; for example, daily handling of rodents to get them used to interacting with humans. This ensures that all BUs and EUs are treated similarly. Second, the experimenter should be blind to the group that experimental units will be assigned to when performing pre-randomisation interventions. For example, when inducing a stroke, brain lesion, or injecting tumour cells into animals, the experimenter should not know which animals will end up in which experimental group. Blinding ensures that all animals are treated similarly and that animals that will be assigned to the treated group do not inadvertently receive lesions that are less severe, for example. Third, it is often useful for experimenters to be blind to earlier observations of the same outcome, as knowing previous results might influence the current assessment, especially for subjective assessments. Fourth, it is often beneficial for the experimenter to be unaware of the results of other outcomes for each experimental or observational unit, as these results may influence the assessment of the current outcome. As was discussed in Section 2.1 on exploratory and confirmatory studies, concealing the results of other outcomes is useful for confirmatory studies, but there may be some advantages to being unblinded for exploratory studies. Fifth, it is necessary to conceal information that can provide the experimenter clues about the treatment groups. For example, if the experimenter knows that animals with identification numbers 1–5 are the controls and 6–10 are in the treated group, then knowledge of the identification number breaks the blinding. Similarly, cage numbers or positions on a microtitre plate may provide the necessary information to identify the experimental groups for all experimental units. Finally, experimenters should not be able to determine which animals belong together in the same group, even if they do not know the corresponding experimental conditions of those groups. For example, experimenters should not know that animals 1–5 belong to one group (call it A) and animals 6–10 belong to another group (B), even if information about whether Group A is the control or treated group is concealed. If differences between groups starts to emerge as the data are collected, then it may be possible to infer that Group A are the controls, and unintentional influences may then begin to affect the subsequent results. This is especially pernicious because the experimenter does not know the treatment groups of the animals and the experiment can be described as blinded, but it gives a false sense that the experiment has been conducted well if the blind can be easily broken. This is why placebo and active pills in clinical trials are identical instead of using red and blue pills, even if researchers do not know which colour corresponds to which group.

It is common to group experimental or observational units from the same experimental conditions together because it makes the experiment easier to conduct. For example, animals in the same cage are often in the same condition, experimental units are often consecutively numbered such that adjacent numbers are usually in the same condition, and glass coverslips from wells in the same condition are placed on the same glass slides. Often what is administratively easier also makes it easier to guess the treatment conditions. Once a hypothesis is half-formed (e.g. the first two coverslips on this glass slide look healthy, maybe these are in the treated condition), future observations may be influenced by this hypothesis. If this occurs, then both the mean and the variance can be biased, although it is usually the mean that receives the most attention. For example, if a researcher suspects that a glass slide contains four wells from the control condition, this could influence the estimated mean. A researcher might also expect that if the four wells on a slide are in the same condition then the values should be similar to each other. This expectation could bias the values towards the slide average, thus reducing the variance of the data. If the coverslips are the experimental units, a reduced variation between coverslips translates into p-values that are artificially small.

It might be hard to achieve statistically optimal arrangements because of practical constraints, and trade-offs will have to be made. Nevertheless, it is important to know where sources of bias can arise and take steps to minimise them where possible and practical.

2.6 Effect type: fixed versus random

The treatment, biological, and technical effects that we have been discussing can be classified as either *fixed* or *random*, and the distinction is important because it leads to different analyses and a different interpretation of the results. Standard statistical tests treat all categorical predictors (factors) as fixed, and so you may have not come across the fixed/random distinction before. Whether the effect of a categorical predictor is fixed or random depends on how it is specified in a statistical model. Thus, the fix/random distinction is not an inherent property of a predictor variable but a matter of how we choose to define it. A fixed effect relates the levels of a factor to the mean of an outcome variable, whereas a random effect relates the levels of a factor to the variance of an outcome. Generally, fixed effects are biologically interesting and test an experimental hypothesis, which is the reason treatment effects are almost always considered fixed [347]. Random effects are usually less interesting such as litter effects, cage effects, differences between incubators, differences between individual rats, but must be taken into account because they affect the outcome.

All categorical predictors can be treated as either fixed or random, but usually one is more appropriate. The choice is often straightforward given the hypotheses of interest

Table 2.3 Deciding between fixed and random effects.

Questions to consider	Fixed	Random
Interested in differences between factor levels?	✓	
Is the factor a treatment effect?	✓	
Are factor levels informative?	✓	
Are the factor levels experimental interventions?	✓	
Are the factor levels specifically chosen?	✓	
Are all levels of the factor included in the experiment?	✓	
Do factor levels come from a population?		✓
Are there many factor levels?		✓
Want to generalise to factor levels not included in the experiment?		✓
Is there nested or hierarchical (sub)sampling?		✓

and the experimental design, but reasonable opinion may differ. Questions to help decide whether a variable is better considered fixed or random are given in Table 2.3.

Suppose we are interested in testing if there are differences between cages on an outcome, rats could be randomly assigned to four cages labelled A, B, C, and D. In this example there is no other experimental variable, only the cage that the rats are in. A standard way to analyse this data would be a one-way ANOVA with four levels, which means that cage is a fixed effect. If significant differences are found between cages, then conclusions can only be made about these four cages, and not about other unobserved cages. Treating cage as a random effect would consider these four cages as being derived from a population of cages and therefore conclusions can be made from these four to the larger population. If rats in cage C had the highest values, there is no reason why in a subsequent experiment rats in a cage also labelled C would also have the highest values, instead of rats in cage B, for example. There is nothing about the letter C on the front of the cage that affects the mean value of rats in that cage, or that can be used to predict the value of rats in other cages also labelled C. The cage labels are therefore said to be uninformative, which is characteristic of random effects. Contrast this with a true fixed effect such as the dose of a drug; if the 50 mg/kg group had higher values than the 0 mg/kg control group, then one would also expect that the 50 mg/kg group would have higher values in a subsequent experiment instead of the 0 mg/kg group. Here, the factor levels are informative. Experiments can have both fixed and random effects and are then analysed with mixed-effects models.

2.7 Factor arrangement: crossed versus nested

When an experiment has multiple factors they can be arranged in one of two ways. The first is a *crossed* or *factorial* arrangement, which occurs when all levels of one factor exist with all the levels of the other factors. This is the most common arrangement in experimental biology and Table 2.4 shows an experiment with two crossed factors. Twenty rats (denoted

Table 2.4 The factor lesion is crossed with the factor drug ($n = 20$).

	No lesion	Lesion
No drug	•••••	•••••
Drug	•••••	•••••

Table 2.5 The factor cage is nested under the factor lesion ($n = 20$).

	No lesion	Lesion
Cage 1	•••••	
Cage 2	•••••	
Cage 3		•••••
Cage 4		•••••

Table 2.6 Alternative display for a nested design where cage is nested under lesion ($n = 20$).

No lesion		Lesion	
Cage 1	**Cage 2**	**Cage 3**	**Cage 4**
•••••	•••••	•••••	•••••

by a dot '•') are randomly assigned to either receive a lesion or not and to be administered a drug or not. The factors are crossed because there are observations for all factor level combinations.

This can be contrasted with a *nested* arrangement where all factor level combinations do not occur. Table 2.5 shows a nested design where the 20 rats are randomly assigned to live in four cages. Cages are nested under the factor lesion as there are no animals that receive a lesion in Cage 1.

⚠ It is a good idea to use distinct names for the levels of the nested factor, as is done in Table 2.5. The alternative is to reuse factor levels so that there is a Cage 1 in the Lesion group, and another Cage 1 in the No lesion group. Even though the labels are the same, these are *not* the same cages. Using distinct factor levels makes the nesting more apparent to you, others, and your statistical software.

The layout of Table 2.5 makes it obvious that some factor level combinations do not occur, but the layout of Table 2.6 makes the nesting relationships clearer.

A third factor arrangement is mentioned here for completeness and is discussed further in Section 2.12. If factors are not nested or crossed they are said to be *confounded*. This occurs when the effect of two or more factors cannot be estimated because levels of one

Table 2.7 The factor lesion is confounded with the factor cage ($n = 10$). It is impossible to separate the effect of the lesion from differences between cages.

	Cage 1	Cage 2
No lesion	●●●●●	
Lesion		●●●●●

factor always correspond to the same levels of another factor. Table 2.7 shows that it is impossible to estimate the effect of both lesion and cage because the No lesion group is in Cage 1 and the Lesion group is in Cage 2. Any observed differences could be due to differences between cages instead of the effect of a lesion. This may appear to be a nested design because of the empty cells, but the difference is that there is no replication of cages at each level of the lesion factor. To make valid inferences one would need to assume that the effects of cage are zero. Moreover, as this assumption cannot be checked, the researcher can only hope that cage effects are absent. Such a design should be avoided.

2.8 Interactions between variables

When there are two or more predictor variables – usually in a crossed arrangement – their joint effect on the outcome may not equal the sum of their individual effects. If this is the case, the variables are said to *interact*. An interaction between variables is a fundamental concept in statistics that many find hard to understand. George Box provides an intuitive and amusing animal breeding example [54, p. 37]. The first variable in Box's example is the presence (+) or absence (−) of a male rabbit. The second variable is the presence (+) or absence (−) of a female rabbit. There are thus four possible combinations of factor levels (−,−), (+,−), (−,+), (+,+), and the results are obvious: bunnies will not be produced if a cage contains neither a male nor a female rabbit (−,−). A single male rabbit (+,−) will not produce bunnies, nor will a single female rabbit (−,+), but placing both a male and a female rabbit in a cage (+,+) will produce bunnies. The effect of 'producing bunnies' is only seen when both factors are at the + level. If two separate experiments are conducted by comparing the empty cage condition (−,−) with the male only condition (+,−), and then comparing the empty cage condition with the female only condition (−,+), one would conclude that neither male nor female rabbits are necessary for producing bunnies. The point is that it is not possible to determine how the system works by studying each variable in isolation.

There are two ways to think about interaction effects, depending on the research question and the type of variables. The first interpretation is useful when both variables are treatment variables applied to the experimental units, such as the application of two drugs. No interaction means that the effect of two factors, call them A and B, are additive. The

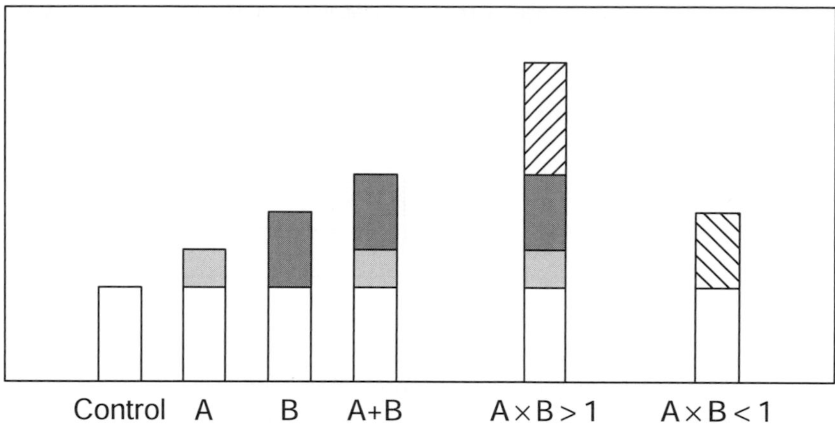

Fig. 2.3 Interaction effects as non-additivity of individual effects. When the effect of *A* and *B* together is additive ($A + B$), there is no interaction. An interaction exists when the combination of *A* and *B* together is either greater ($A \times B > 1$) or less than ($A \times B < 1$) the sum of the individual effects.

effect of *A* and *B* together is simply the effect of *A* on its own *plus* the effect of *B* on its own (Figure 2.3). The white bar in Figure 2.3 represents the control condition without either drug, and the height is the baseline value on some arbitrary outcome. When drug *A* is given the height of the bar is higher, and this can be thought of as the baseline value plus the effect of factor *A* (grey portion of the bar). The same interpretation applies to drug *B*, which has a larger effect than drug *A*. If there is no interaction between the two drugs, the effects are additive; the height of the bar labelled $A + B$ is the baseline value (white), plus the effect of factor *A* (light grey), plus the effect of factor *B* (dark grey). Here, the two effects are stacked on top of each other.

An interaction occurs when the effect of *A* and *B* together is either greater or less than the sum of the individual effects. The bar labelled $A \times B > 1$ shows an example of when the two effects together are greater than the sum of the individual effects, which biologists often refer to as a *synergistic effect* between *A* and *B*. The hatched part of the bar represents the synergistic or supra-additive effect. The combined effect of the drugs are multiplicative instead of additive, with the multiplying factor being greater than one. The bar labelled $A \times B < 1$ shows an example of *A* and *B* together being less than the sum of their individual effects, with the hatched part of the bar showing the combined effect of the two drugs. This relationship could occur if there is a ceiling effect, where factor *B* alone gives the maximum response, so the addition of factor *A* provides no further increase. The effects are still multiplicative, but the multiplying factor is less than one.

A second way to think about interaction effects is that the effect of one factor depends on the level of another factor. Graphically, this is seen as non-parallel lines connecting the experimental groups, which can be formally tested as a 'difference-of-differences'. This interpretation is useful when one predictor variable is a treatment variable, such as a drug, and the other variable is a biological or technical variable. An example is shown in Figure 2.4, where one variable is the presence or absence of a drug and the second variable

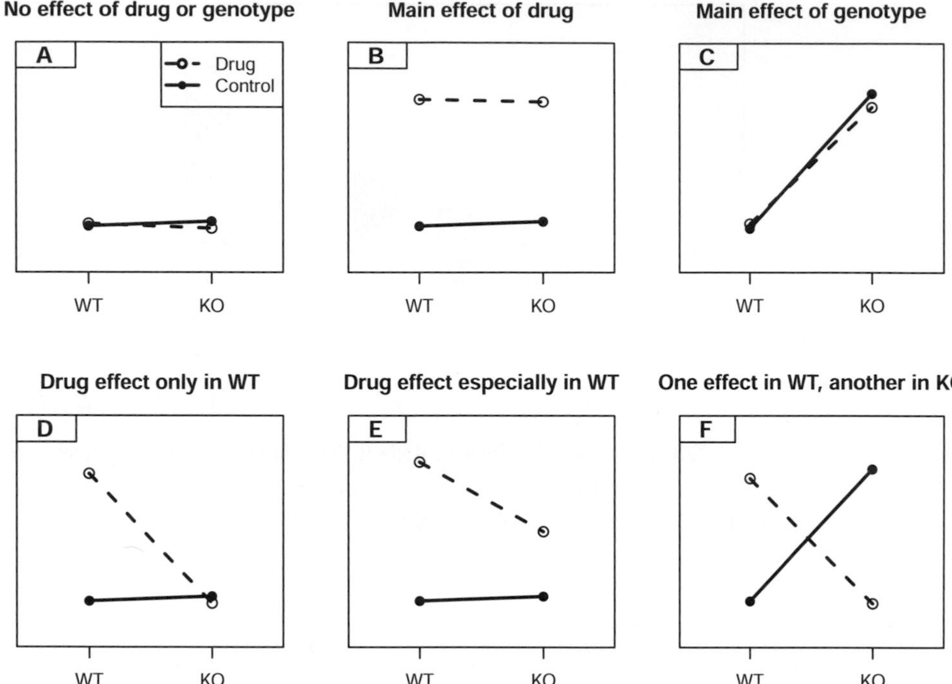

Fig. 2.4 Interaction effects as a difference-of-differences (non-parallel lines). The effect of one factor (drug) depends on the level of another factor (genotype) in the last three panels.

is the genotype – either wild type (WT) or knock out (KO). In Figure 2.4A there is no effect of the drug and no effect of genotype. In Figure 2.4B there is a main effect of the drug, but it is similar in both genotypes. Thus, there is no interaction because the effect of the drug does not depend on the genotype. In Figure 2.4C there is a main effect of genotype but no effect of the drug, and once again no interaction.

In Figure 2.4D the drug only has an effect in the WT animals, and suppose that this was the predicted outcome. Testing whether the interaction is significant tests the research hypothesis but the following incorrect two-step approach is often used [294]. First, demonstrate that there is a significant effect ($p < 0.05$) of the drug in the WT group. Then, show that there is no significant effect ($p > 0.05$) of the drug in the KO group. If both conditions hold, then conclude that these two results support the research hypothesis that the drug only works in the WT animals. The hypothesis of interest is not directly tested with this approach, the conclusion does not necessarily follow, and the form of reasoning is incorrect – a point which has been discussed repeatedly [44, 45, 132, 262, 294]. The correct approach is to test if the effect of the drug in the WT group (Drug:WT − Control:WT) is greater than the effect of the drug in the KO group (Drug:KO − Control:KO), or

$$\overbrace{(\text{Drug:WT} - \text{Control:WT})}^{\text{Drug effect in WT}} - \overbrace{(\text{Drug:KO} - \text{Control:KO})}^{\text{Drug effect in KO}} = 0. \tag{2.2}$$

The test of the hypothesis is based on whether the terms on the left side of the equation are significantly different from zero. If the effect of the drug is the same in both genotypes then the difference-of-differences will be zero; and the degree to which the difference-of-differences deviates from zero represents the differential effect of the drug in each genotype.

A problem with the two-step approach is illustrated in Figure 2.4E. There is a main effect of the drug and an interaction, in that the effect is larger in the WT than the KO group.[6] It could turn out that the Drug:WT versus Control:WT difference is just barely significant, while the Drug:KO versus Control:KO is just on the other side of 0.05. It is incorrect to conclude that the drug only worked in the WT and not the KO mice. If you want to conclude something about the effectiveness of drug in the WT versus the KO groups, the groups need to be compared directly, not via a series of independent tests, the results of which are patched together to arrive at a conclusion. The results of a two-step approach are even harder to interpret if the variance and the sample size of the groups are different.

Another type of interaction is shown in Figure 2.4F. Here, the drug has one effect in WT mice (increases the response), and another in the KO mice. Such effects are less common in biology and harder to interpret. The above discussion also applies to interactions involving more than two variables.

Biologists are often interested in the interaction between genes – called *epistasis* – and between genes and environmental variables. When all genes are measured, the number of possible interactions is enormous, making false positives a problem. For example, with only 20 genes there are already over 1 million ways in which two genes can interact ($2^{20} = 1\,048\,576$), never mind the higher order interactions. There is also some confusion in the literature over definitions and interpretations of epistasis, and Cordell and Phillips provide good reviews [82, 309].

On removable interactions

To further complicate the discussion, we make a distinction between *removable* and *non-removable* interactions [38, 244, 382]. A removable interaction is one that can be nullified by transforming or rescaling the data. An example is the interaction in Figure 2.4E. Log-transforming the outcome variable might remove the interaction because it makes the two lines more parallel.[7] The interaction in the bottom right panel of Figure 2.4F is nonremovable because no monotonic transformation of the data will uncross the lines.

An underlying biological process may have a nonlinear relationship with the measured readout; for example, the expression of a gene and the fluorescence intensity on a microarray chip, or the spatial memory of a rodent and the latency for the rodent to find a hidden platform in the Morris water maze test. Wagenmakers *et al.* provide a good discussion

[6] Brown makes a nice distinction between an 'only for' interaction (the drug works only for the WT animals; Figure 2.4D) and an 'especially for' interaction (the drug works in both genotypes, but especially for the WT animals; Figure 2.4E) [61].

[7] A log-transformation 'pulls in' higher values more than lower values, so the Drug:WT group would become more similar to the other three groups.

and some nice graphs illustrating this point [382], and there is no need to repeat these points here. But why does the distinction between removable and nonremovable interactions matter? If the research hypothesis is about the interaction (e.g. the drug works only, or especially, in the WT animals), then a different conclusion can be reached depending on the scale of measurement. For example, the latency for a rodent to reach the platform in the water maze is measured in seconds, but it is just as reasonable to use the reciprocal of the latency ($1/s$), which is the rate at which the rodent finds the platform.[8] An interaction might be present when using one unit of measurement but not the other. There is no 'correct' scale of measurement, and so removable interactions make it hard to relate the result of the statistical analysis to the underlying biological process. Wagenmakers *et al.* describe some options for probing the true nature of the interaction [382].

2.9 Sampling

Sampling is the process by which one decides which sample material gets included in the experiment, and it takes place at the level of biological units, experimental units, and observational units – and often all three. Sampling implies selecting a subset of items from a larger population, and the main concern is that the items selected are similar to, or representative of, the items that are not selected. For many experiments, sampling biological and/or experimental units does not apply because they are ordered online. When rats are purchased from a supplier there is no expectation that they have been randomly sampled from all the possible rats in the world or even all possible rats from that supplier. In experimental biology, sampling occurs, if at all, at the level of observational units and often after randomisation to treatment groups has occurred. For example, some neurons in a rat's brain will be selected for electrophysiological recording, some cells in a well will be selected for morphological quantification, and some histological slices of an organ or tissue will be selected for measurements. These will often be subsamples or pseudoreplicates but it is still important that they are representative of the population that they are sampled from, and a good way to achieve this is by introducing a random component into the sampling procedure.

Different sampling methods exist and the first and most common method is *simple random sampling* (Figure 2.5). This occurs when each item in the population has the same probability of being selected. For example, 10 000 cells have been plated in a well and 10 of them will be selected with a probability of $10/10\,000 = 0.001$ to measure their morphology. Simple random sampling is straightforward to carry out but the 10 selected cells might be at the edge of the well and none are from the centre. This may be an issue if the cells are denser in the centre but relatively sparse near the edges, and if cell density is relevant for the readout. One way around this is to use a *systematic random sampling* procedure. 'Systematic random' is not an oxymoron because the procedure has both a systematic

[8] Latency data often have a positive skew, which a reciprocal transformation can normalise. Even though latency values are by far the most widely used for the Morris water maze, reciprocal values might be better.

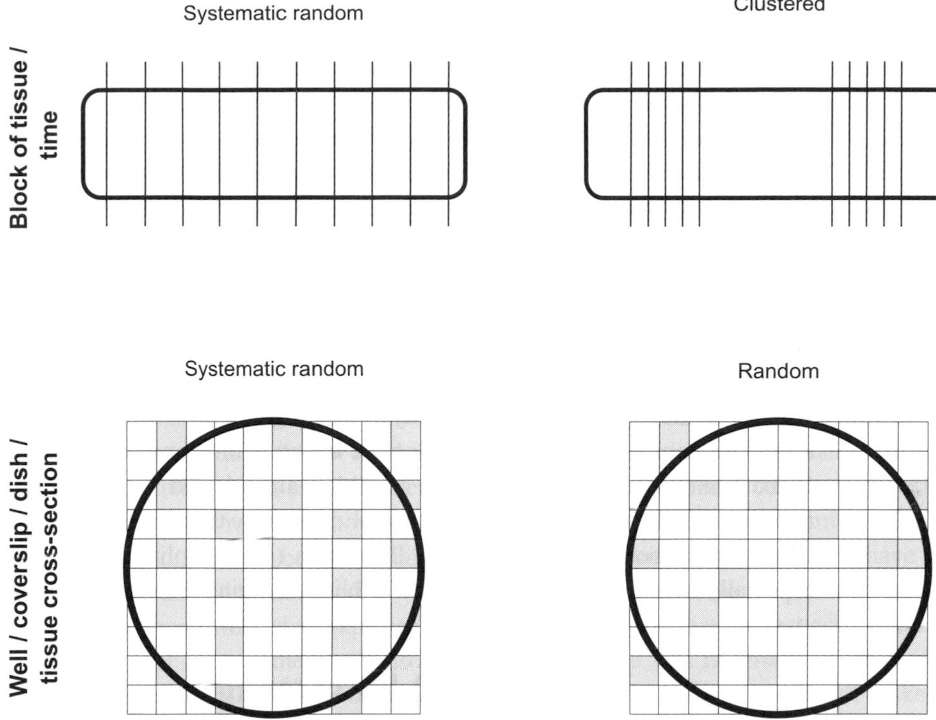

Fig. 2.5 Sampling schemes. Systematic random sampling (left top and bottom) has a random start point and then evenly spaced sampling. Clustering samples together (top right) when the population is homogeneous is often inefficient. Simple random sampling (bottom right) can miss small subgroups.

and random part. Randomness occurs in selecting where or when the first observation or measurement is made, but then subsequent measurements occur systematically, or at fixed intervals in time or space. This method is often used when there are spatial or temporal trends and an even distribution of the samples across time or space is desired (Figure 2.5). One drawback of systematic random sampling is that periodicity in the outcome might be missed. For example, suppose that a single body temperature reading is made every 24 hours for 10 days using a systematic random sampling procedure. The first observation is taken at a random time between 0 and 24 hours (or a more reasonable time-frame such as between 9 a.m. and 5 p.m.) and then every 24 hours thereafter. With such a design, it would not be possible to detect a circadian rhythm in body temperature. Some animals would have all observations near their peak, others near their nadir. Also, additional noise will have been added compared with a design in which all animals had measurements taken at the same time.

The final sampling scheme that we will consider is *clustered random sampling*. If the population is heterogeneous there may be a concern that simple random sampling will miss some subgroups, especially if they form a small proportion of the total population. One may then sample within the defined subgroups, but this is relatively uncommon in experimental biology. It is mentioned to distinguish it from what is occasionally done instead, which is

established however by quantifying the separation between the negative and positive control group – that is, the *assay window*.[9] A threshold can be set before the experiment is conducted requiring the positive controls to be a certain distance from the negative controls, defined by a mean difference, a fixed number of standard deviations, or using one of several statistics that have been developed for this purpose [364, 412, 413]. If the separation between positive and negative controls is not large enough the experiment may be discarded for lack of sensitivity. Basing a decision on the quality of an assay using a statistical test makes little sense – either biologically or statistically. A significant *p*-value does not mean that the experiment is sensitive enough to detect a treatment effect, which may be smaller. We do not need a *p*-value to tell us that the positive controls differ from the negative controls – we knew this before starting the experiment and is why these groups were included!

The expected effect sizes between controls and treatment conditions may vary greatly, and thus the sample size need not be equal. For example, the positive control condition may have a large and robust effect, and so fewer samples may be needed. If the main purpose of the positive control is to confirm that the experimental system can detect an effect if it is present, then few samples may be required. Furthermore, not all control conditions need to be included in the analysis. Usually the main interest is whether the treatment conditions differ from the negative control (and from each other) and it might be preferable to have fewer samples in the positive control condition and more in the negative control condition. We return to the issue of allocating samples across groups when optimal experimental designs are discussed (Section 5.3).

2.11 Front-aligned versus end-aligned designs

In some experiments the treatment is applied to the biological or experimental units for different durations, and the duration of treatment is the experimental factor of interest. Examples include testing the effect of 1, 2, and 3 weeks of exercise, or examining the effect of acute versus chronic treatment of a compound. In such cases, is it better to apply the treatment to all experimental units at the same time at the start of the experiment, and follow them for different lengths of time (Figure 2.6, left), or is it better to stagger the time of application of treatments, and end the experiment for all the EUs at the same time (Figure 2.6, right)? Both options can be a potential source of bias.

With front-aligned designs the biological or experimental units are in the experiment for different lengths of time. For animal studies this means that the animals will be different ages when the data are collected. This is not a problem if the duration of treatments is short, but with longer durations, age effects will be confounded with treatment effects. For cell culture experiments the duration that the cells are in culture will depend on the duration of treatment. A second disadvantage of front-aligned designs is that there may be systematic differences between early and late time points, or events may occur during the study that

[9] See Section 5.1 for more information.

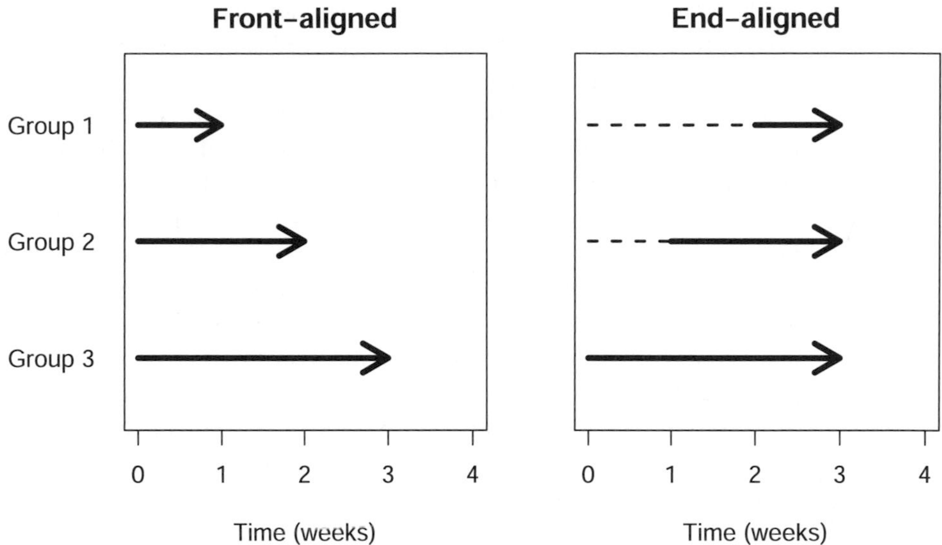

Fig. 2.6 Front- and end-aligned designs for treatments of different duration. In the front-aligned design the treatment is applied to all experimental units at the beginning of the experiment (arrow tails) and EUs are followed for different lengths of time. Observations are made only at the end of the experiment (arrow heads). End-aligned designs start the treatment at different times, but all EUs finish the experiment at the same time. Both options can introduce different types of bias.

will only affect animals that are still in the study. Differences between experimental groups may then emerge that have nothing to do with the treatment. Examples include different animal technicians for the first and last half of the experiment, a new supplier or batch of bedding material, an infection in the colony, or the amount of noise or traffic in the animal house. The same disadvantage applies to cell culture experiments; for example, cells in culture for longer will undergo a greater number of media changes and the frequency of incubator use by others might differ between the beginning and end of the experiment. Some of these events may be unlikely and their effects may be small, but front-aligned designs offer no protection. Moreover, it is often hard to know if such events have occurred or how background variables have changed over time.

A third disadvantage of front-aligned designs is that variations in the duration of sample storage may affect the outcome. It is common to wait until the experiment is complete and all of the samples collected before proceeding to the next step of the experiment, such as histology staining, RNA extraction, or performing a Western blot. Samples collected at earlier time points will usually need to be frozen or kept in a fixative such as paraformaldehyde, and the length of storage will differ between experimental groups, which may or may not be relevant. This is also a potential source of batch effects (see Section 2.12.1) because groups of samples are processed together and they correspond, and are thus confounded with, the experimental groups. Ideally, there would be a control group used at each time point in the above examples, but then the research question is tested with the group-by-time interaction, which is harder to interpret than a main effect of group. These disadvantages can be avoided with end-aligned designs because all experimental units remain in the experiment until it is completed, and any events or changing background variables will affect all of the samples in the same way.

There are some disadvantages to end-aligned designs. The first is that they are often more expensive. All animals will need be housed for the full duration of the experiment and more media and reagents will be required for cell culture experiments. Second, the application of the treatment may be highly variable (treatment error is high), which can introduce a large amount of variability between groups. For example, a fresh concoction of growth factors is made at the beginning of a cell culture experiment and applied once to the groups over the course of the experiment. One group receives the fresh preparation while other groups receive the growth factors after they have been stored in the fridge for different lengths of time, which may affect the potency of the growth factors. The alternative is to make a new batch just before applying it to the cells, but the variations in the preparation of each batch might be large, which could be a source of batch effects. Trade-offs need to be made in choosing a front- versus end-aligned design, and it is a matter of knowing your experimental system, where potential sources of confounding can occur, their magnitudes, and using the best design to minimise these, subject to cost and practical constraints. One factor to consider is that as the duration of the experiment increases, the greater the advantages of an end-aligned design because there is more opportunity for background variables to change or for one-off events to occur in the middle of the experiment.

There is a second type of experiment that requires a choice between a front- or end-aligned design. These are experiments where the interest is in determining the effects of a treatment or experimental intervention at several time points, but observations can only be made at one time point because the animals need to be euthanised or the cells need to be fixed for analysis. An example would be the expression of a gene in the brains of mice at five time points after the application of a compound. One could either inject all mice at the start of the experiment and then euthanise groups of mice at different times (front-aligned). Or, one could stagger the time of injections and then euthanise all of the mice at the same time. The trade-offs are similar to the previous example and it is worth thinking about the pros and cons and making an active decision, instead of using the method that others use.

2.12 Heterogeneity and confounding

Heterogeneity of sample material refers to the 'lack of sameness' between samples. No two people, animals, or cells are identical and sometimes they form distinct groups, classes, or clusters within a set of samples. For example, mice vary in their body weight, but males tend to be heavier on average than females. A sample of mixed-sex mice is therefore heterogeneous. Any biological or technical factor could be a potential source of heterogeneity and it may not always be possible to identify the source. Here, we will only be concerned with heterogeneity that exists between experimental units.

Confounding occurs when treatment, biological, or technical effects cannot be uniquely estimated – the effects are 'mixed up' and cannot be separated. The combination of

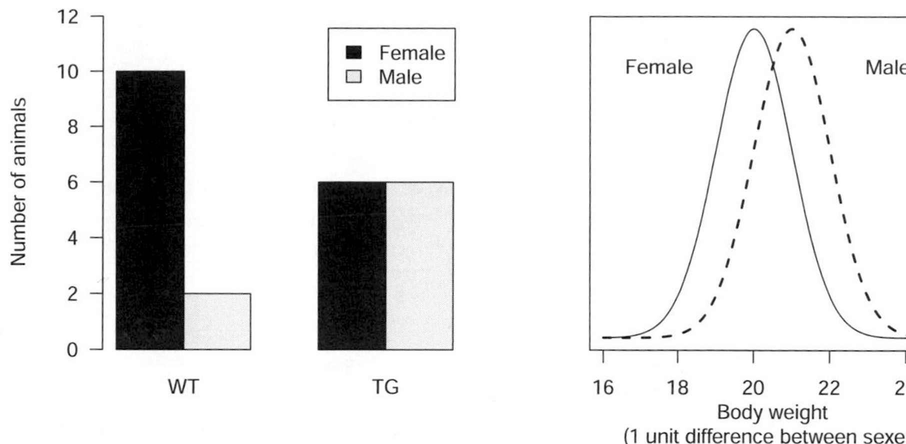

Fig. 2.7 A hypothetical experiment showing that wild-type (WT) animals are 83% female, while transgenic (TG) animals are 50% female (left). Distributions showing a 1 unit (e.g. grams) difference between sexes on body weight (right).

heterogeneity and confounding is a problem because heterogeneity can be mistaken for a treatment effect. An experiment with an all-male treated group and an all-female control group cannot distinguish between treatment effects and sex effects. Similarly, if there is no observed difference we cannot conclude that the treatment effect is zero, because a treatment effect could be counteracted by a sex effect of similar magnitude in the opposite direction. To make any conclusion about the treatment, we would have to assume that the sex effect is zero. Depending on the experiment, this may or may not be a reasonable assumption.

Factors do not need to be completely confounded, even an imbalance between factors can lead to biased estimates. Suppose we are interested in comparing the body weights of wild-type (WT) and transgenic (TG) mice and have a total of 24 mice; 12 males and 12 females. The ratio of females to males differs between genotypes: the WT mice are 83% female (10 female/2 male), and the TG mice are 50% female (6 of each sex; Figure 2.7, left). Also, males tend to be heavier than females and Figure 2.7 (right graph) shows the distribution of weights.

To understand how an imbalance between genotype and sex can lead to incorrect inferences we will perform a simulation where we vary the proportion of females in the WT group and the size of the sex effect. The number of females in the WT group is either 6 (balanced) or 10, and the difference between sexes is either 0, 1, or 2 units. The combination of 10 females and 1 unit difference between sexes is shown in Figure 2.7. In these simulations (the code is not shown), the effect of genotype is set to zero, and we are interested in the number of false positive results when testing the genotype effect, which are defined as the number of p-values below 0.05. Since we know that the genotype effect is zero, any result with a low p-value is known to be a false positive. In these simulations, the sex of the animals was not included in the analysis because we are interested in seeing what happens when an important factor is omitted from the analysis. Sex in this example can represent any biological or technical variable that affects the outcome, but is not taken into account

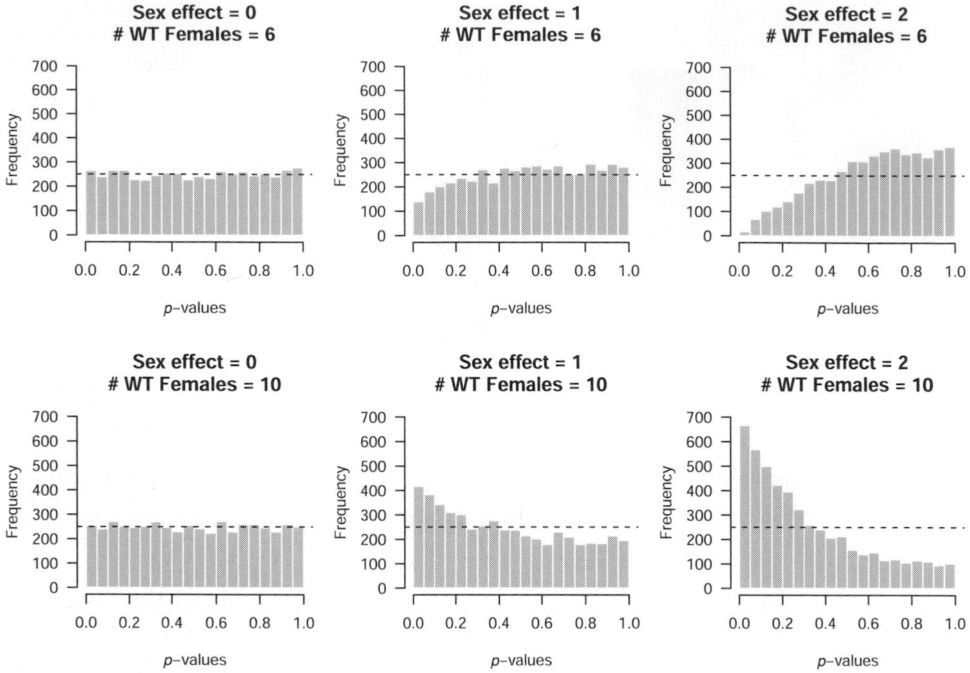

Fig. 2.8 p-value histograms for testing an effect of genotype in 5000 simulations. Different sizes of sex effects and degree of sex imbalance between genotypes are shown. With a large sex effect (right graphs) the p-values are too large (low power) when the sexes are balanced across genotypes (top right) and too small (many false positives) when the sexes are unbalanced (bottom right).

in the analysis. The results of the simulations are shown in Figure 2.8 and are presented as p-value histograms. When there is no effect of sex the histograms should be uniform distributions with the height of the bars at the horizontal dashed line, and this is indeed the case in the top left graph, where the sex effect is zero and the number of females is balanced between genotypes. The height of the left-most bar in each histogram shows the number of p-values from 5000 simulations that are below 0.05. As we move along the first row of graphs, the number of females in each genotype remains the same but the effect of sex gets larger. Note how the p-value histograms shift to the right – there are too few small p-values. We expect to have 5% of p-values below 0.05, but in the top right graph only 0.36% of p-values are below 0.05 (height of left-most histogram bar). We have not invented a way to reduce false positives, but rather excluded a variable from the analysis that affects the outcome. This reduces power because there is excess noise in the data that is unaccounted for.

In the bottom row of Figure 2.8 the proportion of females in the WT group is constant at 83% (as shown in Figure 2.7). As we progress from left to right the histograms are shifted towards smaller values. The middle graph in the bottom row corresponds to the values in Figure 2.7, and 8.3% of p-values are below 0.05, slightly more than the expected 5%. If the effect of sex is larger (bottom right graph) the number of p-values below 0.05 is 13.3%.

From these results we can conclude that when a variable has an effect on the outcome and is not balanced between the groups that one is comparing (genotype in this case), then there will be an excess of significant p-values. This occurs because the effect of sex is correlated with the effect of genotype due to the imbalance between sexes across genotypes, and the greater the imbalance the worse the problem becomes.

When the sexes are equally balanced between genotypes any sex effects can be removed by including sex as a variable in the analysis. Accounting for heterogeneity is harder when imbalance exists because the interpretation of genotype effects is ambiguous when genotype and sex account for the same variation in the outcome (see Section 4.1.1 on partitioning the sum of squares with multiple predictors), but it is still a good idea to include sex in the analysis.

Before discussing sources of heterogeneity we show how heterogeneity and lack of balance can lead to a reversal of effects – known as Simpson's paradox [356]. Figure 2.9A shows a graph with the mean $\pm$SEM (standard error of the mean) for a control and treated group on some outcome. A simple analysis of the treatment effects shows that the treatment increases the value of the outcome compared with the control group ($p = 0.013$). Once again we use sex as a factor that has an effect on the outcome and plot the data separately for males and females (Figure 2.9B). There is a large effect of sex, but the remarkable feature is that the relationship within sex is reversed! For both males and females, the treatment decreases the outcome compared with the control group ($p < 0.001$). How is it that one conclusion is reached when the sexes are analysed together, but the exact opposite conclusion is reached when they are analysed separately – hence the paradox. Suppose this was a clinical trial where a low value of the outcome is considered desirable. Based on the first analysis, one would conclude that, overall, the treatment is harmful, but it is beneficial for males, and it is also beneficial for females. If you were a physician, would you prescribe this treatment?

The first lesson to be learnt is that plotting the mean $\pm$ error bars is one of the worst ways to understand the data. This can be seen by plotting each data point separately (Figure 2.9C), which allows the imbalance to be seen. The solid line shows the overall effect from graph A and the two dashed lines show the sex-specific effects from graph B. The reversal occurs because there are many more treated than untreated males and many more untreated than treated females. The overall effect of the treated group is driven mainly by the effect of sex and not the effect of the treatment. The correct interpretation is that the treatment does indeed decrease the value of the outcome.[10] The second lesson is once again that heterogeneity coupled with lack of balance can be problematic.

The subsections that follow list potential sources of heterogeneity or variation in biological experiments. The main sources of variation depend on the type of experiment but there are still many to consider. As you read the rest of the chapter and consider your own experiments, do not feel overwhelmed by all of the places where unwanted effects can enter. No experiment is perfect, but try to anticipate the major potential sources of variation and design the experiment so that they do not bias the results.

[10] This assumes that people were randomly assigned to treated and control groups. If they were allowed to self-select, this might not be the correct interpretation. See Lindley and Novick for a cogent discussion [239].

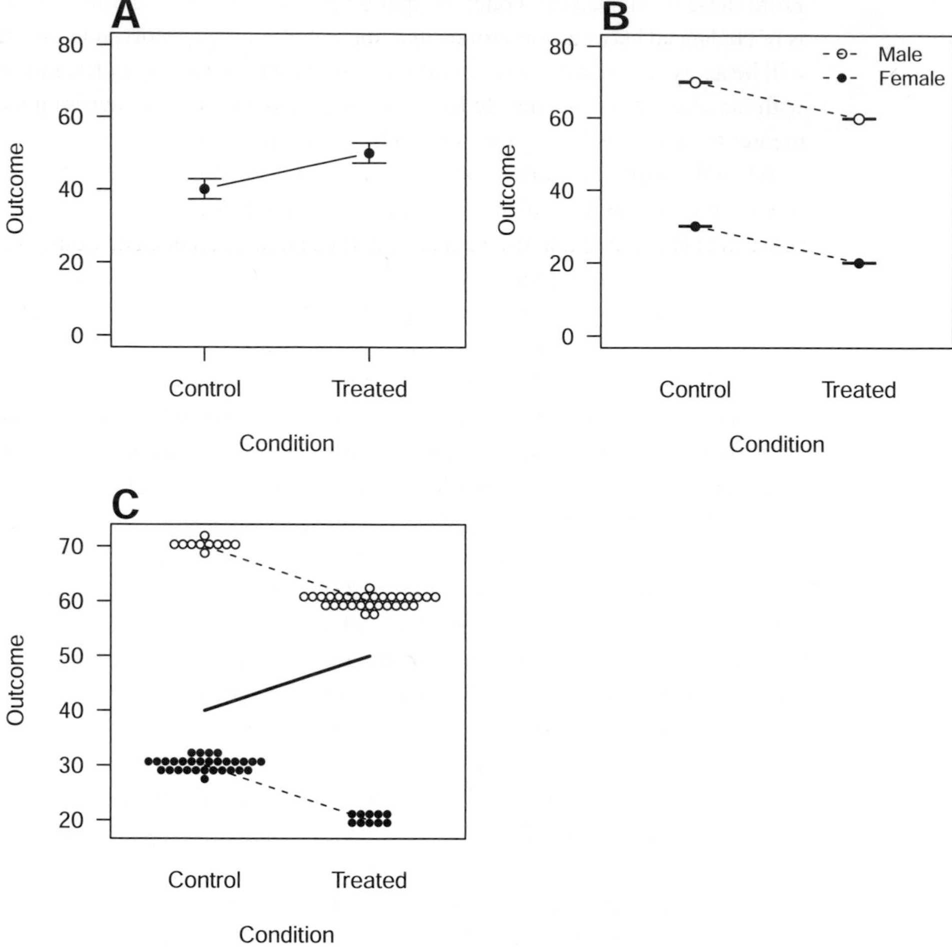

Fig. 2.9 Simpson's paradox. When ignoring the effect of sex, the mean of the treated group is greater than the control group (A). The effect is reversed within each sex (B). The reversal occurs because of the sample size imbalance coupled with a sex effect – most of the males are in the treated group while most females are in the control group (C).

2.12.1 Batches

A *batch* is a generic term for any type of grouping of samples, and we consider three types of batching that occur in biological experiments. The key point is that there may be differences between batches that need to be taken into account.

The first type of batching occurs when samples are grouped during the collection, processing, or acquisition of data. This is usually done for technical reasons or constraints on how the experiment can be conducted. For example, large experiments may need to be conducted – or the samples processed – over several days. This can introduce day-to-day variation in the outcome variables. Some measured outcomes will be more prone to batch effects but all outcomes could be potentially influenced – from behavioural responses to gene expression. Batching and corresponding batch effects could also occur within days if data are collected or samples processed separately in the morning and afternoon.

Another type of batching occurs with reagents, either when purchased from suppliers or made in-house. Suppliers produce antibodies, compounds, dyes, media, and other reagents in batches or lots. Although efforts are made to standardise production procedures there may be differences that affect the outcome variables. Also, consider that even if the production was tightly controlled, the transport, storage, and age of the reagents may differ between batches. It is not always possible to use new reagents. For example, one may need to use a half-bottle of cell culture medium from a previous experiment that has been sitting in the fridge for some time, but is still perfectly fine. Once emptied, a new bottle may be opened and used, but there may be systematic differences from the previous bottle, perhaps in the pH of the media. Reagents are also a potential source of special cause variation – when adding serum or growth factors to the media one might accidentally add 10 μmol instead of 1 μmol, which would affect all samples in that batch.

A final type of batching occurs when different equipment is used. For example, instead of performing qPCR over 2 days to avoid day-to-day variation, it could be done on a single day using two PCR machines, but there could be differences between the machines. Similarly, one could use multiple microscopes, spectrophotometers, incubators, microarray chips (especially those with multiple arrays per chip), next-generation sequencing flow cells, or behavioural testing chambers, and differences between them may propagate to the measured outcomes.

For some of the above examples, differences between batches will be minor and perhaps negligible, but they should not be underestimated. The appreciation of batch effects is probably greatest by those who routinely use '-omics' technologies, and such effects have been described for almost all such technological platforms, including microarrays [14, 15, 227, 303, 403], next-generation sequencing technologies [147, 212], proteomics [16, 162], and SNP arrays[11] [242, 276]. Batch effects are not limited to such high-throughput technologies (although some effects will be technology specific), and need to be considered in the design stage for all experiments.

The simplest way of dealing with batch effects is to not have batches, or at least minimise unnecessary batching. If batches are unavoidable, then ensure they are not confounded with treatment effects; for example, collecting data from the controls on the first day and the treated group on the second day. Aim for a balance between treatments and batches so that an equal number of samples from each treatment group is within each batch. If this is not possible, at least have all possible combinations of effects that you are interested in testing within each batch. For example, if you have one control group and three treatment groups, and the interest is in all possible comparisons between the four groups, ensure that each batch has at least one sample (but preferably more) from each group. There are designs called *incomplete block designs* which can be used when it is not possible to have all treatment groups in all batches (batches are the blocks), but they are not considered here as they are not often required. Lew provides a nice example of interpretation errors that can

[11] Single nucleotide polymorphism arrays for genome-wise association studies.

arise when two experiments (i.e. batches) with different treatment groups but a common control group are combined for a single analysis [235].

2.12.2 Plates, arrays, chips, and gels

Systematic differences may exist between microtitre plates, microarray chips or arrays, electrophoresis gels, flasks, and similar consumables. These differences may be due to the way they were manufactured or how they were handled during the experiment. For example, two microtitre plates cannot physically occupy the same space in an incubator, and gradients in either the average or the variance in temperature or CO_2 from front to back or top to bottom in an incubator may lead to differences in the measured outcome. Once again, having all experimental groups on all plates is a good way to minimise bias.

In addition to differences between plates or arrays, there may be differences within a plate. For example, measured responses can be affected by the spatial location on a microtitre plate, as wells on the edge of a plate can differ from those in the centre. This is often the result of greater evaporation at the edges, which will increase the concentration of dissolved substances. See Section 2.12.8 for a further discussion.

2.12.3 Cages, pens, and tanks

Experiments conducted with whole animals will require some type of housing such as cages, pens, or tanks, and differences between such housing units are often observed. These differences could occur because animals are often not randomised to cages but rather littermates are kept together, and so differences between cages reflect biological differences between litters. Alternatively, data may be collected on a per-cage basis, and the cage might be a proxy for another variable such as time-of-day if circadian effects are relevant. Even if animals are randomly assigned to cages and equal at baseline, cages may develop differently over time. This could be due to the physical characteristics of the housing arrangement such as the position of the cage in the room, lighting and temperature gradients from the top to the bottom of the cage rack, or animals for one experiment are kept in two rooms because of space constraints.

Cages may also evolve differently over time if one cage has a overly dominant or aggressive member. For example, both rats and mice exhibit 'barbering', which is the trimming or plucking of fur or whiskers of cage-mates [26, 60, 181, 207]. Often all but one mouse in a cage has been barbered, which identifies the culprit [207]. It was previously believed that barbering is a normal dominance behaviour, but others have argued that this is not the case [126]. Regardless, it would not be surprising if animals from the barbered and unbarbered cages differ in many ways.

Cage density might also be an important variable to keep constant across all experimental groups. Animals housed at higher densities have been reported to show signs of stress, including reduced growth rate, increased adrenal gland size and concentration of fecal corticosterone metabolites, as well as higher levels of anxiety and barbering [293, 405], although this may be strain specific [210].

There are many other variables that might vary by cage such as ultrasonic vocalisations, sounds and odours, and social transmission of food preferences, which may be hard to control, but may influence the outcomes that one wishes to measure.

2.12.4 Subject/sample characteristics

There are many characteristics or properties that can vary widely between subjects including sex, age, weight or body mass index (BMI), genotype, disease severity, visual acuity,[12] as well as technical aspects such as storage and handling of samples (duration of storage, number of freeze-thaw cycles, and so on). In addition, there are many characteristics that are specific to human samples such as source of tissue (as in tumour samples from different hospitals), medications, and comorbid conditions, which are a particular problem for biomarker studies [277, 315, 322]. Fortunately, many of these can be held constant or are under control of the researcher with animal and *in vitro* experiments. One characteristic that may be hard to control is the genotype of transgenic models of human disease. For example, copy number variations in the transgene have been reported for superoxide dismutase 1 (SOD1) transgenic mouse models of amyotrophic lateral sclerosis (ALS) [7, 346]. Also, transgenic Huntington's disease mice may have a different number of trinucleotide repeats in the transgene, with a higher number being associated with earlier disease onset and death.[13] If treated and control groups differ on these genetic characteristics, it could lead to both false positive and false negative results, depending on the direction of the bias. Sometimes it may only be possible to determine if the groups are similar at the end of the experiment.

Finally, the existence and magnitude of sex differences might be underestimated [314], partly because there is a tendency to conduct experiments with males only [27, 73, 317], and so it is hard to assess how treatment effects differ between sexes.

2.12.5 Litters

Technically, this section should have been included in the previous one as the litter that an animal is from is a subject characteristic, but it is listed separately because litter effects are an underappreciated source of variation in animal studies. Litter effects arise because animals from the same litter are dizygotic twins, they are genetically similar and share prenatal and early postnatal environments, which will tend to make them similar on many characteristics compared with two unrelated animals [159, 164, 222, 415]. Naturally occurring differences between litters are often a large source of variation. In addition, animals from the same litter are often housed, tested, and killed together (i.e. cage effects, order effects) which can introduce heterogeneity that is technical and not biological. When testing for treatment effects it is unnecessary to determine if differences between litters are

[12] Many rodent behavioural tests assume that the animals can see properly, but visual acuity varies between species and declines with age [62, 400].

[13] Huntington's disease is caused by an expansion in the number of CAG trinucleotide repeats in the first exon of the *huntingtin* gene. The number of CAG repeats is unstable and can vary from animal to animal.

due to biological or technical factors, as long as litter effects are not confounded with the treatment effects and litter is included in the analysis.

2.12.6 Experimenter characteristics

Another source of technical variation is the person conducting the experiment. Two people following the same protocol will not perform all tasks in exactly the same way, and this might contribute to the 'secret sauce' phenomenon [80], where one person can get an experiment to work or can obtain better results and another cannot. There might be some unwritten part of the protocol that influences the results or the skill level between experimenters might differ. Ideally, differences between experimenters or technicians will be minor, but if a large experiment needs to be split between multiple experimenters, then the experiment should be designed so that the estimates of the treatment effects will not be confounded with the experimenter effects.

A recent study has shown that the sex of the experimenter can affect how rodents respond to painful stimuli [358]. Rats and mice showed a weaker response to painful stimuli when tested by male experimenters, and the authors hypothesised that stress-induced analgesia was the cause. Differences were also seen for thigmotaxis in the open field.[14] Thus, there are some aspects of the experiment that cannot be removed by better standardisation of protocols or improving skills of the experimenters.

2.12.7 Time effects

It is rarely possible to apply an experimental treatment, to process, or to measure all samples simultaneously, and thus samples have an intrinsic ordering from first to last. This ordering introduces *time* or *order* as a variable that can potentially affect the results, which we refer to as *order effects*. There are five general causes of order effects: cycles, drift, experimenter learning and fatigue, different time lags in multi-step protocols, and one-off events that occur in the middle of data collection. Each are discussed below.

The order of sample collection is important when the measured outcome varies cyclically over time, or is affected by *cyclical events*. A common example are circadian rhythms in many biological processes; for example, corticosterone is a rodent stress hormone with a circadian rhythm. If blood samples are taken first from control animals and then from treated animals, there can be differences in corticosterone levels between groups because of a time-of-day effect. Alternatively, true differences between experimental groups could be reduced or missed altogether if the circadian effect counteracts the treatment effect. The magnitude and direction of the bias will depend on the phase of the circadian cycle and the duration of sample collection. This bias is also reproducible [330]; if the experiment were repeated to verify the findings and the sample collection is the same as the first (controls first, followed by the treated animals), the same circadian effect would again be detected

[14] For the open field test, animals are placed in a large box for a fixed period of time and the amount of locomotor activity is measured, either with infrared sensors or by video tracking. Rodents usually prefer to stay near the walls (thigmotaxis) instead of in the open centre, and this is used as a measure of anxiety.

and misinterpreted as a treatment effect. Here, an 'independent replication' of a bad design offers no protection against false results.

Other cyclical events operating on different time scales are reproductive, seasonal, weekend/work day, and cage cleaning cycles – which may be necessary to either hold constant, or ensure that they are not confounded with treatment effects [292]. In humans, Dopico and colleagues showed that 4000 protein-coding mRNAs in white blood cells and adipose tissue have different expression levels depending on the time of year [100]. This is a problem when sample collection occurs over long periods and can be a source of bias if the proportion of patient and healthy control samples is not constant throughout the year, which would induce partial confounding between time of year and patient group. Circannual gene expression rhythms (and other physiological functions) are also a problem when combining data from different studies, as the date of sample collection is a potential confounder.

The second cause of order effects is *drift*, which is the tendency of experimental systems to change from an initial set of conditions. These are usually gradual changes in background conditions that are assumed to be constant for the duration of the experiment. Drift can be the result of either biological or technical causes including temperature changes, chemical or biological reactions limited by the amount of reactants or the buildup of products, cell viability, electrical gradients across cell or mitochondrial membranes, stress responses, or intensity of fluorescent bulbs. Bland discusses an example of these order effects (from two independent labs) for a homeopathy experiment [48]. Since the order of sample processing was randomised in this experiment, it was possible to detect these effects, adjust for them, and show that there was no effect of the homeopathic treatment.

The third cause of order effects is the *experimenter*. Data collection sometimes requires subjective assessments such as quantifying animal behaviour from recorded videos or determining the degree of pathology in tissue samples. The assessment criteria might change as additional samples are seen during the experiment. For example, the definition of a labelled cell, what constitutes cellular blebbing, or the boundaries of an anatomical region might evolve during an experiment. A person's definitions will become stable with experience and some labs 'calibrate' newcomers by comparing their results to those of a more experienced researcher. Experimenter fatigue is another reason that assessments can change. The effort to scrutinise samples will likely be less during the eighth hour of looking down a microscope than during the first, and this may lead to subtle differences in the estimated values. Experimenter effects are becoming less relevant with the increased use of video and image analysis software that does not require subjective assessments for each sample.

Another seemingly innocent situation where order effects can be important is when a procedure or protocol involves multiple steps and the time to carry out the steps varies. This is illustrated with a hypothetical (and exaggerated) example in Figure 2.10, but is based on several real experiments where such effects were seen. In this experiment, four animals are pre-treated with a compound to test if it inhibits inflammation and another four animals serve as controls. Then all eight animals are injected with a substance that induces inflammation. The procedure to inject all animals with the inflammatory substance takes 1 hour to complete (the first animal is injected at $t = 0\,\text{h}$). Suppose that the inflammatory response peaks 2 hours after the injection of the substance and so collection of blood

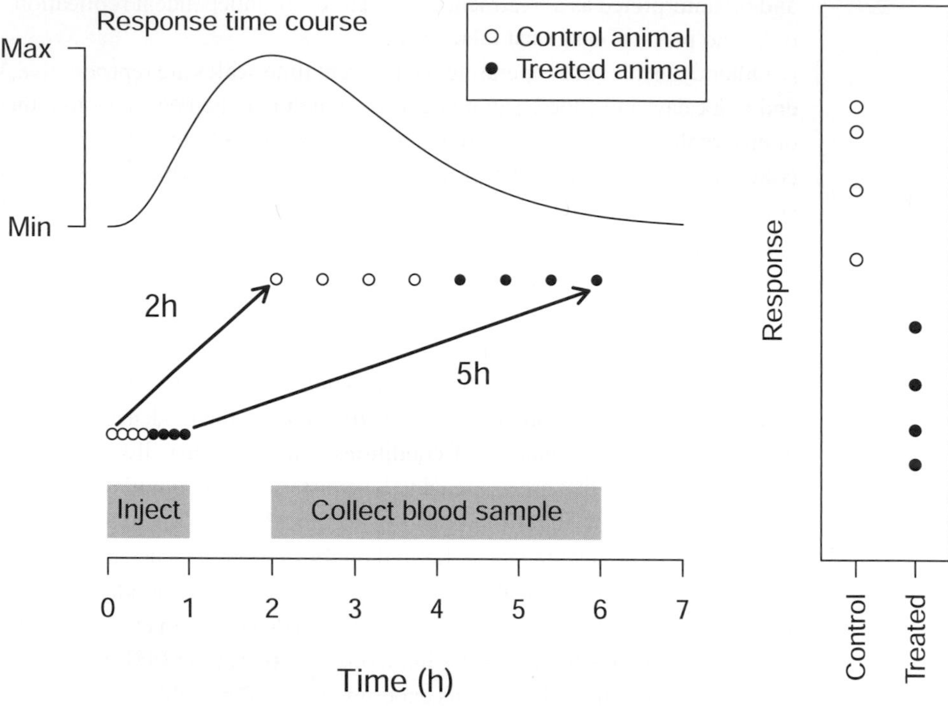

Fig. 2.10 Order effects due to a biological response that varies over time. Four control followed by four treated animals are injected with an inflammatory substance; the procedure takes 1 hour. Two hours after the first injection, blood samples are collected in the same order as the injections, which takes 4 hours. There are 2 hours between injection and collection for the first animal and 5 hours for the last animal. The peak of the inflammatory response is at 2 hours (curve) and then declines. Control animals are sampled near the peak response while treated animals are sampled when the response has subsided, giving the appearance of an effective anti-inflammatory treatment (right panel).

samples begins at $t = 2$ h and takes 4 hours to complete. It is typical that the order of injection is the same as the order of sample collection, and a problem arises when the length of time from injection to collection differs for each animal. For the first animal, it is 2 hours, while for the last animal it is 5 hours (arrows in Figure 2.10) because blood collection takes longer than the injections. The animals in between will have a gradient of time lags between injection and collection, and because the inflammatory response is not constant (there is an increase to a maximal response which then subsides), the measured value of the outcome will be related to the order of sample collection.

A problem arises if all of the controls were injected first, followed by all of the treated animals; it will be impossible to separate the treatment effects from the order effects. The values of outcome are plotted in the right panel of Figure 2.10, and it appears that the anti-inflammatory compound is highly effective. But this conclusion is incorrect and the data points were taken from the height of the time course response curve at the point that observations were made for each animal. This spurious effect would be replicated in a repeat experiment if controls were again injected before the treated animals [330].

The final cause of order effects are *one-off events* that occur while the experiment is underway and only affect samples after the event. Unlike previous causes, which were gradual changes over time, these events introduce a sharp transition before and after the event. Examples include a fire alarm in the middle of a protocol so that incubation or wash times are longer for the later samples, or during a break someone decides to use your microscope to look at their slides and changes the microscope settings, which should have remained constant throughout data acquisition.

Order effects can appear anywhere, they may be due to a one-off event, or stable across replicate experiments. The good news is that the influence of order effects can be taken into account with an appropriate design. For example, randomising or blocking the order of sample collection or processing can prevent confounding order and treatment effects. This is a sensible safeguard even if you do not think order effects are present. Randomising or blocking will not eliminate these effects, but it will enable them to be detected and to be taken into account, making valid inferences possible. There is no statistical fix when order effects are completely confounded with treatment effects. Three options to deal with order effects are:

1. Randomise the order of collection and/or processing.
2. Randomise in blocks. A block consists of one sample from each experimental condition and the samples are processed from the first to the last block. Within each block the order of sample processing is randomised, and this avoids having long sequences of samples from the same condition.
3. Alternate between treated and control groups, or cycle through the groups in a multi-group experiment. This is simpler than blocking and randomising. One drawback is that groups are slightly shifted in time relative to each other. If the sequence starts with the control group followed by the treated group, then for every pair of samples, the control is always slightly earlier in time. This may be a reasonable compromise if it makes the collection of samples easier and less error prone than a method that involves randomisation.

2.12.8 Spatial effects

Another potential source of heterogeneity is the spatial arrangement of samples. Spatial effects arise because objects that are near each other are influenced to a similar extent by background and environmental factors that vary spatially. For example, the level of lighting varies from ceiling to floor in an animal facility. Animals housed in cages at the top of a cage rack will be exposed to brighter light than animals housed at the bottom and the amount of light that rodents are exposed to will vary as a function of the vertical position in the cage racks. The amount of light exposure may or may not be a relevant factor in the experiment. Similarly, there may be temperature, sound, or odour gradients that vary by position in the room and can be a source of cage effects.

Many *in vitro* and molecular biology studies use multi-well microtitre plates, and the arrangement of samples on these plates can be a source of technical artefacts. One type of

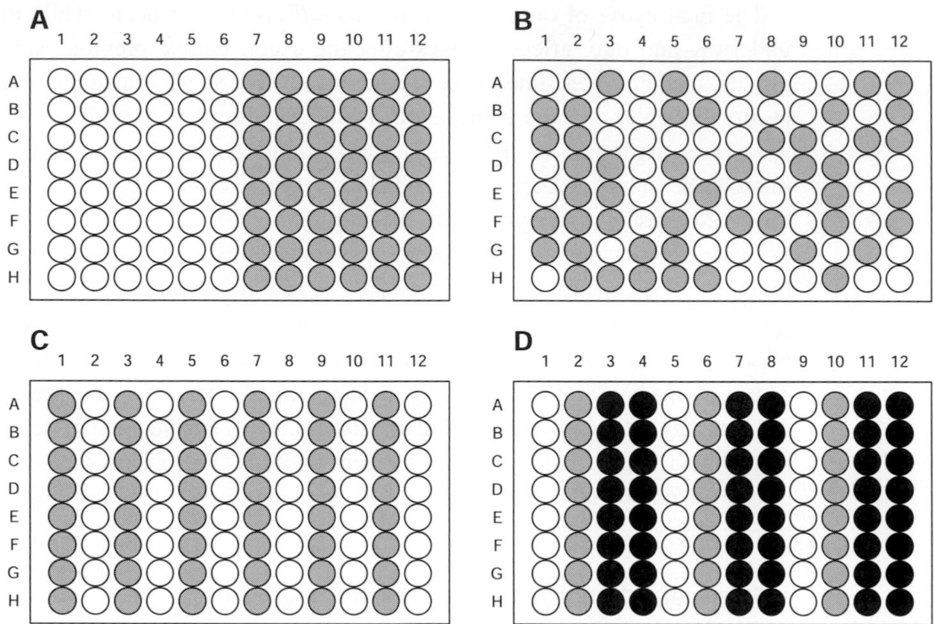

Fig. 2.11 Layouts of 96-well plates. A bad design with control wells (white) on the left half of the plate and treated wells (grey) on the right (A). Completely randomised control and treated wells protects against edge-effects and spatial gradients but may be hard to implement (B). Alternating columns of control and treated wells is a suitable compromise (C). Alternating columns for control and three treatments (D).

artefact is an edge-effect, where wells near the edge tend to differ from wells in the middle of the plate, often because wells near the edge tend to dry out faster, which can change the concentration of substances remaining in the well. This is more of a problem for plates with small wells such as the high density 384- and 1536-well plates. Another type of artefact is a gradient across a plate, with higher values at one side compared with the other. Other artefacts such as stripes and checker-board patterns can also be present, although these are more often seen in automated high-throughput experiments. The layout of samples within plates should be arranged so that valid inferences can be obtained even if these artefacts are present.

Figure 2.11A shows a layout for a 96-well plate with 48 control (white) and 48 treated (grey) wells. This arrangement is problematic because a gradient in the left-to-right direction will be confounded with the treatments; if the right side of the plate has higher values – for technical reasons – it can be mistaken for an effect of the treatment. A positive aspect of this design is that a gradient from top to bottom would not be confounded with the treatments, and there are an equal number of wells on the edges for each treatment condition.

A better layout – from a statistical perspective – is the completely randomised layout shown in Figure 2.11B. Here, gradients in any direction will not be confounded with the treatment effects, and the number of wells on the edges for each treatment is similar. All types of spatial effects can be detected and corrections can be applied. One drawback is that a completely randomised arrangement is often hard to implement and it might be more error prone if the treatments are applied to wells manually, although this would be less of a concern for an automated system. A compromise between what is statistically optimal and what is experimentally feasible is shown in Figure 2.11C. Here, the treatment and control wells alternate by column. This layout provides protection against gradients and edge-effects and is easier to implement.

Figure 2.11D shows a more complex and realistic example with four conditions indicated by different shades of grey and treatments alternating by columns. Having the four experimental conditions in adjacent columns is not ideal because gradients and edge-effects are once again confounded with the experimental conditions. One drawback of the layout in Figure 2.11D is that there are more white and black wells on the edge of the plate compared with the two other conditions. Other suitable layouts exist and there is nothing special about this one; the aim is to find a layout that is easy to implement while also ensuring that any technical artefacts are not confounded with treatment effects.

In addition to spatial artefacts within a plate, plates may differ because of their location in the incubator. There may be temperature, humidity, or CO_2 gradients from top to bottom or front to back. These effects can be a problem if there is an interest in comparing treatment conditions that are located on different plates. The control samples should not be on one plate and the treated samples on another, as it is impossible to separate plate effects from treatment effects. A good rule of thumb is to put experimental groups you are interested in comparing on the same plate. Design layouts can quickly become complex but there is a large biological and statistical literature that discusses how to experimentally or statistically deal with spatial artefacts [236, 249, 258, 414].

These examples used 96-well plates, but the general ideas extend to other situations such as the arrangement of samples under a photographic film for autoradiography, some types of microarrays (e.g. Illumina chips can have up to 12 arrays per chip), and so on. Without randomisation or blocking, it may be hard to determine if differences between experimental groups are due to the treatment or are an experimental artefact. Technical artefacts are often present, and they can often be large. Samples should be arranged so that valid inferences can be made.

2.12.9 Useful confounding

The previous sections emphasised that confounding should be avoided because effects are hard or impossible to estimate. There are situations however when confounding can be beneficial: when there are many technical or biological factors that we are not interested in making an inference about. For example, suppose a large experiment takes two technicians (X and Y) 2 days to conduct, and the experiment has one treated and one control group. A technician effect and a day effect might exist, and the design should control for them. One design would be to have half of the treated and half of the control samples processed by each technician on each day (Figure 2.12A). This would be a three-way ANOVA with condition, technician, and day as the three factors. This design allows all possible main and interaction effects to be estimated. It is a complex design and suppose that interaction effects are unlikely and uninteresting (for example, that the treatment effect is significantly

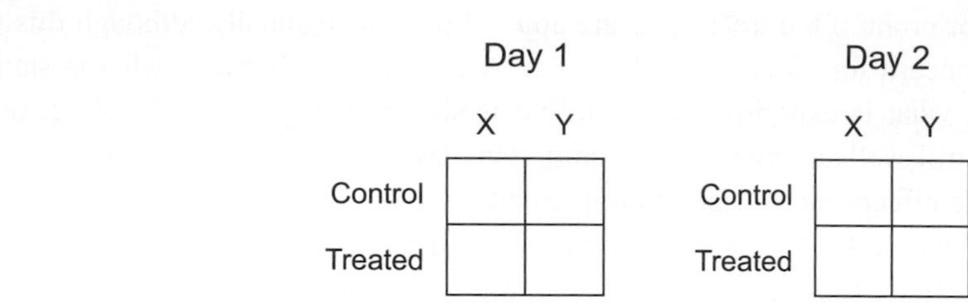

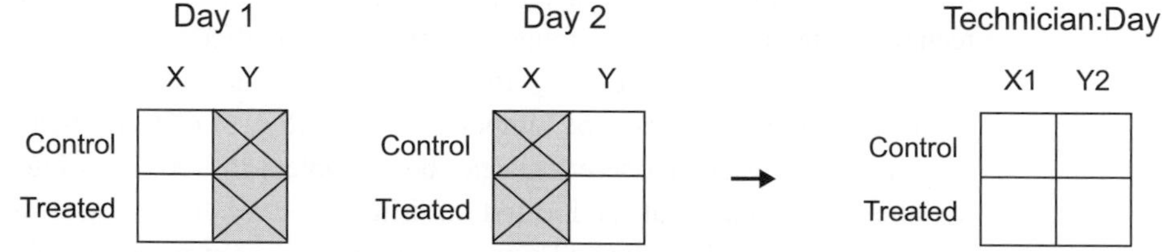

Fig. 2.12 Useful confounding. In the first design (A), the main effect of treatment, technician (X & Y), day, and all interactions can be estimated. Confounding technician and day allows for a simpler design (B), but some effects cannot be estimated. Grey squares indicate no observations.

bigger on the second day, but only for one of the technicians). Another option would be to have half of the control and treated samples analysed by each technician, but technician X only works on the first day while technician Y only works on the second day (Figure 2.12B). Here, we have completely confounded the effect of technician and day.[15] We can think of this as creating a new variable called Technician:Day (T:D for short) which is a two-level factor with levels X:1 (for technician X, first day) and Y:2 (technician Y, second day). The analysis would now be a two-way ANOVA with condition and T:D as factors. This is a simpler experiment to analyse and interpret, and also has fewer parameters to estimate, making the test of treatment effects more powerful. The drawback is that if there is an effect of T:D, then it is impossible to determine whether it is due to how the technicians conducted the experiment or due to splitting the experiment over two days. Furthermore, it is impossible to estimate the technician by day interaction effect.

In real experiments there are many biological or technical effects that could potentially influence the results and it is impossible to take all of them into account as there might be more effects than samples! One must decide which are the major effects that need to be included in the design, and by confounding effects (usually technical) that one is not interested in making inferences about, additional factors can be controlled for without additional experimental or analytical complexity.

[15] Since confounding is a bad thing, the term *aliased* is often used when an experiment is intentionally designed so that some main and/or interaction effects cannot be estimated.

Further reading

Experimental design: *Statistics for Experimenters* by Box, Hunter, and Hunter is a classic and emphasises the distinction between learning and confirming experiments and how statistics and experimental design can be used to learn about and improve systems [56]. Examples are mainly from manufacturing and it covers many topics that are not discussed here such as fractional factorial and response surface designs. There are also some excellent introductory lectures by J. Stuart Hunter from the 1960s on YouTube.[16] *Statistical Principles for the Design of Experiments* by Mead, Gilmour, and Mead has a greater overlap with the contents of this book, and examples are mainly from the agricultural sciences [274]. Many chapters in *A First Course in Design and Analysis of Experiments* by Oehlert are relevant and a free PDF copy is available online.[17]

Designing biological experiments: A great book by Glass (an experimental biologist) that discusses how to validate an experimental system, different types of experimental controls, and how to build and validate a biological model [135].

Technical books: *Design and Analysis of Experiments* by Hinkelmann and Kempthorne [153] and *Statistical Design* by Casella [67] are two excellent books for those who are comfortable with equations.

[16] https://www.youtube.com/watch?list=PL335F9F2DE78A358B&v=NoV1RAq0Uxs
[17] http://hdl.handle.net/11299/168002

3 Replication (what is 'N'?)

I believe sanity and realism can be restored to the teaching of Mathematical Statistics most easily and directly by entrusting such teaching largely to men and women who have had personal experience of research in the Natural Sciences.

Sir Ronald A. Fisher, FRS

Replication is a fundamental concept in both science and statistics and is used in the everyday sense of the term to mean 'doing something more than once'. The 'more than once' part is straightforward, but it is often unclear what exactly needs to be done multiple times, especially when many parts of an experiment can be replicated. In the experimental sciences, there is always a treatment or intervention applied to an entity, which in our case will be a biological entity such as a person, animal, or cell. A basic requirement for replication is to have multiple independent entity–intervention pairs. Suppose that the intervention is a drug given orally to a patient. Each patient–drug pair is considered one replication and provides independent information about the effect of the drug. The effect is then compared with placebo–patient pairs. If the question is 'what is the effect of the drug on patients' then replicating the patient–drug pair and patient–placebo pair enables the question to be addressed.

Other aspects of this experiment could be replicated. For example, we could measure the outcome on each person more than once and replicate the measurement procedure. Or, we could give the drug to the same person multiple times and on each occasion record the outcome. Alternatively, we could even conduct the whole experiment multiple times, say once in England and once in America. Experimenters need to decide what to replicate and often the wrong part is chosen, wasting time and resources. In addition, one occasionally sees that the critical aspect of the experiment is not replicated at all, or only replicated a few times. In such cases it is either impossible to test the hypothesis of interest or the power is so low that the objectives of the experiment are unlikely to be met. A clever statistical analysis cannot fix the problem; it needs to be planned at the design stage.

There are two types of replication. The first is replication that increases the sample size (N) and contributes to testing the experimental hypothesis.[1] It is called *true*, *genuine*, or *absolute* replication by various authors, and when these qualifiers are not used, replication is usually understood to mean genuine replication, and this is the convention followed here. The second type of replication is that which does not increase the sample size and is called

[1] The terms *sample size*, N, and number of *replicates* are treated as synonymous.

pseudoreplication, a *subsample*, or *repeated measurements*.[2] Confusing pseudoreplicates with genuine replicates is a problem in many fields including medical research [9], microbiology [319], ecology [165, 321], plant biology [281], physiology [103], and neuroscience [216].

Replication that increases the sample size is often equated with biological replication (e.g. multiple people or animals), while replication that does not increase the sample size is often equated with technical replication. This is often the case but the terms *biological* and *technical replication* are discouraged because *biological replication does not necessarily equal genuine replication and what might be considered technical replication does not necessarily equal pseudoreplication.* These terms do not capture the important characteristics of the experiment, blur important distinctions, and can be used to inappropriately justify a poor experimental design. Instead, it is better to consider the three aspects that one can replicate in an experiment: the biological unit, the experimental unit, and the observational unit (Box 3.1). These are discussed below and the important point is that only replication of the experimental unit increases the sample size. The term 'unit' refers to a biological entity or sample material and not a measurement unit such as kilograms or seconds.

3.1 Biological units

The *biological unit (BU)* is the entity that we would like to make an inference about, and the purpose of an experiment is to test a hypothesis, estimate some property, or draw a conclusion about biological units. More generally, this can be called the *scientific unit* of interest, but since we are focusing on experimental biology these will always be biological units. Common examples of biological units are people, animals, and cells, and if you want to make a general statement about the effect of a treatment or intervention on a biological unit, it is necessary to replicate the number of such units. For example, you cannot draw a conclusion about the effect of a compound on people in general by observing the effect in one person.

Suppose we are using cell lines from the Cancer Cell Line Encyclopedia (CCLE)[3] and are interested in determining whether breast cancer cell lines proliferate at a different rate than lung cancer cell lines. The hypothesis is about differences between tissues and so it is necessary to use multiple breast and lung cell lines. If one breast and one lung cell line proliferate at different rates, we cannot attribute this to the tissue from which they are derived as no two cell lines are expected to proliferate equally. Suppose instead that we are interested in testing if cancer cells with a *p53* mutation differ in their rate of proliferation from cancer cells with a *KRAS* mutation. Multiple cell lines with these mutations are required

[2] Vaux and colleagues use the term *replication* to refer to pseudoreplication and use the term *repeat* for genuine replication [89, 376, 377]. This reversal of terms from their commonly used definitions may lead to confusion, especially because they were writing for experimental biologists.

[3] `http://www.broadinstitute.org/ccle/home`

Box 3.1 **Types of units to consider**

Biological unit of interest (BU): the entity about which inferences are made. The purpose of the experiment is to test a hypothesis or to estimate a property regarding these units.

Experimental unit (EU): the entity that is randomly and independently assigned to one treatment or another. The sample size (*N*) is equal to the number of EUs. They may correspond to:

1. a biological unit of interest
2. groups of biological units
3. parts of a biological unit
4. a sequence of observations on a biological unit

Ideally, the treatment should be applied independently to each EU, and the EUs should not influence each other. If these conditions do not hold, using a different unit as the EU may be preferable.

Observational unit (OU): the entity on which measurements are taken, which may be different from the experimental and biological units of interest. Increasing the number of OUs does not increase the sample size.

to test this hypothesis. With one *p53* mutant cell line and one *KRAS* mutant cell line it is impossible to distinguish between the effect of the mutations and natural variation between these two cell lines.

3.2 Experimental units

The *experimental unit (EU)* is the smallest entity, unit, or piece of experimental material that is randomly and independently assigned to a treatment condition [67, 114, 153, 274]. Examples include a person, animal, litter, cage or holding pen, fish tank, culture dish, well, or a plot of land. The EU is also called the *unit of allocation* or *unit of randomisation* and ⚠ *it represents the unit to be replicated to increase the sample size (*N*)*. The term *unit of randomisation* makes the defining feature of the EUs clear, but we will use the term EU because it is more common. The EU often corresponds to a biological unit of interest such as an animal, and then the design, analysis, and interpretation of the data are more straightforward (Figure 3.1; top left). However, the EU can also correspond to a collection or group of biological units, such as all mice in a cage if a treatment is applied on a cage-by-cage basis instead of to individual animals (Figure 3.1; bottom left). In addition, the EU can correspond to parts of a single biological unit. For example, individual eyes, patches of skin, or organotypic slice cultures from the same animal, as long as these parts can be randomly assigned to different conditions (Figure 3.1; top right). Finally, an EU can correspond to

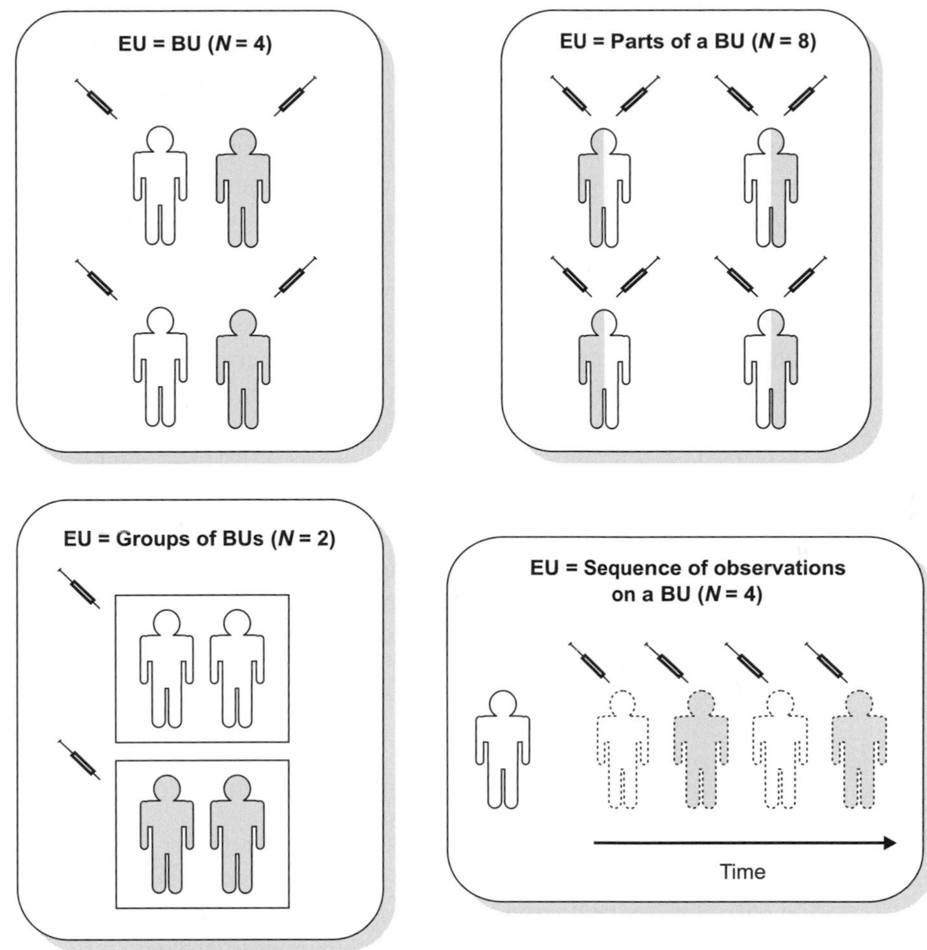

Fig. 3.1 Varieties of experimental units (EUs). The treatments (syringes) are randomly assigned to the EUs and only one measurement is made on each EU. Note how the number of biological units (humans) and experimental units varies across situations. *N* is always the number of EUs. White = controls; grey = treated group.

a sequence of observations on a single biological unit. For example, a period of time is divided into 10 epochs that are randomly assigned to an on-drug or off-drug condition (Figure 3.1; bottom right) [274].

Treatments should be independently applied to each EU

The EU was defined above as the smallest biological entity that is randomly and independently assigned to a different treatment condition. There are two additional requirements for a unit to be unambiguously considered the EU. The first is that the treatment must also be independently applied to each EU. The units that are randomised do not always correspond to the units that have independent applications of the treatment. For example, suppose that 20 rats are randomly assigned to two treatment groups, and are then housed in four cages of five, with rats in the same treatment group housed together. Here, the cages are irrelevant for the treatment assignment; they are only a post-randomisation grouping of biological units for logistic reasons. If the treatment is applied in the drinking water, then it is applied in a common way to all animals in a cage. Recall from Section 2.2 that treatment error is the inability to exactly replicate the application of the treatment to each EU. Since treatments are applied to cages, the treatment error will be similar for all rats in a cage. To take an extreme example, suppose by accident twice the concentration of a compound is put into the drinking water of one cage – all the animals will be affected in the same way. Here, we say that the treatment errors (and thus the experimental errors) are correlated, but an analysis using rats as the EU requires that the errors are independent. If the treatment error is small relative to the variation between rats, then this becomes less of a concern. If we are unwilling to ignore treatment error, then cages should be the EU instead of the rats. Biologists would prefer to have the rats as the EU because the sample size is greater (20 rats versus four cages). A conservative statistician might favour treating the cages as the EUs [67], and a compromise is to divide the rats into a greater number of cages; for example, ten cages of two instead of four cages of five. Reasonable opinion may differ on whether it is better to use the rats or the cages as the EU. Regardless of the choice of EU, it is a good idea to check for cage effects (Section 2.12.3), and possibly to include cage as a variable in the analysis.

EUs must not interfere with each other

The second requirement is that the EUs must not affect or interfere with each other, and a treatment applied to one EU should not affect the outcome of other EUs.[4] For example, suppose rats are randomised to a stress or control condition. Rats emit warning and alarm calls at 22 kHz, and if these ultrasonic vocalisations from the stressed group can be heard by the control animals, then the controls may become stressed as well [63]. If some animals in a cage receive a treatment that alters their behaviour, such as making them more aggressive, this will likely affect the behaviour of the other animals in the cage. In such cases, it is better to use the cage as the EU instead of the animals.

Cells in the same well in an *in vitro* experiment influence each other; they form cell-to-cell connections, some can form gap junctions, and they compete for the same nutrients in the media. When cells undergo necrotic death they release intracellular molecules – so-called damage-associated molecular patterns (DAMPs) – which can affect adjacent cells [195]. Even if cells are randomly assigned to wells by the process of pipetting it is unrealistic to assume that they provide independent information about a treatment effect – which is applied on a per-well basis and not to individual cells – and it is impossible to prove that cells in a well are not influencing each other. It is therefore necessary to use the well as the experimental unit even if measurements can be taken on individual cells in a well.

[4] In the causal modelling literature, this is part of the *stable unit-treatment value assumption* (SUTVA) [337].

Genuine replication consists of independently replicating the application of the experimental treatment or intervention to an experimental unit. There are both choices and constraints on what can be randomly assigned to the treatment groups and how the treatments can be applied. An important step in designing an experiment is to determine what the experimental unit will be. A person is a typical experimental unit because they can be randomly allocated to receive a drug or placebo, the drugs are administered individually, and one person's response to the drug or placebo is unlikely to affect another's response. Similarly, if rodents can be individually randomly allocated to treatment groups, the treatments applied individually, and it is reasonable that the rodents do not affect each other, then rodents are the experimental units. However, if the rodents are pregnant females and the interest is in the effect of the treatment on their offspring, the experimental units are the pregnant females (or equivalently, the litters) and not the offspring derived from them. It follows that the sample size is the number of females, not the number of offspring [219, 222]. This is because pups in the same litter will be randomised together as one group or unit, that is, they cannot be individually randomly assigned to the treated or control conditions. They also receive the treatment together, and it is unreasonable to assume that they do not affect each other *in utero* since they compete for maternal resources. In this case the experimental units (dams/litters) do not correspond to the biological units of interest (offspring).[5] Regulatory authorities do not allow the offspring to be used as independent samples for toxicology studies using this design [167, 297], and it is telling what those charged with protecting the public consider legitimate when there are real consequences for coming to the wrong conclusion. The appropriate experimental unit does not change when the consequences of being wrong are lower. When subsamples (offspring) are treated as genuine replicates in an analysis the sample size is inflated and p-values are inappropriately small.

3.3 Observational units

The final unit is the *observational unit (OU)*, which is also called the *sampling unit* or the *measurement unit* and it is the entity on which measurements are made. It may or may not correspond to the EU or BU and the intuition behind what constitutes N breaks down when the BU, EU, and OU are different entities. For example, in a randomised clinical trial testing the effect of a compound on blood pressure, it is obvious that the sample size should be the number of people, even if blood pressure is measured from both the left and right arm of each person. Here, the experimental unit and the biological unit of interest coincide, and it is clear that N is the number of people and not the number of arms. The two measurements made on each person need to be handled appropriately (e.g. by taking an average), otherwise the amount of evidence would be inappropriately doubled. Returning to the pregnant rodent example, the biological and observational units are the offspring but

[5] This is likely why 91% of studies using the valproic acid model of autism incorrectly considered the offspring and not the pregnant females as the experimental unit and therefore had an inflated sample size [222].

the EUs are the dams, thus the sample size for testing the effect of the treatment is the number of dams and not the number of offspring.

The same principle applies when recording from or measuring properties of cells in cell cultures, slice cultures, or histological sections. Cells are often both the observational and biological units of interest, but rarely the experimental unit. Measuring spine density on multiple neurons per animal is analogous to measuring blood pressure from both arms in that including more arms or neurons on a fixed number of people or animals does not increase the sample size. Similarly, it is usually a well in a microtitre plate that can be randomly assigned to a treatment condition in cell culture studies, making the wells the EUs and not the total number of cells measured.

3.4 Relationship between units

Almost all introductory biology textbooks discuss the hierarchy of life, which starts with atoms at the bottom and progresses through molecules, organelles, cells, tissues, organs, organisms, and populations – all the way to the biosphere. Figure 3.2 shows the region of the hierarchy where most biomedical research takes place – between cells and populations. At the top of the hierarchy are groups of related animals, represented by pregnant female mice (alternatively, litters of mice already born), followed by offspring, tissue sections within offspring, and finally, cells within tissue sections. Note the nesting structure and how one female gives rise to multiple offspring, each offspring provides multiple tissue sections, and each tissue section has many cells. In experiments dealing with multiple levels of biological organisation the sample size may be hard to determine when the aim is to make inferences at one level, experimental manipulations occur at another level, and observations are made at yet another level. Is N the number of litters, offspring, tissue sections, or cells? The sample size can be any of these, depending on the design of the experiment. The biological question of interest determines the design – while taking into account any practical or ethical constraints – and the design determines the appropriate analysis.

Figure 3.2 shows that randomisation can occur at the level of litters, animals, or tissue sections, leading to three different experimental units. Although cells can be randomised, this is rarely done and therefore not shown in the figure. The biological question and constraints on what is feasible determine the entities to randomise. Observations are typically made at the same level as the EU or at levels lower in the hierarchy. Constraints refer to the inability to randomise at the level appropriate to test the hypothesis of interest, usually because groups of biological units will need to be randomised together. As mentioned several times already, a classical example in the preclinical biomedical literature is studying effects of a prenatal intervention on postnatal animals. The interest is in how the prenatal intervention affects the offspring after they are born and we would like the offspring to be the EUs. But it is rarely possible to randomise offspring prenatally to different treatment conditions because the intervention is applied to pregnant females and therefore animals in a litter are randomised together. Here, litters are the experimental units and to increase

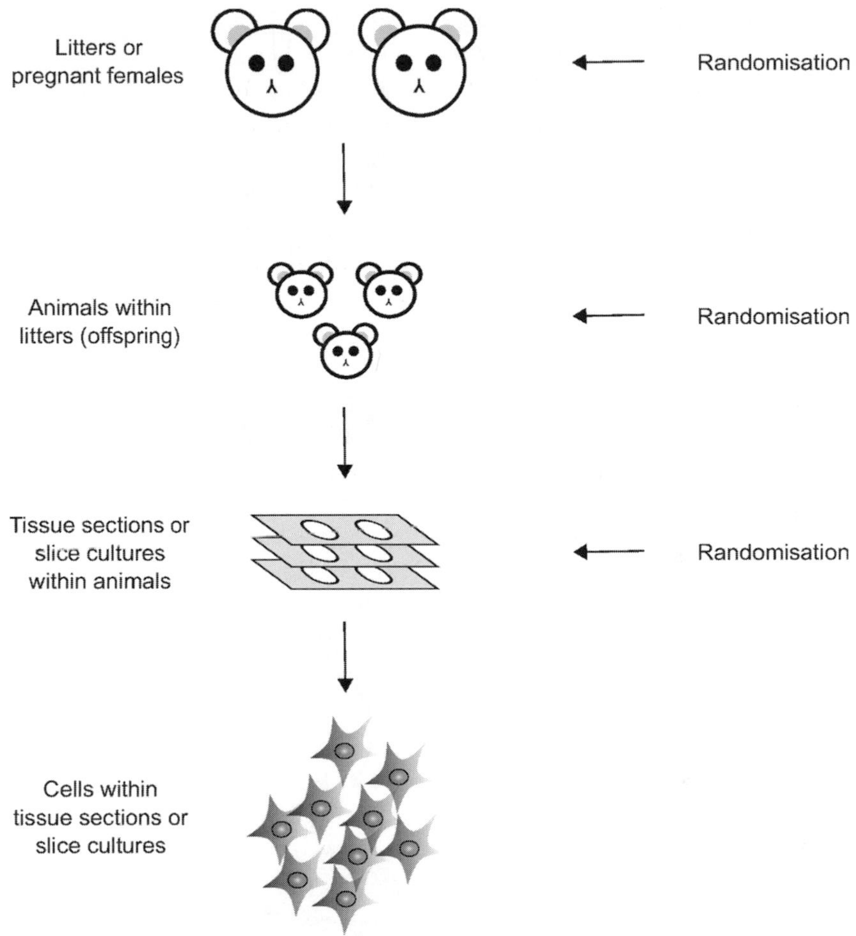

Fig. 3.2 Biological organisation from cells to groups of organisms (litters). Randomisation can occur at multiple levels, and genuine replication occurs only at the level where randomisation is used.

N the number of litters needs to be increased. The same situation can occur lower down the hierarchy. Suppose an electrophysiologist is interested in how a treatment applied to animals affects the electrophysiological properties of cells. Cells are both the biological units of interest and the observational units, but since animals were randomised, N is the number of animals and not the number of cells. A similar situation arises in *in vitro* studies where wells on a microtitre plate are the EUs, but the OUs are cells within a well. Once again, N is the number of wells and not the number of cells.

Things are not always so complex. If the interest is in the effect of a treatment on animals, the animals are randomised to different conditions, and observations are made on the animals, then the BU, EU, and OU coincide and the design and analysis is straightforward. There is, however, one more complication that needs to be considered: *a higher level of biological organisation can influence the outcome measured at lower levels*. For example, consider an experiment where individual mice are randomly allocated to a treatment or

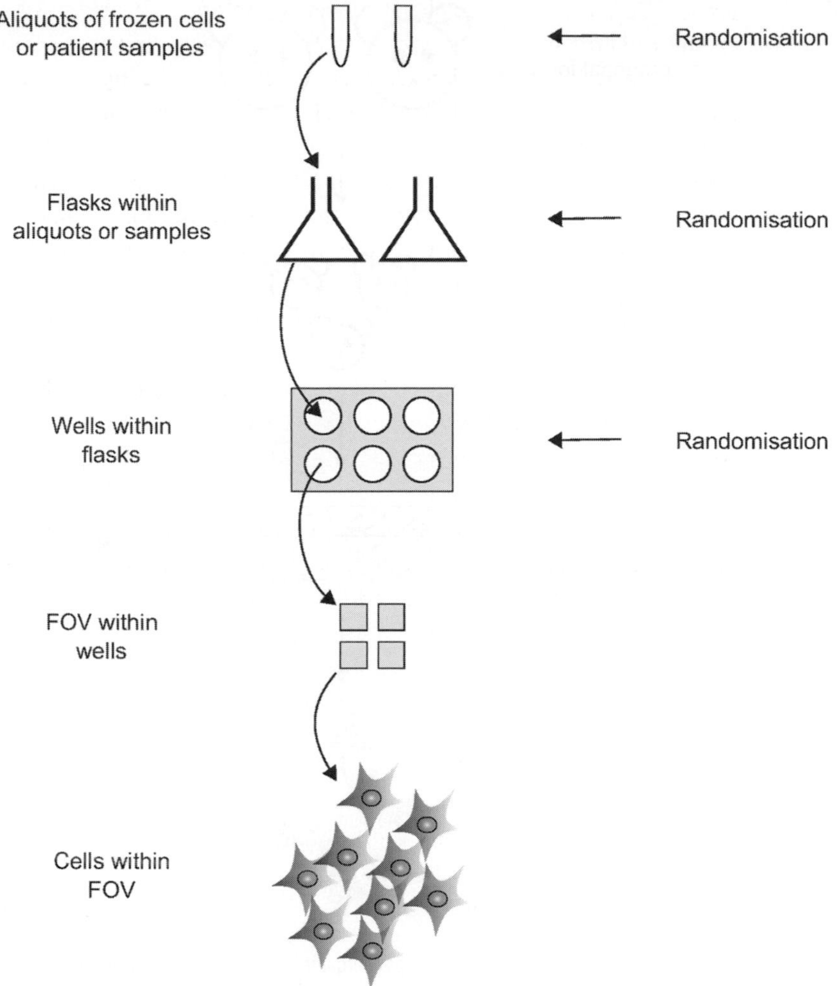

Fig. 3.3 A technical hierarchy from a multi-step protocol. Randomisation can occur at multiple levels, and genuine replication occurs only at the level where randomisation is used.

control group, but the mice are derived from several litters. Since each mouse is randomly assigned, the sample size is the number of mice. A problem arises because animals within a litter will tend to be more alike than animals from two different litters. This means that some litters will have higher values on the outcome variable (on average) while other litters will have lower values. Similarly, observations made on tissue sections from the same animal will tend to be more alike than observations made on tissue sections from two different animals. The same applies to cells within tissue sections. This is a separate issue from correctly identifying the EU; it is about considering which other variables affect the outcome and designing the experiment to take these into account.

In addition to a biological hierarchy, the design of the experiment can impose a technical hierarchy. Figure 3.3 shows how an aliquot of frozen cells is divided into several flasks to grow, cells in each flask are plated down into multiple wells in a microtitre plate, images are taken from multiple fields of view (FOV) in each well, and multiple cells within each FOV are measured. Randomisation can occur at several of the higher levels in the hierarchy, but once cells are within a well, they (usually) cannot be randomised to different experimental conditions.

Given the importance of replication, it is useful to go through several examples with various combinations of BUs, EUs, and OUs. In the figures that follow in this section, the biological unit is represented as a person and the experimental intervention is the application of a drug or a placebo control – indicated with a syringe. In all examples, the application of the treatment to the EUs is done randomly. In figures with both large and small people, the small people are offspring of the larger ones. The people could represent a person, animal, or a cell line. The Eppendorf tubes represent a blood sample or a biopsy taken on the BUs, but they could also represent wells in a plate or flasks. The pair of eyes represent observations or measurements and the number beside them indicates the number of times observations are made.

What constitutes N in the following examples may be at odds with what is considered N in your discipline for some experiments. We return to this point at the end of the section and here only comment that many experiments do not determine N appropriately. The key point in the following discussion can be summarised as *the sample size is where you randomise*.

The designs are summarised in Table 3.2 at the end of this section. Chapter 4 shows how to analyse some of these designs and Table 3.2 provides the page number for the corresponding analysis.

3.4.1 Randomisation at the top of the hierarchy

In the first example (Figure 3.4), the experiment has two people; one is injected with a drug and the other with a placebo. A single blood sample is taken from each person and divided into five aliquots. One measurement is then taken on each aliquot, which could be the concentration of a metabolite or cytokine, and the total number of data points is 10. Presumably the interest is in testing for an effect of the drug. With this experiment, no conclusions can be made about the drug's effect in people. Since the people were randomly assigned to the treatment conditions, the number of EUs and therefore the sample size is two (which does correspond to the number of BUs). The observational units are the aliquots, of which there are 10, but these are subsamples and do not contribute to N.

An example of data that could have been generated from such an experiment is shown in Table 3.1. These data can be entered into statistics software and a p-value calculated, but the result is meaningless because it is impossible to determine if differences are due to the drug or due to natural variation between these two people. We cannot know that there are only two EUs by looking at Table 3.1. Without knowledge of how the experiment was conducted it looks like there are 10 EUs.

The second example (Figure 3.5) is the same as the first, except that instead of dividing the blood sample into five aliquots for each person, a single aliquot is used but five measurements are made. The BU and the EU are still the people and there are 10 data points. In

Table 3.1 Example data corresponding to the experiment shown in Figure 3.4.

Outcome (y)	Condition
9.4	Control
10.2	Control
9.2	Control
11.6	Control
10.3	Control
11.2	Drug
12.5	Drug
12.7	Drug
12.6	Drug
11.7	Drug

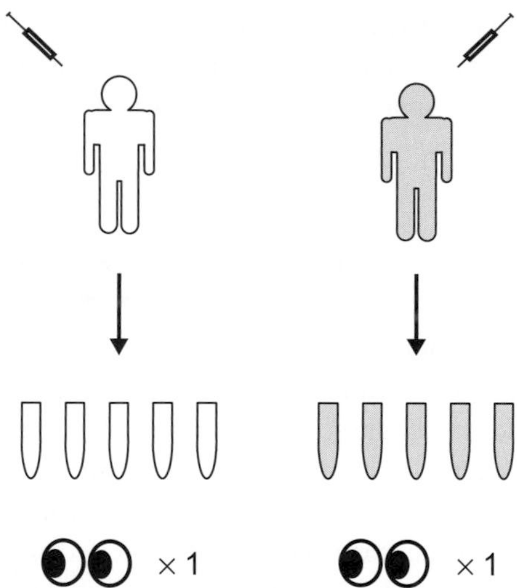

Fig. 3.4 Two people are injected with either a drug or placebo; five aliquots are taken per person, and one measurement is taken per aliquot. BU = person (2); EU = person (2); OU = aliquot (10); total number of values = 10.

both this and the previous example, the measurements would be considered 'technical replication' but they occur at different levels or steps in the protocol. The variability between values will likely be greater in the first example because the variability between aliquots will usually be larger than multiple measurements on the same aliquot. The variability in the second experiment is only measurement error. Having multiple aliquots per person and multiple measurements on each aliquot is useful for understanding where sources of variability arise, but they do not contribute to the sample size.

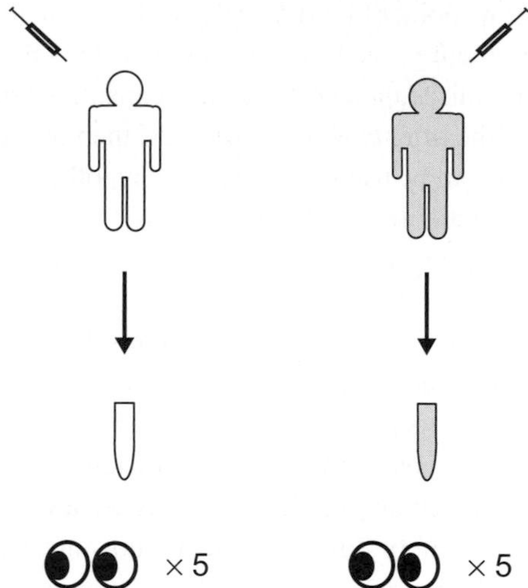

Fig. 3.5 Two people are (randomly) injected with either a drug or placebo; one aliquot is taken per person, and five measurements are taken per aliquot. BU = person (2); EU = person (2); OU = aliquot (2); total number of values = 10.

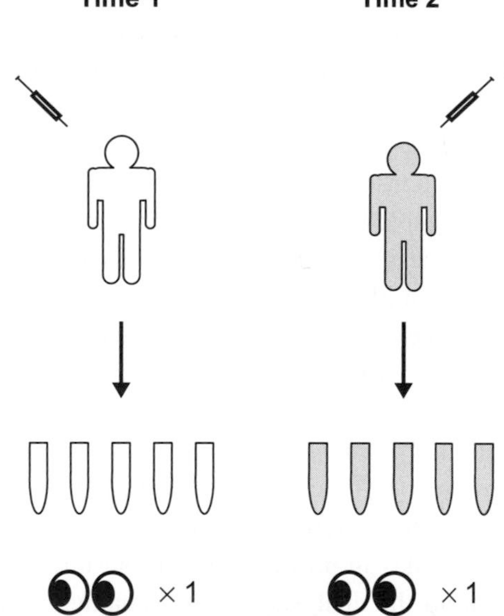

Fig. 3.6 One individual is (randomly) injected at two time points with either a drug or placebo; five aliquots are taken per time point, and one measurement is taken per aliquot. BU = individual (1); EU = time points (2); OU = aliquots (10); total number of values = 10.

The third example (Figure 3.6) has only one person, and they are injected with either the drug or placebo at one of two time points. Which condition they get at any time point is randomly chosen and the time between the two injections is long enough so that any effects of the drug have washed out and that there are no carry-over effects. A carry-over effect would occur if a treatment applied at an earlier time point has an effect at a later time point.

At each time point a blood sample is taken from the person, divided into five aliquots, and one measurement is taken on each aliquot (the OU). The person is the biological unit and the two randomised time points can be considered the EUs. If the interest is in determining the effect of the drug *in this person only*, then observations at two time points provide two values which can be used to assess this hypothesis, but the experiment is poorly designed because the outcome variable is likely not constant across time (e.g. circadian effects as well as changes at smaller and longer time scales) and the treatment effect is confounded with these fluctuations. In other words, changes across time cannot be distinguished from changes due to the drug. The aliquots are subsamples and do not contribute to the sample size. Note how such a design can lead to results that consistently mislead. Suppose the placebo injection is given first at 9 a.m. and a blood sample taken soon after. The drug is injected at 4 p.m. on the next day following the same protocol. If the outcome is blood glucose levels then one might expect higher levels at 9 a.m., soon after breakfast, then at 4 p.m., shortly before dinner. If the aliquots are inappropriately treated as genuine replicates one could perform a t-test with two groups of five and would find a significant result even if there is no drug effect. If the procedure was repeated exactly on another occasion (placebo in the morning and drug in the afternoon), the same misleading results would be replicated [330]. Replicating a poorly designed experiment (no randomisation to time point) and incorrectly determining the EU (the 10 aliquots instead of the two time points) has only provided more misleading evidence.

The experiment in Figure 3.6 is *not* a repeated measures or longitudinal design, which would have only one randomisation at the beginning of the experiment and multiple observations taken over time. The biological unit in Figure 3.6 is randomised twice to different treatment conditions and measured once at each time point.

The next example (Figure 3.7) is an improvement over the previous one and is an example of a N-of-1 design. There is still only one person (the BU) and he[6] is randomly assigned to receive either a placebo or drug injection at one of 10 time points (five of each). Only one blood sample is taken at each time point and one measurement taken on each sample (one OU per EU). A valid statistical test can be done as there are 10 EUs, and even though there may be daily fluctuations in the measured outcome, these will tend to average out over the different time points. An important point is that statistical inferences can only be made about *this person* (EU), and cannot be used to get an idea about the drug's effect in people in general. One may argue that this person is representative of some population that we would like to make an inference about, but this is a non-statistical generalisation; it does not follow from the analysis, and the smallness of the p-value does not provide greater evidence about what might happen in other people. Note also that this is not a repeated measures design, which requires that the treatment condition is constant over time.

In the next example (Figure 3.8) there are five people and both the drug and placebo are applied to each person at the same time. Suppose that the people's eyes are randomly assigned to receive either the drug or placebo. To make this example less gruesome, assume that the drug and placebo are not injected but applied topically, and that the aliquot represents a swab of lacrimal fluid. In this example, the eyes are the experimental units because

[6] The BUs in all the examples are drawn as men because my female BUs looked like men with skirts.

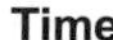

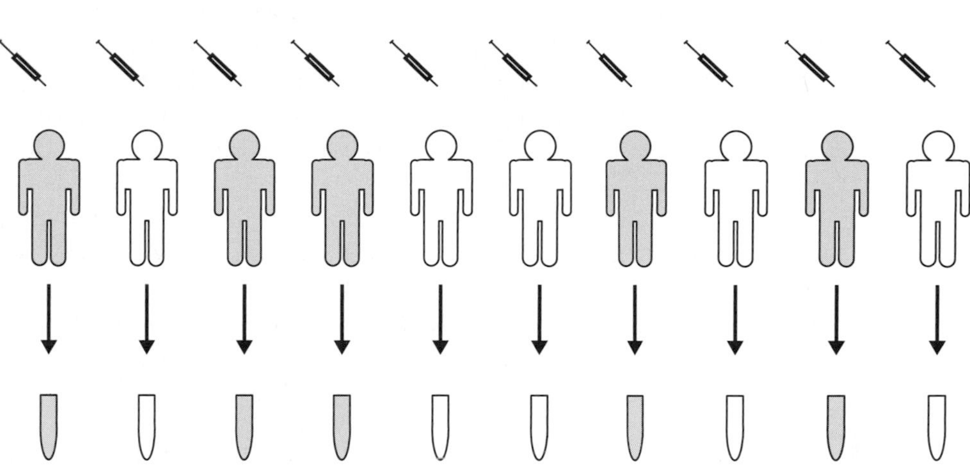

Fig. 3.7 One person is (randomly) injected at 10 time points with either a drug or placebo; one aliquot is taken per time point, and one measurement is taken per aliquot. BU = person (1); EU = time points (10); OU = aliquots (10); total number of values = 10.

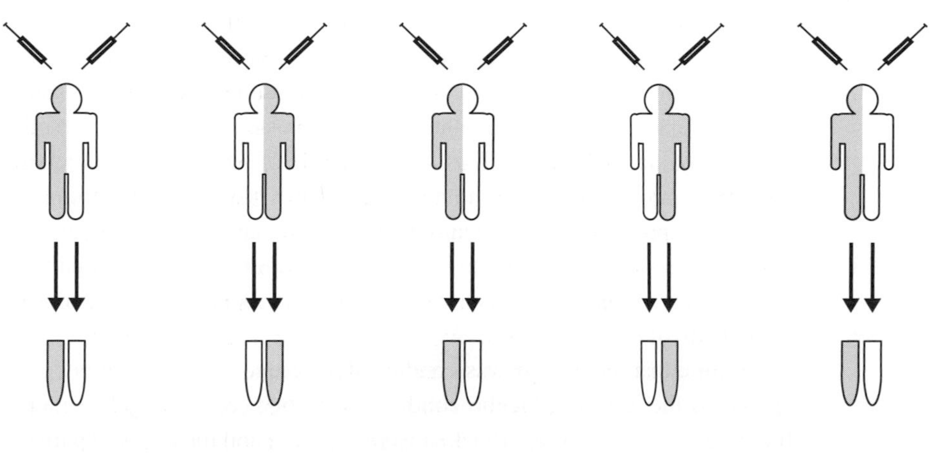

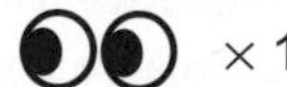

Fig. 3.8 The left and right eye from five individuals are (randomly) applied with either a drug or placebo; one aliquot is taken from each eye and one measurement is taken per aliquot. BU = individuals (5) or eyes (10); EU = eyes (10); OU = aliquots (10); total number of values = 10.

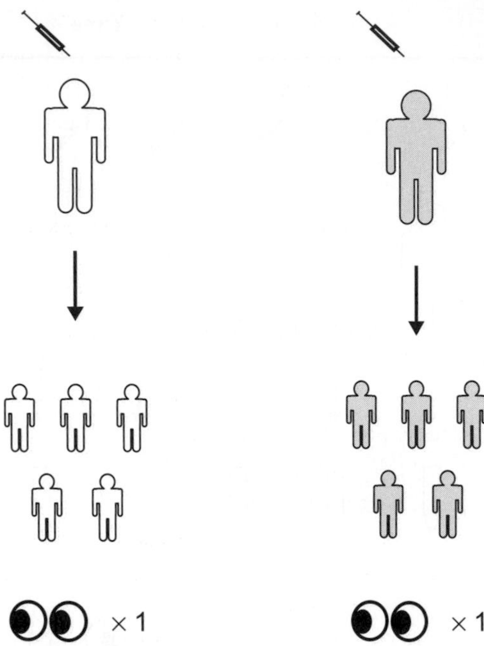

Fig. 3.9 Two pregnant females are (randomly) injected with either a drug or placebo; each have five offspring and one measurement is taken per offspring. BU = offspring (10); EU = pregnant females (2); OU = offspring (10); total number of values = 10.

they are randomly assigned to the experimental conditions and N is therefore equal to 10. This is an example of where the EU is a part of a biological unit and the observational unit is the swab (aliquot). Note that the 10 eyes were not assigned to the treatment groups in a completely random manner because they were randomised *within* each person. Once one eye of a person is assigned to either the drug or placebo condition, the other eye is assigned to the remaining condition. This is an example of a randomised block design, and a valid analysis can be performed with a paired-sample t-test. An assumption of this experiment is that the application of the treatment to one eye has no effect on the other eye. If the drug enters systemic circulation and can affect the other eye, then this paired design is unsuitable. This is a biological consideration that may make this design undesirable, even though statistically it is valid.

Assume that the design was conducted differently and that 10 people are randomly assigned to the drug or placebo condition, and both eyes of each person receive the same treatment. One swab is again taken from each eye and measured separately. In this case the person is the EU, even though we have measurements from 20 eyes. Eyes are 'technical replicates' in this example because units that are randomised together do not contribute to N. There are twice as many OUs than EUs, and one option for the analysis would be to average the two values for each person.

In the next example (Figure 3.9) two people (assume pregnant females even though they appear as males) are randomly assigned to be injected with the drug or placebo and are therefore the experimental units. Suppose that the interest is not in the effect of the drug on these people but on their offspring, which are the biological units of interest (smaller people in the figure). One measurement is taken on each BU and thus the BU and OU coincide, but differ from the EU. This is an example where treatments are applied to groups of biological units and the sample size is the number of groups and not the number of BUs. Recall the second version of the previous example when pairs of eyes were randomised together (as a group) because people were randomly assigned to the drug or placebo conditions – the EU was the number of people and not the number of eyes. Similarly, the offspring in the present example correspond to the eyes in the previous example in that they do not all contribute to N because multiple offspring do not constitute replication of the treatment to an experimental unit.

The design of this experiment is identical to that of Figure 3.4; there are only two experimental units and the offspring are subsamples and do not contribute to N. In Figure 3.4, however, the BUs were the people and so the aliquots were easily identified as subsamples. In this example the BUs are the subsamples, making it less obvious that they are not genuine replicates. Although we can put numbers into a computer and get numbers back, the result is meaningless for testing the effect of the drug. In addition, the treatment effects cannot be separated from natural variation between the two adults, and how this propagates to their offspring. This error of considering the biological or observational unit as the experimental unit is common in the biomedical literature.

For the next example (Figure 3.10), four people are randomised to either the drug or placebo condition at the beginning of the experiment, and three measurements are taken on each person at different times. This is a repeated measures design, and whether the treatment is applied once at the beginning of the experiment (e.g. a single injection as shown in Figure 3.10) or continuously throughout the experiment (multiple injections) is irrelevant for determining the number of experimental units. This example is simpler than previous ones because people are the BU, EU, and OU; the main question is whether the multiple measurements on each person contribute to the sample size. When testing the effect of the drug, they do not; the sample size is four and the number of time points is irrelevant. The key difference compared with the example in Figure 3.7 (other than having multiple people) is that each person receives only one treatment during the experiment.

3.4.2 Randomisation at the bottom of the hierarchy

The example shown in Figure 3.11 is a case where the experimental unit is part of a biological unit. There is only one person (BU) from which a blood sample is taken and divided into 10 aliquots. The drug or vehicle control are randomly applied to the 10 aliquots and one measurement is taken on each aliquot (one OU per EU). The experimental units are the aliquots and a valid statistical test can be performed to assess if the drug has an effect. Similar to the example in Figure 3.7, inferences about the effect of the drug can only be made about this person and inferences about other people is a non-statistical generalisation. If the blood sample was divided into 20 aliquots instead of 10, no further information is gained about the drug's effect in other people, but this does increase the sample size and power to detect the treatment effect in this person. This may seem like cheating; how can

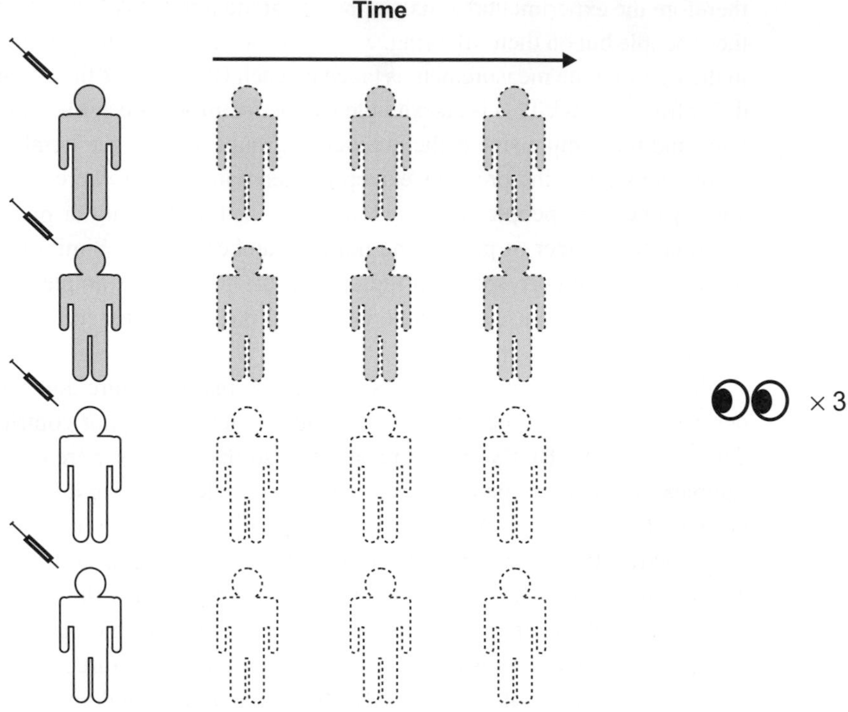

Fig. 3.10 Four people are (randomly) assigned to the drug or placebo condition and a single observation is made on each person at three time points. This is an example of a repeated measures design. BU = person (4); EU = person (4); OU = person (8); total number of values = 12.

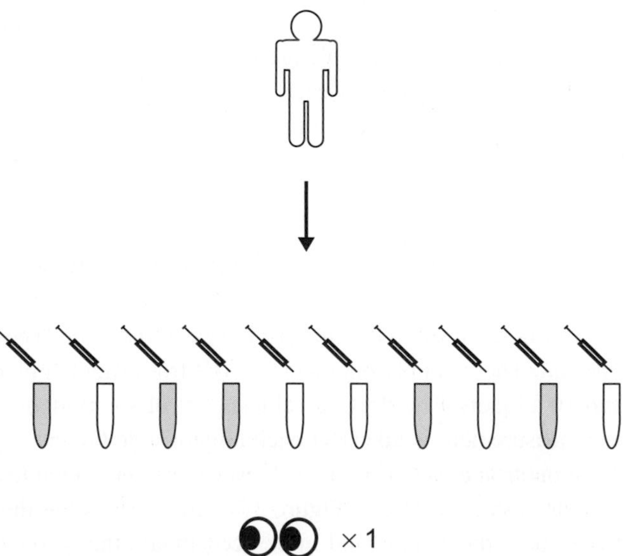

Fig. 3.11 Ten aliquots are taken from one person and (randomly) injected with either a drug or placebo, and one measurement is taken per aliquot. BU = person (1); EU = aliquots (10); OU = aliquots (10); total number of values = 10.

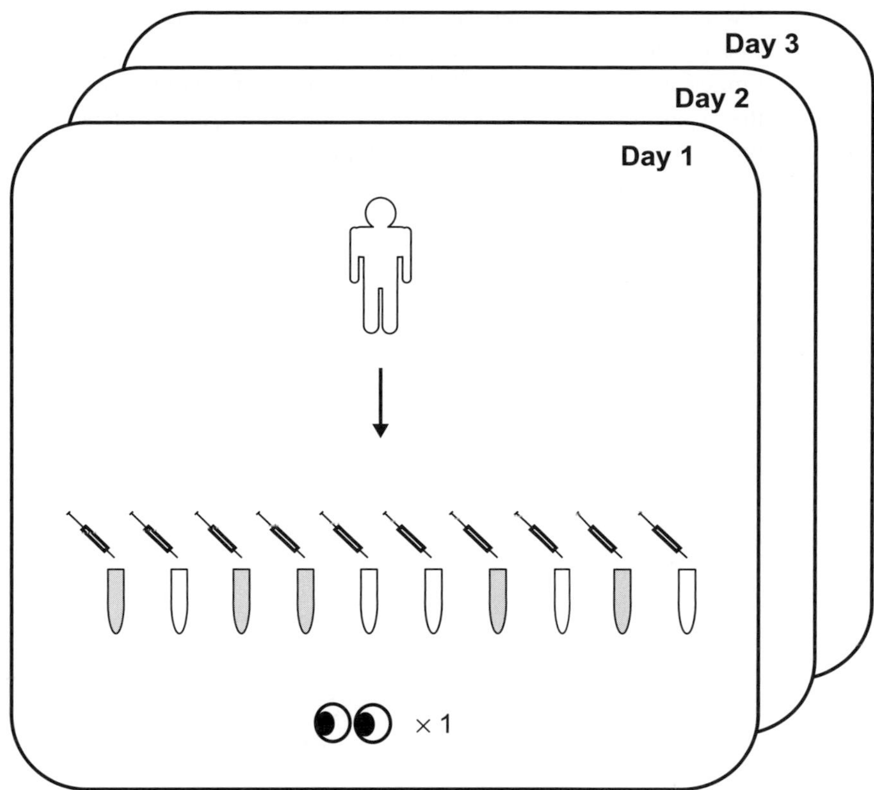

Fig. 3.12 Ten aliquots are taken from one person and (randomly) injected with either a drug or placebo, and one measurement is taken per aliquot. This whole procedure is then repeated on 3 days. BU = person (1); EU = aliquots (10 per day = 30); OU = aliquots (10 per day = 30); total number of values = 30. Alternatively, if the interest is in the consistency of the effect across several days, BU = person (1); EU = mean of the 5 aliquots per group on each day (2 groups per day × 3 days = 6; the individual aliquots are now considered pseudoreplicates or subsamples); OU = aliquots (10 per day = 30); total number of values = 30.

one take a fixed amount of sample material, and obtain more information by dividing it into a greater number of aliquots? The reason is that the application of the treatment to the sample material (aliquot) has been independently replicated more times. There is aliquot-to-aliquot variation in the measured response and the comparison is between aliquots with and without the drug. With more aliquots the estimated mean of each group is more precise. Note how this differs from taking more observations on an aliquot – the application of the treatment has not been replicated and so further information is not obtained about the treatment effect. The 'person' in this example could also represent a pool of multiple samples. For example, in primary cell culture experiments it may be necessary to combine cells from several animals into one large pool to obtain enough cells. Cells from this pool are then placed into different wells and a treatment applied to the wells.

The next example (Figure 3.12) is the same as the previous one but the whole experimental procedure is replicated on three separate days. There is still only one biological unit (the person), 10 EUs per day (aliquots), and one measurement is taken on each aliquot. The previous example was a valid analysis of the treatment effect, even though it was limited to only one person. What does this additional replication across days provide? If the experimental system is sensitive to the many details of how it is carried out, then repeating the whole procedure on multiple days provides further information in a way that using 30 aliquots on a single day does not. It provides an estimate of the consistency of the effects across the different experimental runs (days). This approach is common in cell culture experiments where the person represents either primary cells derived from a person or animal, or a cell line vial that has been thawed, with the aliquots representing flasks or wells in a microtitre plate. Replicating the whole procedure multiple times establishes that the effect can be reproduced and was not the result of some peculiar feature of the first attempt.

If this experiment is conducted on just 1 day (as in the previous example; Figure 3.11) the EU is the number of aliquots, which is 10. It follows then that if the experiment is repeated on 3 days, the number of EUs is $10 \times 3 = 30$. This is indeed the case and a valid statistical test can be performed, with a sample size of 30. We can, however, decide to perform another equally valid analysis by considering the multiple aliquots within days as the OUs, which do not contribute to the N. This is a scientific judgement about the relevant unit that we would like to make inferences about. For example, suppose on Day 1 the mean of the five drug aliquots is 22% higher than the mean of the control aliquots. Treating the aliquot as the EU would allow for a valid statistical test of whether 22% is unusually large, and it is the variation between the aliquots that provides the 'noise' beyond which the signal of 22% needs to stand out. Suppose on the next 2 days the mean difference is 5% and 12%, which gives an overall mean difference of 13% over the 3 days ($(22 + 5 + 12)/3 = 13$). By shifting the focus of our inference to the day, the variation between aliquots is no longer the relevant noise to test if the overall mean difference of 13% is unusually large (nor is the number of aliquots relevant). It is the variation in the size of the treatment effect from day to day. The values of 22, 5, and 12 have a standard deviation of 8.544, and so we can ask if 13% is unusually large given this day-to-day variation. The sample size is now only three – 10 times smaller than if we consider the aliquot as the EU. The power is greatly reduced and is why some may prefer the first analysis.

A difficulty with *in vitro* studies is that the results often depend on the specific circumstances that vary each time the experiment is carried out. This may be hard to detect unless there is an experimental condition that is meant to be identical across many experiments. Examples can be seen in Figure 1 of Lovell, which shows negative control data for over 400 Ames tests [246], and Figure 2 in Adler *et al.*, which shows negative control data from bone marrow chromosomal aberration assays over several years from two laboratories [4]. These data sets show that repeating the exact same experimental procedure can produce variable outcomes, despite efforts to standardise protocols. This is why replicating the entire experimental procedure multiple times is recommended for cell culture studies [89, 216, 376, 377], and why this information is required in the *Nature* journals' new checklist [3].

Although valid statistical inferences can be made for a cell culture study carried out on a single day with a single biological replicate, the homogeneity of the experimental material

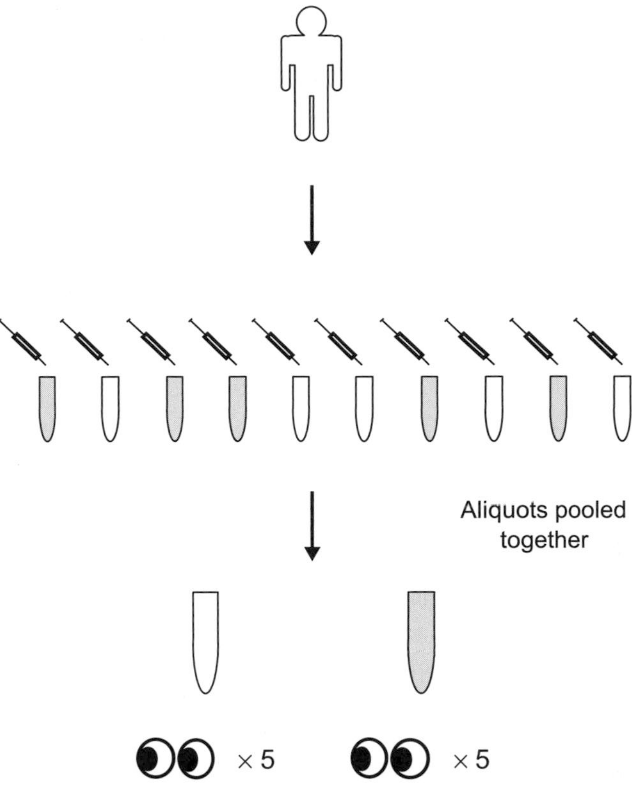

Fig. 3.13 Ten aliquots are taken from one person and (randomly) injected with either a drug or placebo. Aliquots from the same condition are then physically pooled and five measurements are taken per pooled sample. BU = person (1); EU = aliquots (initially 10, but then pooled into 2); OU = pooled aliquots (2); total number of values = 10. The correct number of EUs for the analysis is 2.

is so great and the conditions under which the experiment is run are so narrowly defined that it is hard to know what will happen if the experiment is conducted again. It is important to establish that the phenomenon is robust enough to survive multiple replications of the entire experimental run or protocol. For this reason, we recommend that *in vitro* experiments are repeated on multiple days, and the number of wells, aliquots, or culture dishes within a day are treated as subsamples. The number of replicates can be increased by conducting the experiment on more days. There will be exceptions, and it is the responsibility of the researcher to indicate what was done and justify using aliquots (or similar) as the EUs. Arguing that a valid analysis is used is insufficient justification, one would need to argue why a less interesting and less relevant hypothesis is tested.

The next example (Figure 3.13) has only one person and a blood sample that is divided into 10 aliquots that are randomised to the drug or vehicle control conditions. Suppose that to obtain enough sample material for later analyses it is necessary to pool the samples from the five aliquots in each condition into one larger aliquot (the OU). Then, five measurements are taken on the two pooled samples (larger aliquots). There were 10 EUs

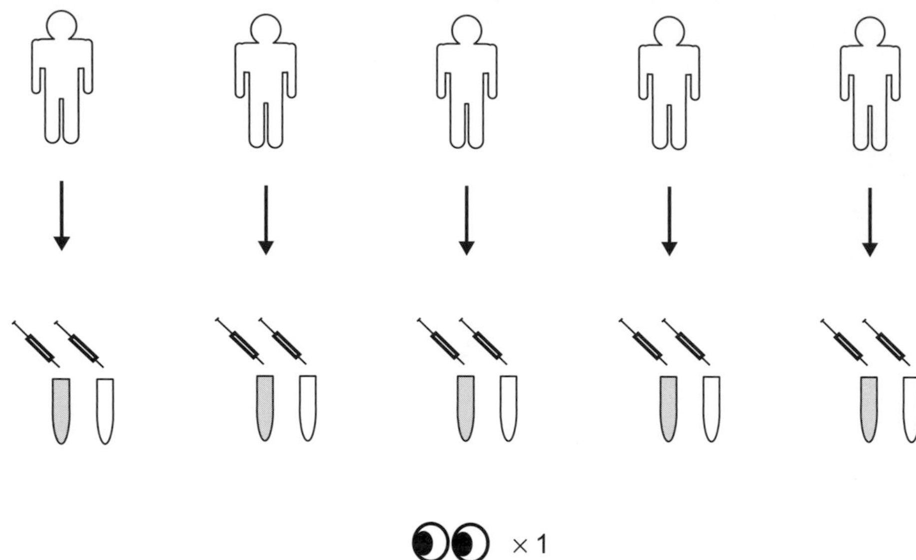

Fig. 3.14 Two aliquots are taken from five people and (randomly) injected with either a drug or placebo, and one measurement is taken per aliquot. BU = person (5); EU = aliquots (10); OU = aliquots (10); total number of values = 10.

(small aliquots) and 10 values at the end of the experiment, but pooling after the application of the experimental treatment has removed the information on the variability between the EUs that is required for a valid statistical test. The variability between EUs (original aliquots) will be larger than the variability between the five measurements on the pooled aliquots. Thus, the precision will be inappropriately low and the p-values artificially small. The lesson is that one should not pool experimental units after the treatment has been applied. If pooling sample material is necessary, then it should be done before applying the experimental interventions, and ensure that there are enough pooled EUs.

The above advice does not apply when samples are pooled for processing but can be individually distinguished afterwards. For example, next-generation sequencing experiments often add unique DNA 'barcodes' to cDNA derived from multiple experimental units. cDNA from the EUs are physically pooled or multiplexed during sequencing, but the barcodes enable one to distinguish the EU that a piece of cDNA is from, and so the variability between EUs can still be determined.

In the next example (Figure 3.14), a blood sample from five people is taken and divided into two aliquots. The drug is randomly added to one aliquot and the vehicle control to the other; one measurement is taken on each aliquot. Here, we have replication of biological samples and thus statistical inferences can be made about people in general, or at least to people similar to those in the experiment. The aliquots are still the EU and OU and note how this design differs from that in Figure 3.11. There are 10 aliquots in both designs and here one can address questions about other people, whereas in Figure 3.11 one is limited to inferences about the effect of the drug in only one person.

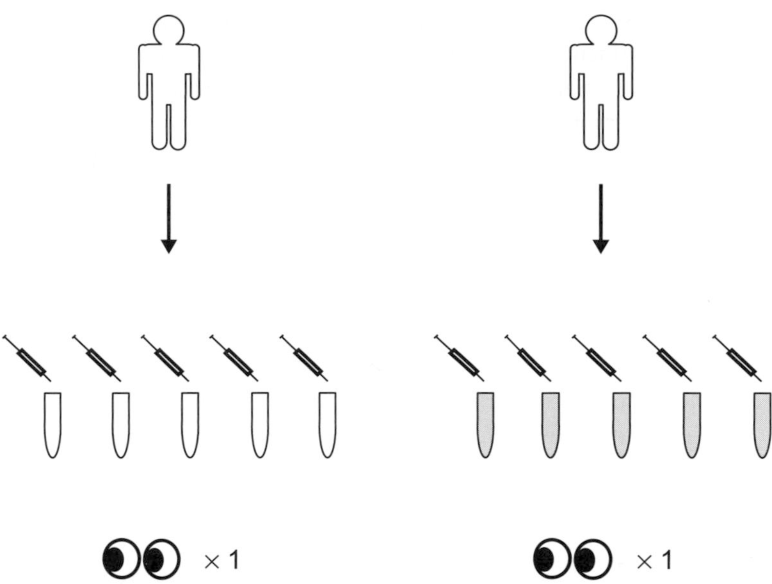

Fig. 3.15 Two people are (randomly) chosen to be in the drug or placebo condition. Five aliquots are taken per person, injected with drug or placebo, and one measurement is taken per aliquot. BU = person (2); EU = person (2); OU = aliquot (10); total number of values = 10.

There are two ways that the 10 aliquots can be randomised to the drug or vehicle groups. The first is to take the 10 aliquots and randomly divide them into two groups of five. The problem with this approach is that two aliquots from the same person can be both assigned to the drug group, or both to the placebo group. The second method avoids this by performing the randomisation *within* each person by assigning one aliquot from a person to either the drug or placebo condition, and the remaining aliquot to the other condition. The difference between assigning all of the aliquots completely at random or assigning them randomly within each person is an important experimental design decision that also affects the analyses. It is better to assign within people because this achieves a nice balance between the treatments and the people. In this example the people are *blocks*, which are discussed in Section 2.4. By using blocks, known sources of variability such as person-to-person variability can be removed, making it is easier to detect treatment effects. This design is called a randomised block design and is the same as the example in Figure 3.8. The data in Figure 3.14 could be analysed with a paired-samples t-test because there is a clear pairing of aliquots within people. To increase the sample size in a randomised block design the number of blocks (people) should be increased.

The next example (Figure 3.15) has two people; one is randomised to the drug condition and the other to the placebo condition. Five aliquots are taken from each person, all aliquots receive the same treatment, and one measurement is taken from each aliquot. In the previous examples, the unit that was randomised (person or aliquot) was also the unit that directly received the drug or placebo. In this example, the people are randomised, but treatment is applied to the aliquots. This is an interesting situation because we expect the variability between aliquots to be greater compared with applying the treatment to the person and then taking multiple aliquots as in Figure 3.4. Indeed, this variability between aliquots within a person was previously considered suitable for a sensible analysis (e.g. Figure 3.11). In this example, the people are the BUs and the question is whether we could count the aliquots as the EU, even though they were not randomised. The people should be considered the EU and not the aliquots, partly because it was the people that were randomised, but also because the aim of such an experiment is (we can assume) to make conclusions about the effect of the drug on people in general, and so the number of people needs to be replicated. The aliquots are best thought of as OUs and do not contribute to the sample size. With only two people it is impossible to separate the effect of the treatment from pre-existing differences between these two people. Even if more people are included, it would be preferable to have both the drug and placebo condition applied to aliquots within each person (as in Figure 3.14) because the person-to-person variation can be removed.

In the next example (Figure 3.16), the large people represent parents (they can be either male or female) and each parent has two offspring. The treatment is applied to the offspring any time after they are born, including in old age. There are three randomisations that can be used in this experiment. First, one offspring from each parent is randomly assigned to receive either the drug or placebo, and then their sibling receives the remaining treatment (Figure 3.16A). Randomisation occurs *within* the litter, and this ensures that the litters and treatment conditions are balanced, such that both the placebo and the drug are applied once to animals from each litter. The offspring are the EUs, BUs, and OUs, and so the analysis is straightforward. This is a randomised block design once again (compare with Figure 3.8 and 3.14) and has the advantage that the variation between families is irrelevant because the comparison is done within each family.

The second method keeps offspring from the same family together during randomisation so that offspring from the same family receive the same treatment (Figure 3.16B). The treatment however is applied *individually* to each offspring. Compare this example with Figure 3.9, where the offspring were also randomised together, but the treatment was applied to all offspring in a family *at the same time* (since the treatment was applied to the pregnant females). In both examples offspring from the same family are randomised together, but differ in whether the treatment is applied simultaneously to all offspring in a family or to each offspring individually. Determining the EU in the present case is more ambiguous, but the offspring can be considered the EU because there is replication of the experimental intervention to a biological entity. When the treatment is applied once to all offspring, the treatment errors will tend to be correlated (treatment errors are discussed in Section 2.2), while they will be uncorrelated when treatment is applied to the offspring individually.

In Figure 3.16A the variables family and treatment are said to be *crossed*, while in Figure 3.16B family is *nested* under treatment. Crossed and nested factors are discussed in Section 2.7. Crossing is preferable to nesting, and so the first method of randomisation

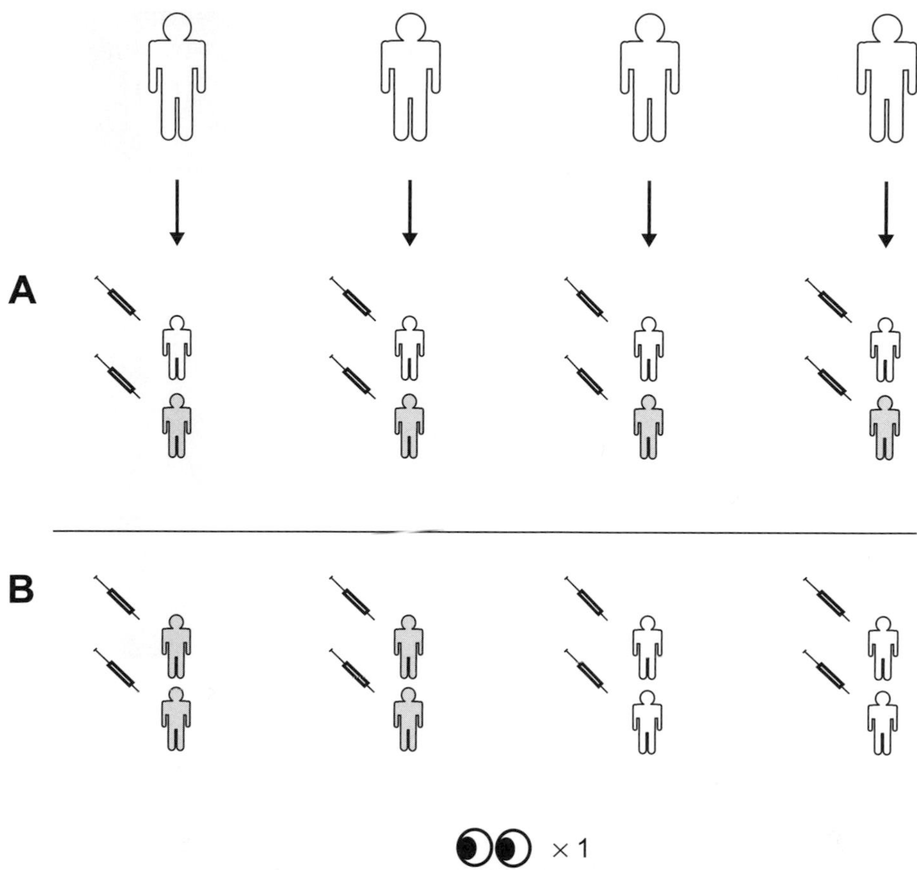

Fig. 3.16 Four adults each have two offspring. In (A), one offspring from each adult is (randomly) injected with either a drug or placebo, and one measurement is taken per offspring (randomisation occurs *within* families). In (B), offspring from the same family are (randomly) injected with either a drug or placebo, and one measurement is taken per offspring (randomisation occurs *by* family). The first method of randomisation is preferred. BU = offspring (8); EU = offspring (8); OU = offspring (8); total number of values = 8.

should be used if possible.[7] If crossing is not possible, then it is necessary to include multiple families in the nested experiment, and also include family as a variable in the analysis. Otherwise, we have the situation shown in Figure 3.15, where it is impossible to distinguish treatment effects from variation between two units higher in the biological hierarchy. In Figure 3.15, the people were treated as the EUs and the aliquots (analogous to the offspring in this example) were treated as subsamples. In the current example, however, the smaller units are treated as the EUs, and the difference relates to the hypothesis that we are interested in testing. In Figure 3.15, the hypothesis related to the effect of the drug on people, while in the current example the interest is in the effect on the offspring. The

[7] Briefly, the test for a treatment effect is more powerful with a crossed design.

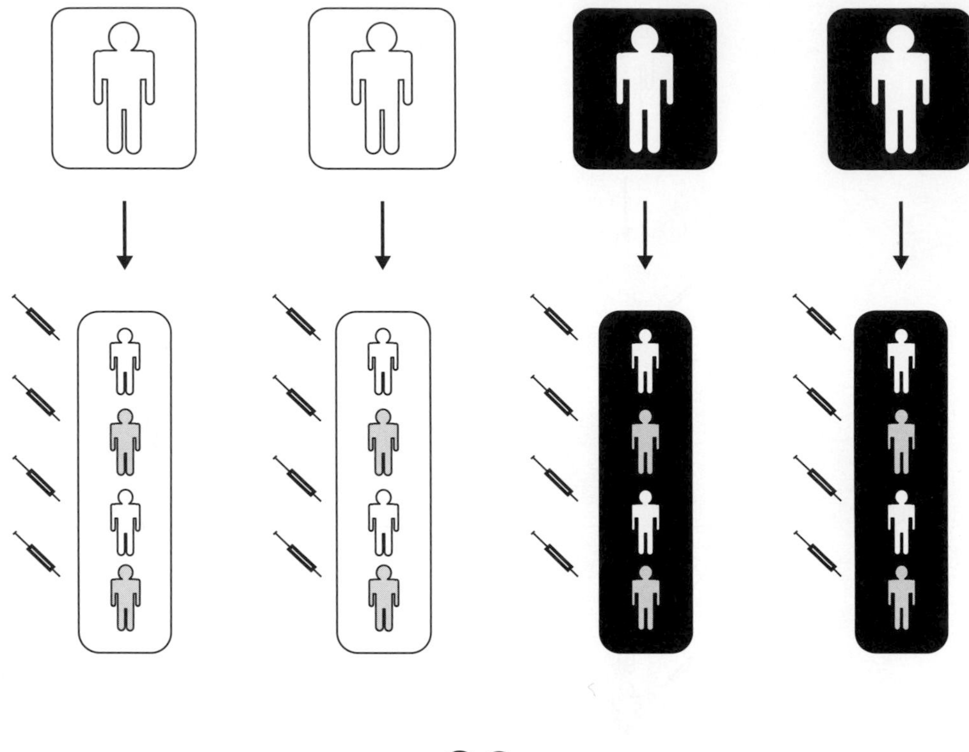

Fig. 3.17 Four pregnant females are (randomly) assigned to live in one of two housing conditions (light and dark boxes) and each have four offspring. The offspring are (randomly) injected with either a drug or placebo, and one measurement is taken per offspring. When testing for the effect of parental environment on offspring: BU = offspring (16); EU = pregnant female or litter (4); OU = offspring (16). When testing for the effect of the drug: BU = offspring (16); EU = offspring (16); OU = offspring (16); total number of values = 16.

randomisation in Figure 3.16B muddies the conceptual waters and should be avoided if possible.

There is also a third method of randomisation where the familial structure is ignored and the eight offspring are randomised to the drug or placebo conditions (not shown in the figure). If there are no family effects on the outcome variables, then this method is suitable. If the outcome differs between families, however, then this method can lead to an imbalance between family and treatment condition, making inferences more difficult.

3.4.3 Randomisation at multiple levels

The example shown in Figure 3.17 is more complex because there are two experimental interventions at different levels in the hierarchy and therefore two types of experimental unit. The four large people are pregnant females and they are randomly assigned to one of

Box 3.2 Key points about replication

1. Determine what the experimental and observational units are, and note how they relate to the biological unit of interest.
2. Replicate the EU to increase *N*.
3. If there are multiple OUs for each EU, or if multiple measurements are taken on each EU, then this must be accounted for in the analysis (e.g. average values for each EU or use a hierarchical model).
4. Does replication of the EU address a scientifically relevant question; can the results be generalised to something of interest? If not, replicate at a higher level (e.g. replicate the entire experimental procedure multiple times in a cell culture experiment).
5. When reporting results, make it clear what the EU is, the number of EUs, whether the OU was different, and how multiple measurements or subsamples were handled.

two conditions, indicated by the light and dark boxes. In this example, the females could be rats and the boxes could be housing environments. There is genuine replication of the treatment (housing environment) so testing for group differences is possible. The offspring from these females are housed with their mother and are randomly assigned to receive either a drug or vehicle injection. One measurement is taken on each of the 16 offspring. Assume that the interest is in the effect of two experimental variables on the offspring, which are the biological units of interest. The first experimental units are the adult females, which were randomly assigned to the housing conditions. There are four EUs for testing the effect of housing. The second type of EU is the offspring, which were randomly assigned (within females) to receive the drug or vehicle injection, and $N = 16$ when testing for a drug effect. A design with two (or more) types of EU is called a *split-unit* or *split-plot* design.

A split-unit design can be thought of as two experiments in one. The first experiment is testing the effects of housing using four groups of animals. Each female and her offspring are randomised together and so constitute four independent replications of the treatment to the sample material. The offspring are considered subsamples when testing for housing effects and this part of the experiment resembles the design in Figure 3.9. The second experiment is testing the effect of the drug and resembles the design in Figure 3.14, where randomisation occurred within blocks. Here, the four offspring belonging to the same family are a block. This split-unit design can be considered a completely randomised design at the level of pregnant females and randomised block design at the level of animals within females.

The above examples should cover most situations in experimental biology (summarised in Table 3.2), but given the complexity of biological experiments there will be cases where one has to think about how the underlying principles apply. In most situations the BU, EU, and OU are clearly defined, although reasonable opinion may differ in some circumstances. Box 3.2 summarises the points about replication to consider when designing an experiment.

Table 3.2 Summary of examples. The final column indicates the page number where the example is analysed with R. CRD = completely randomised design; RBD = randomised block design; SU = split-unit; ANOVA = analysis of variance; IS = independent samples; PS = paired samples, RM = repeated measures.

Figure	BU	EU	OU	Comments	Design name	Test	R-code
3.4	Individual	Individual	Aliquot	Bad design	–	–	–
3.5	Individual	Individual	Aliquot	Bad design	–	–	–
3.6	Individual	Time point	Aliquot	Bad design	–	–	–
3.7	Individual	Time point	Aliquot	Valid design	CRD	IS *t*-test	p. 144
3.8	Individual/eyes	Eyes	Aliquot	Valid design	RBD	PS *t*-test	p. 171
3.9	Offspring	Pregnant dam	Offspring	Bad design	–	–	–
3.10	Individual	Individual	Individual	Valid design	RM-ANOVA	RM-ANOVA	p. 181
3.11	Individual	Aliquot	Aliquot	Valid design	CRD	IS *t*-test	p. 144
3.12	Individual/Day	Aliquot	Aliquot	Valid design	RBD	PS *t*-test	p. 171
3.13	Individual	Aliquot (small)	Aliquot (pooled)	Bad design	–	–	–
3.14	Individual	Aliquot	Aliquot	Valid design	RBD	PS *t*-test	p. 171
3.15	Individual	Individual	Aliquot	Bad design	–	–	–
3.16A	Offspring	Offspring	Offspring	A is better	RBD	PS *t*-test	p. 171
3.17	Offspring	Pregnant dam	Offspring	Effect of housing	SU (CRD)	SU ANOVA	p. 175
		Offspring	Offspring	Effect of drug	SU (RBD)	SU ANOVA	p. 175

3.5 How is the experimental unit defined in other disciplines?

When authors in other disciplines define the EU, they expect a certain amount of shared knowledge about the data or the experiment from their readers, which can mislead an unwary reader from another discipline. We discuss how the experimental unit is defined in other fields and how those experiments parallel the designs in this chapter because it can provide further insights.

In agricultural experiments, the EU is a piece of land – called a plot – and it contains many plants. Each plot of land is randomised to treatment groups or factor-level combinations, such as with and without fertiliser. These experiments often use blocking to account for spatial variations in soil quality or drainage. The outcome is often the total yield of the crop from each plot, and the contribution of individual plants is not measured. The scientific unit of interest is the plot because a farmer wants to know what happens to the yield when he takes a piece of land and does X versus doing not-X, which requires multiple plots of land. How the individual plants react is irrelevant. The plants in different plots are analogous to cells in different wells in a microtitre plate. In both cases, the plants and cells are randomised together to the treatment conditions, the treatment is applied in a common way, and it is likely that adjacent plants and cells influence each other. The difference is that a cell biologist may be interested in the cell-level data, but even so, the hypothesis must be tested at the well level.

Some clinical trials randomise whole hospitals or clinics to treatment conditions and all patients within a hospital receive the same treatment. For example, patients in hospitals A, B, and C are the controls while patients in hospitals D, E, and F are in the treated condition. These experiments are called *cluster-randomised trials*, where the hospital or clinic represents a cluster of patients that are randomised together. Cluster-randomised trials are used when it is hard or undesirable to assign patients to treatment conditions; for example, if the treatment is a novel surgical intervention and only some hospitals have the facilities to perform the new surgery. It is better if all hospitals have both control and treated patients – that is, if hospital and treatment are crossed – and randomising clusters of patients is a less preferred but sometimes necessary design. In the analysis of cluster-randomised trials the experimental unit is sometimes the patient, especially when the treatment is applied directly to the patient (for example a drug), and when the interest is in drawing a conclusion about patients. This is one of the few fields where a less appropriate analysis is conducted because it is hard or impossible to get enough hospitals to have reasonable power. As you might expect, there is some debate about the appropriate unit of analysis for these studies [99].[8] All agree that the cluster variable should be included in the analysis, and that increasing the number of clusters instead of the number of patients per cluster is beneficial.

If, however, the treatment is applied to all patients simultaneously or in a common way, such as group therapy by a psychologist in each hospital, then the hospital is the appropriate experimental unit. Similarly, if the intervention is not applied to patients but to the doctor

[8] There is a nice series of short articles on cluster-randomised trials in the 'Statistics Notes' section of the *British Medical Journal* [9, 46, 47, 186–188].

or the clinic, such as introducing a new procedure to be followed, then the EU is the cluster and not patients, even if the outcome is recorded on the patients.

In many educational studies new teaching methods can only be applied to whole classes. Thus the classes are randomised to treatment conditions, treatments are applied in a common way to all students in a class, and it is likely that students affect each other. For example, a single disruptive student may hinder learning for the whole class. For these reasons the classes and not the students are the EUs [180].

In manufacturing experiments, there may be no scientific units of interest at the start of the experiment that are randomised to different conditions as we have been doing. Instead, raw materials are combined to produce the units of interest and therefore the focus is on the independent production of EUs. Experimental manipulations can occur either at the level of the raw materials or at a later part of the manufacturing process. For example, if we are baking a cake, we could vary the ingredients, such as the amount of water (low versus high) and sugar (low versus high) added. The EUs are the independently prepared cake mixes. It would be inappropriate to make one cake mix at each combination of water and sugar content, divide these into smaller portions and consider the portions as the EUs. The portions are just subsamples. However, even if we have a single cake mix prepared, we can divide it into several portions and randomly assign each portion to be baked at one of two temperatures. Because we are randomising the portions to different treatment conditions, the portions *might* be considered the EUs. But if there are only two ovens, and all of the portions are baked at the same time, the process of baking is like applying a treatment in a common way to all the EUs. There might be differences between the ovens other than the temperature setting, and so the portions should not be considered EUs; there is no way of separating the effect of temperature from any other differences between the ovens. If there are several ovens and one portion is placed in each, then the portions can be considered the EUs. A valid experiment can still be conducted if there are only two ovens, and the solution is to repeat the experiment several times (possibly on different days) by making a new cake mix from scratch, dividing into two portions, and randomly assigning the portions to the ovens. This is a randomised block design where the blocks are days, that is, independent preparations of the cake mix followed by the baking procedure. This last example is analogous to repeating a cell culture experiment several times on different days. The entire procedure is repeated and the size of the treatment effect is compared against the variability of the effect from each experimental run (day).

4 Analysis of Common Designs

The first principle is that you must not fool yourself, and you are the easiest person to fool.

Richard Feynman

. . . the function of significance tests is to prevent you from making a fool of yourself, and not to make unpublishable results publishable.

David Colquhoun, FRS

This chapter discusses how to analyse common experimental designs. The focus is on correctly specifying the model so that it reflects the design and interpreting the output. Data analysis is a large topic and three decisions were made to keep this chapter concise. First, 'nicely behaved' data sets are used where the following are known to be true:

1. The outcome variable is normally distributed.
2. The variances are equal across groups.
3. The errors are independent.
4. There are no outliers.
5. There are no missing data.
6. The designs are balanced (equal number of samples in each group).

The first three points are the usual assumptions for standard statistical tests. The fourth and fifth points ensure that we do not have to consider unusual features of the data. The final point is relevant for designs with multiple factors. When the groups are unbalanced, the factors become correlated with each other, and the results (p-values) become sensitive to choices about how the model is defined.

The second decision was to only describe designs that are frequently used in experimental biology. Thus, fractional factorial, incomplete block, Latin square, and other designs that are commonly covered in books on experimental design are not discussed.

The third decision was to limit the discussion to ANOVA-type models and output. There are two traditions in frequentist data analysis. The first is the ANOVA tradition, which started in agronomy and spread to other experimental disciplines. It focuses on partitioning sources of variation, counting degrees of freedom, and ensuring that F-statistics and p-values are calculated with the correct error term. This is what we discuss in this chapter. The second is the regression tradition, which is more often associated with observational studies and focuses on estimating parameters, effects sizes, and confidence intervals. The two approaches are mathematically identical for the designs that we discuss; they differ only in how the output from an analysis is presented [76]. We will mostly use ANOVA methodology because of its close association with the experimental sciences and because it forces one to think more about the relationship between the experimental design and the analysis.

The R code is integrated throughout the chapter and most of the discussion is relevant even if you are not using R as the output resembles other statistical packages.

4.1 Preliminary concepts

Before discussing the designs, three preliminary concepts are reviewed. The first is *sum of squares (SS)* – what it is and how to calculate and partition it. This relates to a question often asked by students when introduced to analysis of variance: 'Why are we analysing variance when I am interested in the difference between group means?' The second concept is *degrees of freedom* and using them to check if a model is correctly specified. The final concept is how *multiple comparisons* lead to more false positives and methods for controlling the overall error rate.

4.1.1 Partitioning the sum of squares

Partitioning the sum of squares is central to the analysis of variance. Variation in the outcome variable is the result of:

1. treatment effects,
2. biological effects,
3. technical effects, and
4. various types of errors.

The aim is to partition the total variation in the outcome (which equals 100%) and attribute it to the three types of effects. Then, whatever variation remains is attributed to error. For example, suppose 20% of the variation in the outcome is due to the effect of the treatment, 30% is due to differences between sexes, and 15% is due to the day the experiment was run, which leaves $100 - 20 - 30 - 15 = 35\%$ of the total variation unexplained and thus attributed to the error term. The treatment is said to 'explain' or 'account for' 20% of the variance in the outcome. The data below will make the idea concrete. This example is a two group experiment with four observations per group. y is the outcome variable and x is the grouping factor with levels A and B.

```
> y <- c(6, 2, 3, 1, 4, 8, 7, 9)
> x <- factor(rep(c("A", "B"), each=4))
> data.frame(y, x)
  y x
1 6 A
2 2 A
```

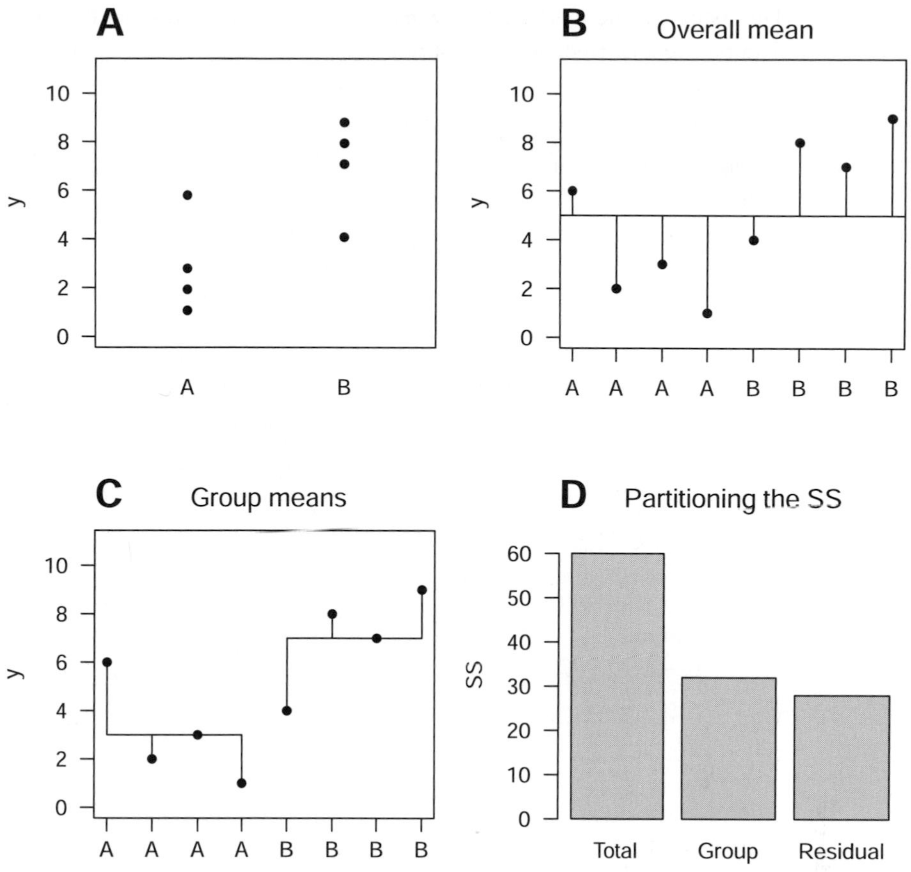

Fig. 4.1 Partitioning the sum of squares (SS). A data set with two groups (A). The total sum of squares is equal to the squared lengths of the vertical lines in (B). The squared lengths can also be calculated from the group means, and this represents the variation remaining in the data after taking the experimental groups into account (C). Panel (D) shows how the total SS is partitioned into the part attributed to Group and to the residuals.

```
3 3 A
4 1 A
5 4 B
6 8 B
7 7 B
8 9 B
```

The data are plotted in Figure 4.1A and the question is whether the means of the groups are different. In Figure 4.1B, the data points are spread out along the x-axis for a clearer visualisation and the horizontal line is the overall mean of the data. The vertical lines represent the distance from each point to the overall mean, and the sum of squares is calculated by taking the length of each vertical line, squaring it, and then adding them all together.

This is called the *total sum of squares* (TSS) and it represents the total variability in the data before any predictor variables are included. The TSS is equal to 60 and is calculated in the R code below.

```
> mean.y <- mean(y)
> tss <- sum((y - mean.y)^2)
> tss
[1] 60
```

The distances are squared because the sum of the unsquared distances always equals zero, since the lengths of the vertical lines below the mean exactly balance the lengths of the vertical lines above the mean. The R code below shows that when each value of y is subtracted by `mean.y`, some differences will be negative and some positive, and they perfectly balance such that they sum to zero. This can be checked by not squaring the values before summing them.

```
> # mean differences are positive and negative
> y - mean.y
[1]  1 -3 -2 -4 -1  3  2  4
>
> # sum without squaring equals zero
> sum(y - mean.y)
[1] 0
>
> # squaring the deviations makes them positive
> (y - mean.y)^2
[1]  1  9  4 16  1  9  4 16
```

Squaring a negative number makes it positive, and so the sum of all of the squared values will be greater than zero.[1] The total sum of squares is therefore a measure of how far the data are spread around the overall mean; if the data are far from the mean, then the vertical lines in Figure 4.1B (and their squares) will be larger. You may recall that the standard deviation and variance also measure how far data are spread around a mean. What is the connection with the TSS? The TSS is the numerator of the equation for the standard deviation and variance. Dividing the TSS by $n - 1$ gives the variance, and taking the square root of the variance is the standard deviation.

In addition to the total sum of squares, the sum of squared distances from the *group means* can also be calculated (Figure 4.1C). This value is known as the *residual sum of*

[1] A question often asked is why the absolute values of the differences are not used, which removes the minus signs? The main reason is that it is easier to differentiate equations with a square (remember the chain rule from secondary school calculus!) than when an absolute operator is used – an important consideration in the pre-computer era when these methods were developed. Methods that use absolute values exist, but are not discussed here.

squares (RSS) because it represents the variability remaining after the predictor variable (Group) has been included; it is the leftover or residual variability. The code below calculates the mean for Group A and Group B, uses these to calculate the RSS for each group separately, and then combines the values to get the overall RSS.

```
> mean.A <- mean(y[1:4])
> mean.A
[1] 3
>
> mean.B <- mean(y[5:8])
> mean.B
[1] 7
>
> # Residual SS
> rss.A <- sum((y[1:4] - mean.A)^2)
> rss.B <- sum((y[5:8] - mean.B)^2)
> rss <- rss.A + rss.B
> rss
[1] 28
```

The total and residual sum of squares can now be used to calculate the *reduction* in variability due to the predictor variable (Group) by subtracting the total SS from the residual SS. This represents the variability in the outcome that is attributed to the predictor variable.

```
> # SS due to Group
> ssx <- tss - rss
> ssx
[1] 32
```

If the above terms are rearranged, the following relationship holds: `tss = ssx+rss`. In other words, the total SS is the sum of the SS due to the predictor plus the residual SS. More generally, Eq. (4.1) shows the relationship between the total SS, one or more predictors, and the residual SS. The form of the equation is identical to the fundamental experimental design equation (Eq. (2.1), p. 53). The total variation in the outcome is the sum of the treatment, biological, and technical factors (predictors), plus the error or residual term:

$$\text{Total} = \text{Predictor(s)} + \text{Residual}. \tag{4.1}$$

The values of sums of squares cannot be directly interpreted as being large or small, and so the proportion or percentage of the TSS that a predictor variable accounts for determines the importance of the predictor. In this example, Group accounts for just over half of the total variation in the outcome and appears to be an important predictor. Partitioning the TSS into the part attributed to Group and the residual can be seen in Figure 4.1D. The heights of the bars labelled Group and Residual sum to the height of the first bar. The question now arises: did Group account for a significant proportion of variation in the outcome, or was this reduction due to chance? Predictor variables will always account for some variation in the outcome, even if it is only noise, and we need to test if the variation accounted for is larger than expected by chance.

Partitioning the SS with multiple predictor variables

The previous example had only one predictor variable but many experiments have multiple predictors, which makes partitioning the SS complicated when the cross-tabulated predictors have an unequal number of samples, such as the following layout where 20 samples are unequally distributed across the four cells instead of having five in each cell.

	Factor 1	
Factor 2	3	7
	7	3

Such a design is said to be *unbalanced* and the predictors are correlated with each other or *nonorthogonal*.[2] This is a problem because the sum of squares can be partitioned in several ways, leading to different conclusions about the importance of the predictors.[3] The results can vary dramatically depending on the degree of imbalance and method of partitioning. This has generated some confusion and anxiety, but many are unaware of this issue and use

the default settings of their statistical software.

The following discussion only applies when there are two or more predictor variables and when they are correlated. In balanced designs, the variance of the outcome can be uniquely attributed to each predictor variable, meaning that there is only one way to partition the sum of squares, making the interpretation of the results straightforward. For nonorthogonal designs the order that the predictor variables are entered into the statistical model is important for determining the order in which effects are tested.

Figure 4.2 illustrates these points. The boxes represent the total variation in the outcome (total sum of squares). The three circles represent the main effect of factor A, the main effect of factor B, and the AB interaction. The area of the circles represents the proportion of variance in the outcome accounted for, denoted by the lower-case letters inside the circles. The area outside of the circles but inside the box is the variation in the outcome that is not accounted for by any of the factors and represents the residual sum of squares. The diagram on the left in Figure 4.2 shows the case where A and B are uncorrelated. This situation is advantageous because the total sum of squares is equal to the area of the circles plus the residual sum of squares (TSS $= a + b + c +$ RSS). Also, calculating the proportion of total variance that each factor accounts for is simple, it is the area of the circle divided by the area of the box.

[2] The terms correlated and nonorthogonal (and uncorrelated and orthogonal) are used interchangeably, but they have slightly different meanings [328].

[3] These difficulties do not arise if cell frequencies are proportional to the marginal frequencies (row and column totals), even if there is an imbalance. Such cases will not be considered here.

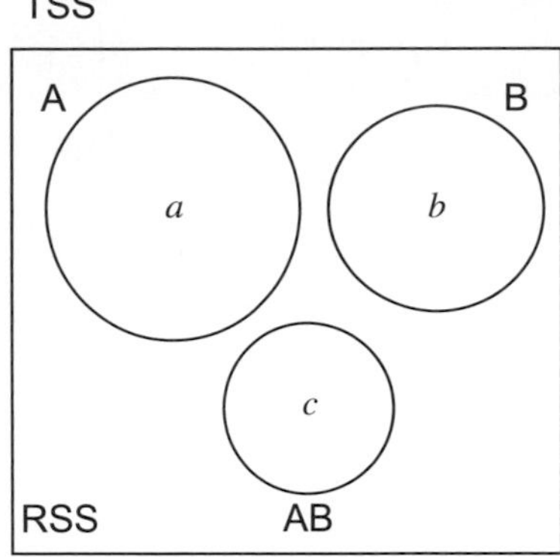

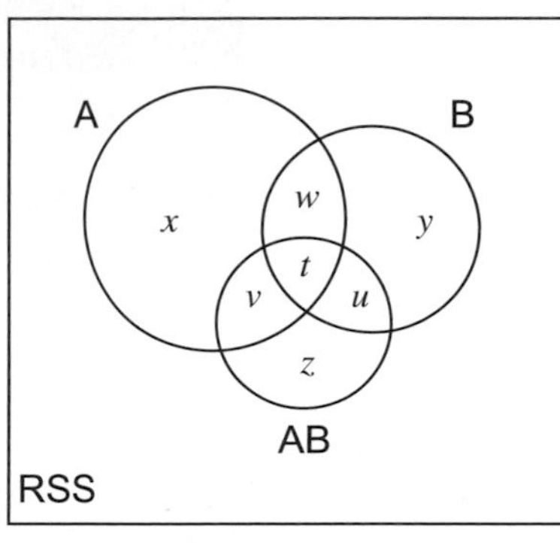

Fig. 4.2 Partitioning the sum of squares with two factors. In the left diagram A and B are orthogonal and in the other diagram they are correlated and thus account for overlapping variance.

Things get complicated, however, when the predictor variables are correlated (Figure 4.2, right diagram). The correlation means that the proportion of variance that the factors account for is not unique, denoted by the overlapping circles. There are multiple ways to calculate the sum of squares and thus multiple ways to attribute the variation in the outcome to the predictors. This raises the question of which method is correct or better. Three methods for partitioning the SS will be described (called Type I, II, and III sum of squares) before we address this question. Table 4.1 summarises the discussion that follows and the basic points are:

Type I: Each predictor variable is tested in the order that it appears in the model and the test is for the additional variation that the predictor explains.

Type II: Each predictor is tested after removing the variation due to the other predictors. Order does not matter.

Type III: Each predictor is tested after removing the variation due to the other predictors, plus higher order interactions. Order does not matter.

The top half of Table 4.1 shows the results for uncorrelated predictors. The right hand side of the R model formulae are shown to indicate the order that the predictors appear in the model, and the interaction between A and B is indicated with a colon (:).

For orthogonal designs the order that the variables enter the model and the SS Type makes no difference for partitioning the sum of squares; for example, the proportion of variance accounted for by factor A is always a.

The bottom half of the table is more complicated. The sum of squares for the main effect of A and B, differs depending on the SS Type and the order that the variable appears in the model. For example, when factor A is entered first, the Type I SS calculates the proportion of variance that A accounts for as the sum of the areas x, w, t, and v, which corresponds to the area of circle a in the orthogonal design. The proportion of variance accounted for by B is then the sum of the areas of y and u – the key feature is that the areas in common to both

Table 4.1 Partitioning the sum of squares with orthogonal and nonorthogonal designs. The letters refer to the circle areas in Figure 4.2.

		SS Type		
R model syntax	**Predictors**	**I**	**II**	**III**
Orthogonal				
`~ A + B + A:B`				
	A	a	a	a
	B	b	b	b
	AB	c	c	c
`~ B + A + B:A`				
	B	b	b	b
	A	a	a	a
	BA	c	c	c
Nonorthogonal				
`~ A + B + A:B`				
	A	$x+w+t+v$	$x+v$	x
	B	$y+u$	$y+u$	y
	AB	z	z	z
`~ B + A + B:A`				
	B	$y+w+t+u$	$y+u$	y
	A	$x+v$	$x+v$	x
	BA	z	z	z

factor A and B (w and t) are not included. So the test for factor B is based on the *unique* variance that has not already been accounted for by factor A. Similarly, the proportion of variation accounted for by the interaction is equal to z, which excludes regions v, t, and u. The interaction therefore only includes variation that has not been accounted for by either factor A or B. Type I SS is also called a *sequential* sum of squares because the predictor variables are tested one at a time in the order in which they appear in the model, and tests are for the additional variance accounted for by each variable, after removing the variance accounted for by the previous variables. The same is true with the second nonorthogonal model, where B is entered first. The effect of B is the sum of regions y, w, t, and u (corresponding to the area of b in the orthogonal design), the effect of A is then the sum of x and v, and the interaction once again is the area of z.

With Type II SS (also known as a *hierarchical* SS), each main effect is tested after removing the variance accounted for by the other main effects. So when testing for the effect of A, only regions x and v are used, and the regions shared with B (w, t) are excluded. Similarly, when testing for the effect of B, only regions y and u are used and the regions shared with A (w, t) are excluded. The interaction once again accounts for only the variance in the outcome that has not been accounted for by either A or B. With Type II SS the order that the factors were entered into the model does not matter.

A Type III SS (also known as a *marginal* or *unique* SS) resembles a Type II in that when testing for the effect of A, the variance accounted for by B (w, t) is first removed. But in addition, the variance accounted for by the interaction effect (v) is also removed, leaving only region x to represent the proportion of variance accounted for by A. Similarly, when testing for the effect of B, the variance accounted for by A (w, t) and the interaction is first removed (v), leaving the region y. Finally, the interaction accounts for only the variance in the outcome that has not been accounted for by either A or B (z), which again is the same as the Type I and Type II SS.

The area of regions w and t in Figure 4.2 will be large if the two predictor variables are highly correlated. It could happen that each predictor is highly significant when tested on its own, but when both are included in the model, the p-values for both are large with a Type II or III SS. Although both predictors account for a large proportion of the variance in the outcome, they mostly account for the *same* variance. Thus for Type II and III SS only the (small) unique variance of each variable is tested (regions x and y). With a Type I SS, the predictor entered first will have a small p-value while the other predictor will have a large p-value, and the interpretation of variable importance will depend on the arbitrary ordering of the variables.

There are several points to consider. First, the test for the interaction is always the same regardless of SS type and order of predictor entry. Second, the order of variables is not important for Type II and III SS because each main effect is adjusted for the other main effects. Third, if the interaction is not included in the model, then Type II and III methods will give the same results for the main effects of A and B because the only difference between Type II and III SS is whether the effect of the interaction is removed before testing main effects. Finally, the same principles apply when there are more than two predictor variables, but are harder to represent with Venn diagrams. For example, if there was a third variable, C, then the full model could be written as

```
> outcome ~ A + B + C + A:B + A:C + B:C + A:B:C
```

A Type I SS tests each term from left to right to see if it explains additional variance not accounted for by the previous terms. A Type II SS tests for the variance accounted for by A that is not also accounted for by B or C. A Type III SS further removes the effect accounted for by A:B and A:B:C when testing for the effect of A.

Which type of SS should be used? It makes no difference if the predictor variables are orthogonal or if the scientific interest is only in the interaction, as all methods give the same result. Type I SS is rarely used, partly because it ignores the other factors in the model, thereby not making full use of a design with multiple factors. The main choice is between Type II and III. Type II is more powerful, especially when there is no interaction. It can be seen in Figure 4.2 that the variance accounted for by factor A is the area of regions x and v for a Type II SS, and is larger than x on its own, which is what a Type III SS uses. However, if there is an interaction, then the interpretation of the main effect is difficult regardless of the SS type. There is no agreement on the Type II versus III debate and recent discussions can be found in the following references [150, 211].

The above discussion might have made ANOVAs seem more complex than your first introduction to them. Introductory statistics books and courses often only consider balanced designs. The examples that follow also use balanced designs but you should be aware of issues surrounding unbalanced designs. These points are not specific to R and are the result of having multiple ways to partition the sum of squares when predictor variables are correlated. *The lesson here is that in designed experiments the correlation of the predictor variables is largely under control of the experimenter and by planning an experiment with an equal number of samples in each cell, none of these difficulties arise*. Missing values may occur, disrupting a carefully planned design, but this will induce only a small correlation between the predictors. The higher the correlations, the more the results (i.e. *p*-values) will differ depending on the options chosen.

A final point is about the default settings that R uses. For models fit using `aov()` the `summary()` and `anova()` functions use Type I SS. To obtain Type II and III SS, the `Anova()` function (note the capital ‘A’) from the `car` package can be used.

```
> model <- aov(outcome ~ A*B) # example model
> summary(model) # Type I
> anova(model) # Type I
> car::Anova(model) # Type II
> car::Anova(model, type="III") # Type III
```

4.1.2 Counting degrees of freedom

The concept of degrees of freedom (df) is important but somewhat abstract and Drăghci [101, pp. 231–240] gives an excellent explanation, which is loosely followed here. Df are determined from the sample size and must be calculated correctly to obtain a valid *p*-value. In a real analysis, we do not calculate the df, the statistical software does this, but the model needs to be specified correctly. However, calculating df ‘by hand’ enables us to check that the results of an analysis make sense.

There are several equivalent ways of describing degrees of freedom. The first is *the number of items in a system that are free to vary given a set of constraints*, and in statistics it is *the number of observations that are free to vary*. For example, suppose a rat’s weight is measured three times. The values are 270, 269, and 271 g, with a mean value of 270 g. Calculating a mean is a constraint because three numbers can no longer take any value; once the first two numbers have been defined, the final number can only be one value so that the mean of the three is equal to the calculated value. For example, in the equation $(270 + 269 + x)/3 = 270$, x can only be equal to 271. Therefore the number of df is $3 - 1 = 2$. More generally, if n is the number of observations and c is the number of constraints, then $df = n - c$. Admittedly, this common definition provides no insight about why degrees of freedom are important or what has been gained by determining that there are two of them.

A second definition is that df are *the number of additional measurements beyond what is strictly required to estimate a quantity of interest*. If the interest is the body weight of

Box 4.1 Calculating degrees of freedom in statistical models

- The total df is always the number of experimental units (N) minus one.
- For a categorical predictor with t levels df $= t - 1$.
- For a continuous predictor (with only a linear term included) df $= 1$.
- For interactions multiply the dfs of the respective predictors. For example, the interaction of a categorical and continuous predictor is df $= (t - 1) \times 1$.
- The residual or error df is the total df minus all other dfs.

a single rat, only one measurement is required. Since three measurements were taken in this example, the extra two measurements correspond to two degrees of freedom. More generally, if n is the number of observations and c is the minimum number of *required* observations, then df $= n - c$, the same as the first definition.

A third definition is that df are *the number of independent values available to estimate error*. If only one measurement is taken, there is no way to estimate the uncertainty in that measurement. If two measurements are taken, then the first can be thought of as estimating the body weight while the second can be thought of as estimating the error in the first measurement. Similarly, a third measurement is another estimate of the error, and so on for further measurements. In practice, the average of the three measurements are used as the estimate of body weight, but as we saw in the first definition, once the mean of the three measurements is calculated, only two of the values are free to vary and the third is completely determined. Thus, even though there are three measurements, there are only two independent estimates of error. This also fits with the second definition: if only one measurement is required to estimate the quantity of interest, then the other two measurements are available to estimate the error. This definition is especially relevant for estimating the correct error term in statistical models and why we bother to calculate them.

A fourth definition is that df are *the number of observations minus the number of parameters*, where a parameter is a value estimated from the data such as the mean of a group or the slope of a line. If the mean body weight of the rat is the only parameter estimated, and three measurements are taken, then df $= 3 - 1$, consistent with the other calculations.

In a statistical analysis the total df is equal to the sample size minus one ($N - 1$), and with every parameter estimated, a df is subtracted from the total. By examining the df from the output of an analysis we can determine whether the model is correctly specified. The key thing to look for is that *the residual df can never be greater than the number of experimental units*.[4] Box 4.1 shows the rules for calculating the degrees of freedom.

Now that df have been defined, let us return to the data shown in Figure 4.1 and calculate the dfs. Equation (4.2) shows the relationship between the total df, residual df, and the df for one or more predictor variables. This equation is identical to Eq. (4.1) when we were discussing the sum of squares. Not only does the total SS equal the sum of the predictor

[4] Some statistical software refer to the residual df as the *error* df.

and residual SS, but so does the total df:

$$\text{Total df} = \text{Predictor(s) df} + \text{Residual df.} \tag{4.2}$$

For the data in Figure 4.1, there are eight samples and thus the total df equals $8 - 1 = 7$ (Box 4.1). The Group factor has two levels (A and B), and the df for this predictor is the number of levels minus one ($2 - 1 = 1$). Substituting these values into Eq. (4.2) gives:

$$8 - 1 = (2 - 1) + \text{Residual} \tag{4.3}$$
$$6 = \text{Residual.}$$

Thus, the residual df is six. It is useful to compare the values we calculated above with the results of an ANOVA. The code below uses the aov() function and then the results are displayed as an ANOVA table using the summary() function.

```
> simple.mod <- aov(y ~ x)
> summary(simple.mod)
            Df Sum Sq Mean Sq F value Pr(>F)
x            1     32    32.0    6.86   0.04
Residuals    6     28     4.7
```

The column called Sum Sq shows the sum of squares. The values of 32 for x and 28 for the residuals corresponds to our earlier calculations. The df are also the same as we just calculated.

The Mean Sq column displays the *mean squares* (MS), which are calculated by dividing the SS by the df in the same row. Thus, for the residuals we have $28/6 = 4.7$. The MS is an intermediate value used to calculate the F-statistic, shown as F value in the next column of the above output. To calculate the F-statistic, divide the MS for a predictor variable by the residual MS, which is equal to $32/4.7 = 6.86$. A large F-statistic indicates that a large proportion of the variation in the outcome is attributed to the predictor variable. In other words, a large F-statistic suggests that the null hypothesis of no treatment effect is false. The F-statistic, treatment df, and residual df are used to calculate the p-value, which is equal to 0.04. In the past one would refer to a table in the back of a statistics book to obtain the p-value, but we can calculate it 'by hand' using the pf() function. The arguments are the F-statistic, the df for the treatment factor (df1), and residual df (df2). The pf() function calculates the area under a part of a curve and we need to include the lower.tail = FALSE argument to indicate that the area in the upper tail needs to be calculated.

```
> pf(6.86, df1=1, df=6,  lower.tail = FALSE)
[1] 0.0396308
```

The p-value is the same as calculated with the aov() function (rounded to two decimal places). Calculating p-values by hand, given F-statistics and dfs, is useful for checking results reported in publications.

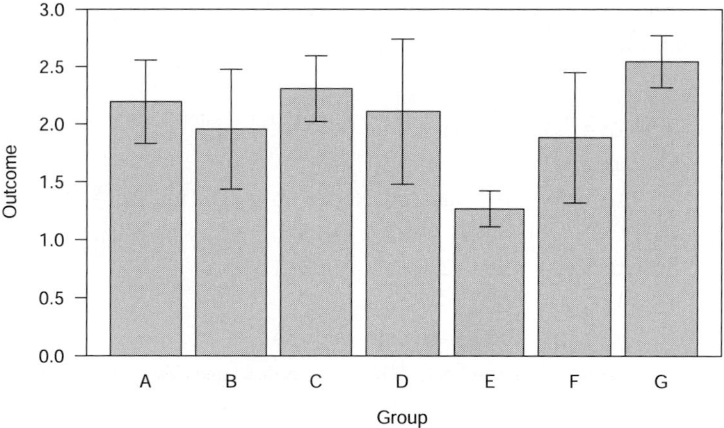

Fig. 4.3 A randomly generated outcome variable with equal means across the seven groups.

4.1.3 Multiple comparisons

Recall from Chapter 1 (Section 1.4) that a *p*-value is the probability of obtaining more extreme results, given that no effect exists. α is the probability of incorrectly claiming that an effect is there when none exists, that is, a false positive. α is set by the researcher and should not be confused with a *p*-value, which is calculated from the data. Setting $\alpha = 0.05$ means that if there is no effect, 1 in 20 tests will incorrectly produce a significant result. α is the *per-comparison* error rate, which applies to a single comparison. When multiple hypotheses are tested, the probability that *at least one* of the comparisons will be a false positive is greater than α. To illustrate this point the data in Figure 4.3 were randomly generated with the same mean and variance for each of the seven groups.

```
> set.seed(123)
> y.rand <- rnorm(7*5, 2) # 7 groups with 5 samples each
> g <- gl(7, 5, labels=LETTERS[1:7]) # grouping variable
>
> library(sciplot)
> par(las=1)
> bargraph.CI(g, y.rand, xlab="Group", ylab="Outcome",
+             ylim=c(0,3))
> box()
```

An overall ANOVA is not significant ($p = 0.51$), but the difference between Group E and G catches our eye and so is compared with a *t*-test. The *p*-value is small (0.002) and it seems reasonable to believe that the difference between the groups is real. One might argue that only one statistical test was done (excluding the overall ANOVA) and so there is no issue with multiple comparisons.

```
> # overall anova
> summary(aov(y.rand ~ g))
            Df Sum Sq Mean Sq F value Pr(>F)
g            6   4.92   0.820     0.9   0.51
Residuals   28  25.52   0.911
>
> # t-test between two groups
> t.test(y.rand[g=="E"], y.rand[g=="G"], var.equal=TRUE)

Two Sample t-test

data:  y.rand[g == "E"] and y.rand[g == "G"]
t = -4.661, df = 8, p-value = 0.00162
alternative hypothesis: true difference in means is not equal to 0
95 percent confidence interval:
 -1.910910 -0.645876
sample estimates:
mean of x mean of y
  1.26685   2.54525
```

This line of thinking ignores that groups E and G were chosen *after* the data were examined and they happened to be the groups with the lowest and highest mean. If other groups had the lowest and highest mean, then they would have been chosen. Many tests are implicitly conducted, even though only one t-test was used. Comparing the two most extreme groups out of seven possibilities has a higher false positive rate than if only two groups are present. One approach to keep the number of false positives under control is to *predict* the two groups that will be different *before seeing the data*. This is called an *a priori* comparison but suffers from two problems. The first is that it depends on the honesty of the scientist – not necessarily honesty to the scientific community but honesty to oneself. This is what Feynman was referring to in his quote at the beginning of this chapter. After seeing that groups E and G are different it is too easy to fool oneself by thinking, 'Well, I didn't pick this comparison beforehand, but it makes perfect sense. I probably should have defined some *a priori* comparisons, and I if had, I would have picked this one, so everything is OK.' Unfortunately, *post hoc* rationalisations do not control the false positive rate. The second problem is that if many *a priori* tests are defined, the issue of multiplicity applies once again.

The second and more common approach to control false positives is to acknowledge that the per-comparison error rate is not useful when there are multiple comparisons and treat the set of comparisons as a family of tests. The error rate across the family of tests can then be controlled at or below some specified level. This new error rate is called the *familywise*

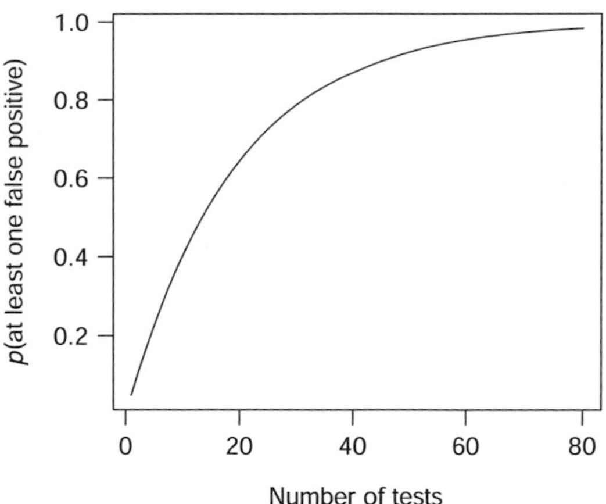

Fig. 4.4 Probability of at least one false positive result when the per-comparison error rate is 0.05.

error rate and will necessarily be more stringent than the per-comparison error rate. Some experiments may have several families of tests, and the error rate for all the tests can also be controlled, and is called the *experimentwise* error rate. The error rate for multiple tests that are independent of each other can be calculated with the following equation:

$$\begin{aligned} p(\text{at least one false positive}) &= 1 - p(\text{no false positives}) \\ &= 1 - (1 - \alpha)^m \\ &= 1 - (0.95)^m, \end{aligned} \tag{4.4}$$

where α is the per-comparison error rate, usually set at 0.05, and m is the number of tests that are conducted. When there is only one comparison, $m = 1$, and the probability of a false positive is 0.05. If two hypotheses are tested the error rate is $1 - 0.95^2 = 0.0975$, and if 10 hypotheses are tested, it is 0.40. Figure 4.4 shows how the probability of obtaining at least one false positive increases as the number of tests increases. Referring again to Figure 4.3, there are 21 pairwise comparisons that can be conducted with seven groups, and so the probability of at least one false positive is $1 - 0.95^{21} = 0.66$, which is much higher than the per-comparison error rate of 0.05.

Most biologists would agree that the number of false positives reported should be controlled, hence the widespread use of corrections for multiple testing. In actual practice, however, error rates are rarely controlled in any meaningful sense. The conventions regarding which error rates should be controlled (per-comparison, familywise, or experimentwise) are arbitrary and without any real justification [113, 333]. There is no agreed definition of what constitutes a family of tests, and the correction is critically dependent on this choice. Furthermore, corrections do not take into account researcher degrees of freedom (transformations of the data, variables to include in the model, outcomes to report, and so on) and researchers can try one of the many correction methods and can choose the one with the lowest p-value. These are considered 'silent' or 'hidden' multiplicities that are hard to control [39, 40]. In addition, correction for multiple testing increases the number of false negatives, and there is no reason why the false positive rate should be controlled or fixed (usually at 0.05) for all experiments while allowing power to drop to unreasonably low levels [144, 284–286].

The main problem is that in the frequentist approach to statistics the p-value tries, unsuccessfully, to serve as both an error rate and as evidence against the null hypothesis (small p-values indicate that the observed results are inconsistent with the null hypothesis) [137]. The frequentist solution to the problem of multiple comparisons is to try and control the error rate by increasing the required evidence for rejection (require smaller p-values). In a legal setting, this is equivalent to requiring more evidence than usual to convict a defendant because there are multiple trials and the court wishes to keep the number of innocent people sent to jail below 5%. Why should the evidence required to convict a person depend on how many other people are on trial?

Several methods are described below for controlling the familywise error rate, where the family is all 21 pairwise comparisons between the seven groups. *Fisher's least significant difference (LSD)* is commonly seen in publications as a *post hoc* test and many mistakenly believe that it corrects for multiple testing.

Fisher's LSD is the same as conducting separate t-tests between all groups, with the exception that Fisher's LSD uses data from all groups to calculate the within group standard deviation, whereas a t-test uses only data from the two groups being compared. Fisher's LSD tries to control the number of false positives by requiring the overall ANOVA F-test to be significant before testing for group comparisons. If the overall ANOVA is not significant, then pairwise comparisons are not conducted. If the overall ANOVA is significant, then pairwise comparisons are conducted, but *there is no adjustment for the number of comparisons*. The logic is that if the group means are the same, then in only 5% of the cases will the overall ANOVA be significant. Using a significant overall result as a go/no go criterion for follow-up pairwise tests thus offers some protection against false positives, but it is not enough, especially when the number of comparisons is large.[5] Most statistics software presents the output for all possible comparisons regardless of the significance of the overall ANOVA; it is left to the user to notice if the overall ANOVA is significant or not. Another problem when used in biological research is that often one or more control groups are included in the analysis and so the overall ANOVA will always be significant (if the mean of the negative control group is the same as the positive control group, then something went wrong with the experiment), and so Fisher's LSD provides no control of the false positive rate. Fisher's LSD therefore cannot be recommended as a method to control the number of false positives. It is only described below so it can be compared with other methods.

Fisher's LSD can be calculated with R using the `pairwise.t.test()` function and setting `p.adjust="none"`. The argument `pool.sd=TRUE` indicates that all seven groups are used to calculate the within group standard deviation. If this is set to `FALSE`, then the within group standard deviation is calculated using only the two groups being compared. This is equivalent to manually calculating a t-test between all possible comparisons. Pooling results in better estimates of the within group standard deviation but assumes that the standard deviations are similar in all of the groups – the homogeneity of variance assumption.

[5] The approach controls the false positive rate only if there are three groups [231].

```
> # Fisher's LSD
> pairwise.t.test(y.rand, g, p.adjust.method = "none",
+                 pool.sd=TRUE)

Pairwise comparisons using t tests with pooled SD

data:  y.rand and g

  A    B    C    D    E    F
B 0.70 -    -    -    -    -
C 0.85 0.56 -    -    -    -
D 0.89 0.80 0.74 -    -    -
E 0.14 0.26 0.10 0.17 -    -
F 0.61 0.91 0.49 0.71 0.32 -
G 0.56 0.34 0.70 0.48 0.04 0.28

P value adjustment method: none
```

The table of numbers in the above output are the p-values; redundant values are not shown and indicated with dashes. The p-value for the comparison of group E with G is 0.04, more than 10 times larger than calculated earlier with a t-test. The reason is that this analysis used the pooled estimate of the within group standard deviation and groups E and G have smaller variances than the average (look at the error bars in Figure 4.3). The pooled estimate is therefore larger, making the differences between these two groups harder to detect. Setting the argument `pool.sd=FALSE` will give the same p-value as calculated with the t-test. To control the familywise error rate for all 21 comparisons with Bonferroni's method, use `p.adjust.method="bonferroni"`. Bonferroni's method is conservative (makes the p-values too large) but it is easy to understand. If $\alpha = 0.05$ is the per-comparison error rate, then to control the error rate for m tests the new significance threshold is $\alpha/m = 0.05/21 = 0.0024$. Alternatively, 0.05 can be used as the threshold for significance and the p-values multiplied by m. Holm developed a less conservative method that is preferable to Bonferroni's and it can be used by setting `p.adjust.method="holm"`.

```
> pairwise.t.test(y.rand, g, p.adjust.method = "bonferroni",
+                 pool.sd=TRUE)

Pairwise comparisons using t tests with pooled SD

data:  y.rand and g

  A   B   C   D   E   F
B 1.0 -   -   -   -   -
```

```
C 1.0 1.0 -   -   -   -
D 1.0 1.0 1.0 -   -   -
E 1.0 1.0 1.0 1.0 -   -
F 1.0 1.0 1.0 1.0 1.0 -
G 1.0 1.0 1.0 1.0 0.9 1.0

P value adjustment method: bonferroni
```

As Colquhoun explained in the quote opening this chapter, the purpose of significance tests is to prevent a researcher from making a fool of themselves by claiming that an effect exists when none is present [81]. When multiple p-values are calculated the probability that at least one is a false positive increases. Hence the need to use corrections for multiple testing. The trade-off is that as the false positive rate is being held constant the false negative rate increases. In some situations controlling the false positive rate is of less concern, for example when conducting a screening experiment. If the aim is to find active compounds in an assay, why should a compound be penalised more heavily if it is tested in a group of 10 000 others compared with 100 others. The aim of a screening experiment is not to proclaim to the world that active compounds have been discovered but to select compounds for further experiments. It is often preferable to rank the compounds and select those that show some effect for the next experiment (or as many of these as can be afforded), possibly using additional criteria for selecting and ranking [221].

A digression on statistical models and classical tests

Standard textbooks rarely mention that t-tests are special cases of ANOVAs and that there is no difference between regression and ANOVA, even though they appear in different chapters, have different equations, are under different menus in statistical software, and we are told that they are for different types of data. ANOVA, regression, and t-tests are all examples of statistical models that can be represented as

$$\text{Data} = \text{Prediction} + \text{Error}. \tag{4.5}$$

The data are represented as the combination of predicted values (the treatment, biological, and technical factors) and the error, which represents the part of the data that cannot be predicted perfectly. Note the parallels with the fundamental experimental design equation (Eq. (2.1)).

Throughout this chapter statistical models are used to analyse all examples. Statistical models are similar to scientific models such as a transgenic mouse model of Parkinson's disease or signal transduction pathways found in every biology textbook. They are all a *simplified version of some aspect of reality but capture the important or relevant features and can be used to describe, represent, explain, predict, visualise, and understand phenomena.* Models can be thought of as maps, which capture some features but exclude others. A good model, like a good map, contains only the relevant features for the problem at hand.

A map of the London Underground is useful if you plan to use the Tube, but terrible for navigating the streets on foot, and the reverse is true for a street map. Thus, it is best not to ask whether a model is right or wrong (although some may be so bad that calling them 'wrong' is being charitable), but rather is it useful, suitable, or appropriate (or not). All models have assumptions, usually simplifying assumptions; for example, assume that the earth is a perfect sphere, or that the data are normally distributed. Inferences and decisions will be poor if based on inappropriate models or assumptions that do not hold.

In this chapter we fit models to data instead of 'doing tests'. Mathematically, there is no difference between these approaches, but as a philosophy of data analysis, there is a large difference. Why focus on statistical models? First, they provide a unified framework for data analyses instead of a 'cookbook' this-data-goes-with-this-test approach. Most of the commonly used statistical tests (e.g. t-test, ANOVA, regression, Wilcoxon, and so on) were developed by the 1950s, and some much earlier (William Gosset developed the t-test in 1908). One of the advances in statistics has been demonstrating how many of the classical tests are specific examples of more general linear models. It is because of academic inertia that students still learn many separate tests instead of how to fit models to data. In addition, if one takes the cookbook approach, then the first question asked is whether the test is correct, to which the answer is always 'no'. Since a test or statistical model is an approximation of reality it is not correct, but a model may be suitable for a given data set and purpose to which it is put, but this is something different. Suppose that we have cell count data. The values are whole numbers and bounded below by zero because it is impossible to have negative counts. Strictly speaking, a t-test is not 'correct' because it assumes that data are unbounded and can take any value from minus infinity to positive infinity. But a t-test may be suitable if the counts are far away from zero and approximately normally distributed (and the variances in each group are similar, there are no other relevant variables that need to be included, and so on).

A second reason for focusing on models is that statistical inference depends on the model being good, and by this we mean approximately true.[6] We can never know all the factors that affect the outcome variable, but we can be reasonably certain of the important drivers in designed experiments, especially highly controlled experiments conducted in laboratories. Output from an analysis such as p-values, confidence intervals, and predicted values will be of little value if they are derived from a poor model, and if the focus is on fitting a good model (instead of calculating a p-value) then it is less likely that results from bad models will be reported.

Third, it is easy to expand one's analytical skills by learning to fit other – often more general – models. Everything you know about modelling data is relevant for this incremental extension to your knowledge. Compare this with learning a new statistical test, which will likely have a different name, use different notation, and perhaps have different assumptions to be checked. It may not be clear how it relates to other tests and the rest of your statistical knowledge.

[6] Purely predictive models need not make any claims about representing the true data-generating mechanism, their purpose is to make the best predictions and this may entail dropping a variable that is known to affect the outcome but has little predictive value.

Finally, focusing on models forces one to think about how the biological question can be translated into a statistical question; in other words, how a mental or conceptual model relates to a mathematical model, which can then be tested against the data. Competing models can be compared to see which is better supported by the data, making the connection between the science and the analysis closer. McPherson writes 'statistical models are not mathematical constructs of statisticians but are the translation of the ideas and knowledge of investigators into a statistical form' [272].

The connections between an ANOVA, t-test, and a regression analysis are shown below using the data from Figure 4.2 (p. 129). The output from the earlier ANOVA analysis is shown again below.

```
> summary(simple.mod)
            Df Sum Sq Mean Sq F value Pr(>F)
x            1     32    32.0    6.86   0.04
Residuals    6     28     4.7
```

Next, the output from the t.test() function assuming equal variances (var.equal=TRUE) is shown.

```
> t.test(y ~ x, var.equal=TRUE)

Two Sample t-test

data:  y by x
t = -2.619, df = 6, p-value = 0.0397
alternative hypothesis: true difference in means is not equal to 0
95 percent confidence interval:
 -7.73772 -0.26228
sample estimates:
mean in group A mean in group B
              3               7
```

The p-value for the t-test ($p = 0.0397$) is the same as the ANOVA analysis above, the degrees of freedom is equal to the residual df from the ANOVA, and if the t-statistic is squared ($-2.619^2 = 6.86$), it equals the value of the F-statistic.

Next, the summary.lm() function presents the results of the ANOVA model we fit earlier as regression output.

```
> summary.lm(simple.mod)

Call:
aov(formula = y ~ x)
```

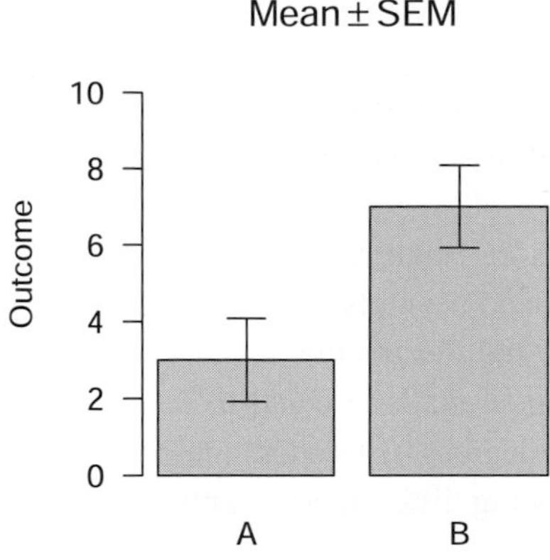

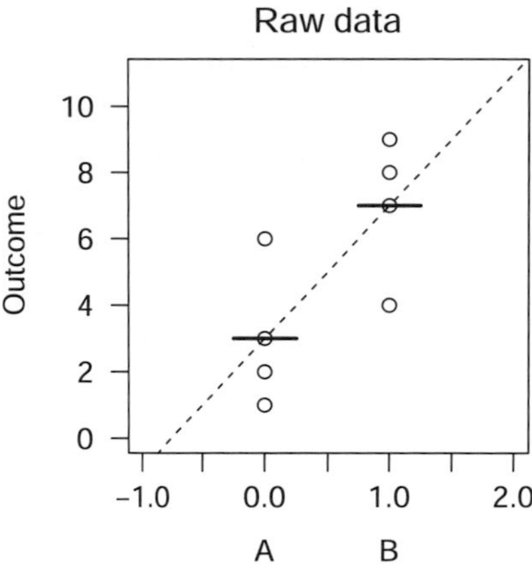

Fig. 4.5 The graph on the left is a typical bar graph with the error bars representing one standard error of the mean (SEM). The graph on the right plots the raw data, the mean of each group (solid lines), and a regression line (dashed line). The factor levels A and B were recoded as 0 and 1, respectively. Note how the regression line passes through the mean of the two groups. The mean of Group A is the intercept and the difference between group means is the slope of the regression line.

```
Residuals:
   Min     1Q Median     3Q    Max
 -3.00  -1.25   0.00   1.25   3.00

Coefficients:
            Estimate Std. Error t value Pr(>|t|)
(Intercept)     3.00       1.08    2.78    0.032
xB              4.00       1.53    2.62    0.040

Residual standard error: 2.16 on 6 degrees of freedom
Multiple R-squared:  0.533,Adjusted R-squared:  0.456
F-statistic: 6.86 on 1 and 6 DF,  p-value: 0.0397
```

The output looks different, but focus on the coefficients table. The first line is the `Intercept`, and recall from secondary school mathematics that the intercept is the location on the y-axis that the regression line passes through when $x = 0$. The estimate of the intercept is 3, which happens to be the mean of Group A. We calculated this earlier as `mean.A` and is given in the t-test output above. The second row of the coefficients table (`xB`) is the slope of the regression line (dashed line in Figure 4.5). The estimate is 4, and is the difference in group means.

```
> mean.B - mean.A
[1] 4
```

These convenient results occurred because the group labels A and B are converted to 0 and 1 by R (as in Figure 4.5). Recall that one way to calculate the slope of a line is the change in y over the change in x. Since the change in x is one unit (going from zero to one), the slope is the change in y (because of division by 1), and is equivalent to the difference in group means.

The t-value of `xB` is 2.62, and is the same value of the t-statistic from the t-test (the sign is different, but this is arbitrary and depends on whether Group A was subtracted from Group B or the other way around), and the p-value is the same once again. The last line of the regression output contains an F-statistic equal to 6.86, which is the same as the ANOVA analysis and has the same degrees of freedom and the same p-value. Thus, three tests that are usually thought of as being different are identical.

4.2 Background to the designs

For each of the examples below, the discussion follows the same pattern: background and motivation to the research question, a description of the experiment, a description of the data, the design equation with degrees of freedom, and, finally, the results and interpretation. The discussion assumes familiarity with model fitting in R (if not, see Section A.14, p. 375).

A summary design table lists the main features of the design. The treatment, biological, and technical effects display the variable names, whether they are fixed or random, and the levels of the factors. N is always the number of experimental units and the notes section is used for comments to explain the design. In addition, for each example the equation linking the data to the predictor variables and the error is displayed, along with the degrees of freedom. The degrees of freedom are calculated according to the rules in Box 4.1.

4.3 Completely randomised designs

The defining feature of completely randomised designs (CRD) is that all experimental units can be independently and randomly assigned to all treatment conditions or factor level combinations.

4.3.1 One factor, two groups

In Section 4.1, starting on p. 124, we used a simple one factor design with two groups to illustrate the concept of partitioning the sum of squares and counting the df, and so do not discuss another example here. There is only one treatment effect called ‘Group’ with the levels A and B. This design and analysis can also be used for the data shown in Figures 3.7 (N-of-1 design) and 3.11 (experimental unit is part of a biological unit).

Design summary

Data:	Simulated example
***N*:**	8
Outcome:	y
Treatment effects:	Group (fixed): levels = {A, B}

$$\begin{array}{ccccc} \text{Outcome} & = & \text{Group} & + & \text{Error} \\ (8-1) & & (1) & & (6) \end{array}$$

4.3.2 One factor, multiple groups

Suppose we are interested in the effects of an anti-depressant on rodent behaviour and we randomised 20 rats to four doses of fluoxetine: 0, 60, 180, or 240 mg/L given in their drinking water [214]. The outcome is the total immobility time in the forced swim test, which measures depressive-like behaviour in rodents. The greater the immobility time the greater the depressive phenotype, and anti-depressants are known to decrease immobility time.

Design summary

Data:	`fluoxetine` data set in the `labstats` package
***N*:**	20
Outcome:	Immobility time on the forced swim test
Treatment effects:	Dose (fixed): levels = {0, 80, 160, 240}
Notes:	Dose is treated as both a continuous and categorical variable

Dose is categorical:

$$\begin{array}{ccccc} \text{Outcome} & = & \text{Dose} & + & \text{Error} \\ (20-1) & & (3) & & (16) \end{array}$$

Dose is continuous:

$$\begin{array}{ccccc} \text{Outcome} & = & \text{Dose} & + & \text{Error} \\ (20-1) & & (1) & & (18) \end{array}$$

The first few lines of the data are shown below, along with a summary. The data are plotted in Figure 4.6 and a dose-dependent effect can be seen.

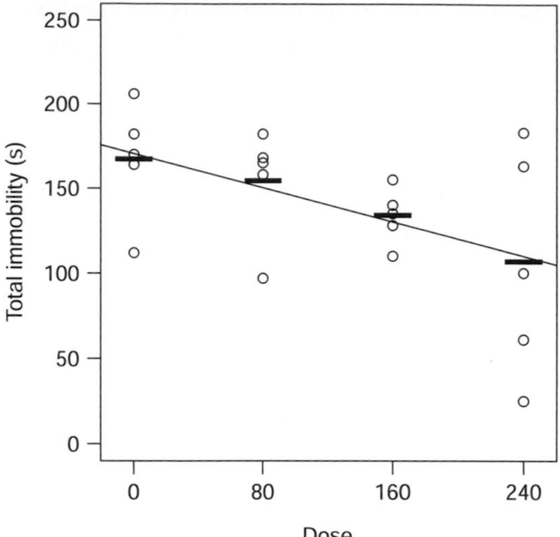

Fig. 4.6 One factor design. Horizontal lines are the group means and the thin line is the regression line.

```
> library(labstats)
> head(fluoxetine)
  dose time.immob
1    0        182
2    0        112
3    0        206
4    0        170
5    0        164
6   80        158
>
> summary(fluoxetine)
      dose          time.immob
 Min.   :  0    Min.   : 25
 1st Qu.: 60    1st Qu.:112
 Median :120    Median :156
 Mean   :120    Mean   :140
 3rd Qu.:180    3rd Qu.:168
 Max.   :240    Max.   :206
```

This data set will be analysed in two ways. The first treats dose as categorical factor, which leads to a one-way ANOVA and is the most common analysis for such an experiment. The second analysis treats dose as a continuous variable, leading to a regression analysis.

The ANOVA model is fit in the usual manner with the `aov()` function. Since dose is a continuous variable in the `fluoxetine` data set, we need to let R know that it should be a factor for this analysis by specifying `factor(dose)` in the function call.

```
> crd.mod1 <- aov(time.immob ~ factor(dose), data=fluoxetine)
> summary(crd.mod1)
             Df Sum Sq Mean Sq F value Pr(>F)
factor(dose)  3  10420    3473    1.98   0.16
Residuals    16  28043    1753
```

The output format is the same as before with sum of squares, mean squares, df, and F-statistics. The p-value for dose is not significant and therefore we might conclude that the dose–response observed in the figure is consistent with chance. The ANOVA model is a general test for the equality of the four group means (the null hypothesis) and this analysis can detect any type of departure from the null.

We are, however, interested in a specific pattern: a linear dose–response relationship. As a general rule, if you are interested in detecting a specific relationship, then a focused hypothesis test for that relationship is more powerful than a general test that can detect all possible relationships. R is unaware that the four categories have an inherent order and therefore does not use this information. Even though the rats were randomised to the doses, dose need not be a categorical factor in the analysis; it can be a continuous variable. With a single continuous variable this analysis becomes a linear regression, but as was mentioned before, there is no real distinction between regression and ANOVA. Since dose is already a numeric variable in the `fluoxetine` data set, the following code represents the regression model.

```
> crd.mod2 <- aov(time.immob ~ dose, data=fluoxetine)
> summary(crd.mod2)
            Df Sum Sq Mean Sq F value Pr(>F)
dose         1  10161   10161    6.46   0.02
Residuals   18  28303    1572
```

The result of this analysis is now significant ($p = 0.02$)! Why did this happen and what is the correct analysis? First, as discussed above, *correctness is not a property of models*. We should ask instead if the models are suitable and whether one is better than the other. Let us first understand why the p-value is smaller when dose is continuous. The ANOVA analysis has 3 df for dose and 16 for the residuals while the regression analysis has 1 and 18. The difference occurs because estimating four means requires 3 df while estimating the slope of a straight line only requires one. The ANOVA model has 10 420 SS for dose while the regression model has slightly less at 10 161. Thus, the ANOVA model accounts for more of the variation in the outcome (the SS is larger), but to do so, the ANOVA model required two more df. Recall that one definition of df is the number of observations minus the number of parameters. The ANOVA model estimates four parameters (four group means) while the regression analysis estimates two (slope and intercept). A model with more parameters will always fit the data better because it has greater freedom, but it is more complex. The question is whether the extra complexity is worth it. This can be addressed in several ways and here we test if the additional complexity provides a significantly better fit; in other words, does it account for an appreciable amount of variation in the outcome. Figure 4.6 shows that the regression line is close to the means of the four groups and therefore describes the data well. Estimating a separate mean for each group is unlikely to provide a better fit, and the two models can be formally compared with the `anova()` function.

```
> anova(crd.mod2, crd.mod1)
Analysis of Variance Table

Model 1: time.immob ~ dose
Model 2: time.immob ~ factor(dose)
  Res.Df   RSS Df Sum of Sq     F Pr(>F)
1     18 28303
2     16 28043  2     259.4 0.074  0.929
```

The output displays the two models, the residual df (`Res.Df`) and residual SS (`RSS`), which are identical to the values calculated previously. The difference in df (`Df`) and SS (`Sum of Sq`) between the two models is also shown. We see that the ANOVA model accounted for more variation in the outcome (`Sum of Sq = 259.4`) but that this was not a significant improvement ($p = 0.929$).

Both models are appropriate for this experiment, but the regression analysis is preferred for several reasons. The first, which we have already seen, is that it is more powerful. Second, the regression provides a simpler and more informative interpretation. In the code below the results of the regression model are summarised with `summary.lm()`, which outputs the intercept and slope of the regression line. The `coef()` function prints only the table of coefficients and the `confint()` function outputs the 95% CI for these estimates.

```
> coef(summary.lm(crd.mod2))
            Estimate Std. Error  t value    Pr(>|t|)
(Intercept)  170.440 14.8368131 11.48764 1.01541e-09
dose          -0.252  0.0991326 -2.54205 2.04365e-02
>
> confint(crd.mod2)
```

```
                2.5 %       97.5 %
(Intercept) 139.26901 201.6109876
dose         -0.46027  -0.0437301
```

The estimate for dose is −0.25, which is the slope of the line in Figure 4.6. This tells us that for every mg/L increase in fluoxetine the immobility time decreases by 0.25 s, with a 95% CI between 0.04 and 0.46 s – providing a quantitative relationship between the experimental manipulation and behaviour.

There is no biology in the results of the ANOVA analysis, all it tells us is that the group means are unequal ($p < 0.05$). To get an idea of how they are unequal we need to look at a graph or do additional calculations in the form of contrasts or *post hoc* tests. Tukey made a similar point half a century ago regarding the conclusions that a psychologist and physicist would reach when conducting an experiment that records how much a spring stretches when weights are suspended from it. The physicist would establish a quantitative relationship between weight and the length of the spring (Hooke's Law), whereas a psychologist would conclude 'when you pull on it, it gets longer' [370]. Biologists tend to fit models and make conclusions in the same way as psychologists ('fluoxetine makes rats do something different') but it is usually better to determine the quantitative relationship between variables, even if it does not become a law.

Another advantage of the regression analysis is that it is easier to compare results across studies. With an ANOVA one can compare p-values and the proportion of variance accounted for by the predictor variable – usually expressed as the coefficient of determination (R^2). Since R^2 is a unitless number, it is harder to meaningfully compare across studies. It is easier to compare slopes, and the values can be formally combined with a meta-analysis. The analysis of this data is described in more detail in reference [214] and is not repeated here.

4.3.3 Two factors, crossed

Suppose that there are three poisons and four treatments to test. We could do three separate experiments, one for each poison, where we test the four treatments. Alternatively, we could do four separate experiments, one for each treatment, where all three poisons are used. These experiments are inefficient because they will be smaller than one large experiment that tests all treatments with all poisons. This is one motivation for using a factorial design.

The data for this example are originally from Box and Cox and are contained in the `boot` package [55]. Box and Cox provided little context for this experiment and we do not know if the purpose was to find the best treatment for a given poison, or to find the best overall treatment. It was probably known before the experiment that the poisons had different effects.

In this experiment, 48 animals (rodents presumably) are randomly assigned to one of three poisons (1, 2, 3) and to one of four treatments (A, B, C, D). There are two crossed factors with $3 \times 4 = 12$ factor level combinations, and with four animals in each cell. The outcome is the survival time.

Design summary

Data:	`poisons` data set in the `boot` package
***N*:**	48
Outcome:	Survival time (units of 10 hours)
Treatment effects:	Poison (fixed): levels = {1, 2, 3}
	Treatment (fixed): levels = {A, B, C, D}

Outcome	=	Poison	+	Treatment	+	Poison:Treatment	+	Error
(48 − 1)		(2)	+	(3)	+	(6)	+	(36)

Even though poison contains numbers as category names, the `summary()` function below indicates that it is a factor (the factor levels are given, not means and other numeric summaries).

```
> data(poisons, package="boot")
```

```
> summary(poisons)
      time          poison treat
 Min.   :0.180    1:16   A:12
 1st Qu.:0.300    2:16   B:12
 Median :0.400    3:16   C:12
 Mean   :0.479           D:12
 3rd Qu.:0.623
 Max.   :1.240
```

The data are plotted in two ways, each of which allows some relationships to be seen more clearly (Figure 4.7). The graph on the left shows the survival time by poison, grouped by treatment. Note how the error bars are larger in groups with higher means.[7] This pattern is common with survival or time-to-event data and a reciprocal transformation can often make the variances similar across groups. The reciprocal of survival time is the rate of death; this is calculated below and is plotted in the right graph in Figure 4.7. The transformation stabilised the variances and now lower values indicate better survival. Unlike the first graph, the *x*-axis is now the treatment and the grouping variable is poison. With the

[7] Since the sample size is the same in each group, the error bars can be directly compared to judge the within-group variability. This cannot be done when sample sizes differ because the error bars are a function of both the variability and the sample size.

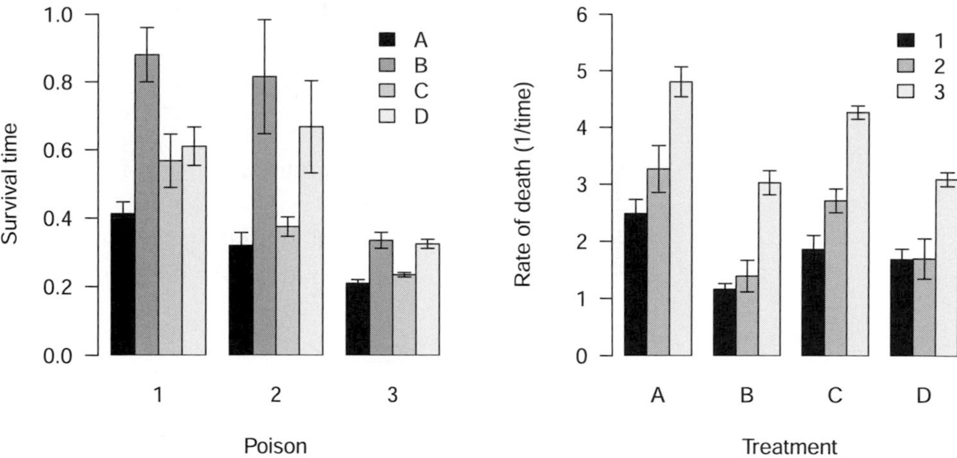

Fig. 4.7 A two-way factorial design. The graph on the left uses survival time as the outcome. The graph on the right swaps the *x*-axis with the grouping factor and uses the death rate (reciprocal of survival time) as the outcome. Error bars are SEM.

left graph it is easier to see how the treatments compare within each poison, whereas with the right graph it is easier to see how the three poisons compare within each treatment. As always, it is useful to plot the individual data points, but are not shown here to save space. The code below generates the graphs in Figure 4.7.

```
> # reciprocal transformation
> poisons$rate <- 1/poisons$time
>
> par(mfrow=c(1,2),
+     las=1)
> bargraph.CI(poison, time, treat, data=poisons,
+             legend=TRUE, xlab="Poison", ylab="Survival time",
+             err.width=0.05, ylim=c(0,1))
> bargraph.CI(treat, rate, poison, data=poisons,
+             legend=TRUE, xlab="Treatment", ylab="Rate of death
+             (1/time)", err.width=0.05, ylim=c(0,6))
```

An ANOVA can answer three basic questions about these data: (1) Are the treatments equally effective? (2) Are the poisons equally toxic? (3) Do the treatments have the same effectiveness for all poisons? These questions correspond to the two main effects and the interaction between treatment and poison. The analysis below uses the rate data because variances are similar across groups. Both main effects have small p-values and we can conclude that the treatments are not equally effective and that the poisons are not equally toxic. The interaction p-value is 0.39, indicating that the data are consistent with the hypothesis that the treatment effects are the same for all poisons.

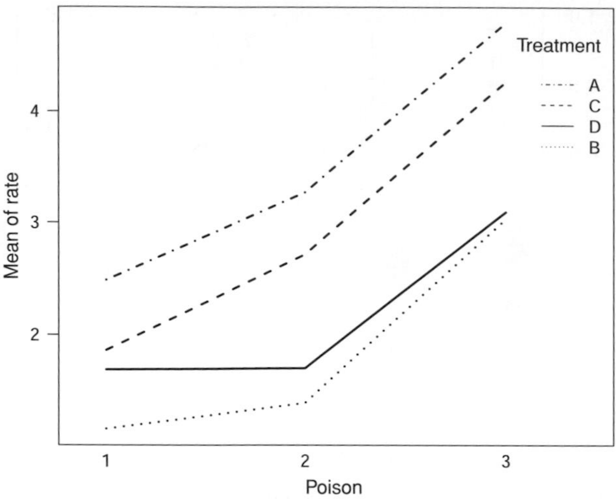

Fig. 4.8 Interaction plot. A zero interaction would have completely parallel lines.

```
> mod.2way <- aov(rate~treat*poison, data=poisons)
> summary(mod.2way)
             Df Sum Sq Mean Sq F value  Pr(>F)
treat         3   20.4    6.80   28.34 1.4e-09
poison        2   34.9   17.44   72.63 2.3e-13
treat:poison  6    1.6    0.26    1.09    0.39
Residuals    36    8.6    0.24
```

It can be hard to detect interaction effects (or lack thereof) with bar graphs like those in Figure 4.7. Figure 4.8 shows an alternative graph that plots the group means for each treatment connected by lines. *The absence of an interaction manifests itself as parallel lines or line segments*, which appears reasonable (although treatment D has a slightly different pattern). The p-value for the interaction ($p = 0.39$) indicates that the lines do not deviate enough from parallel to reject the null hypothesis. The graph is created with the `interaction.plot()` function, which lacks a `data` argument and so the `with()` function is used.

```
> par(las=1)
> with(poisons, interaction.plot(poison, treat, rate, lwd=2))
```

The results from the overall ANOVA allowed us to answer three general questions, but from the numeric results we cannot determine which poison is the deadliest or which treatment is the most effective. There are still many unanswered questions and there are other analyses that can be conducted, some of which are questionable.

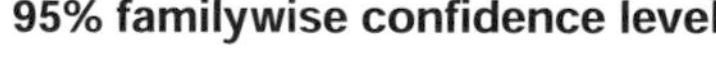

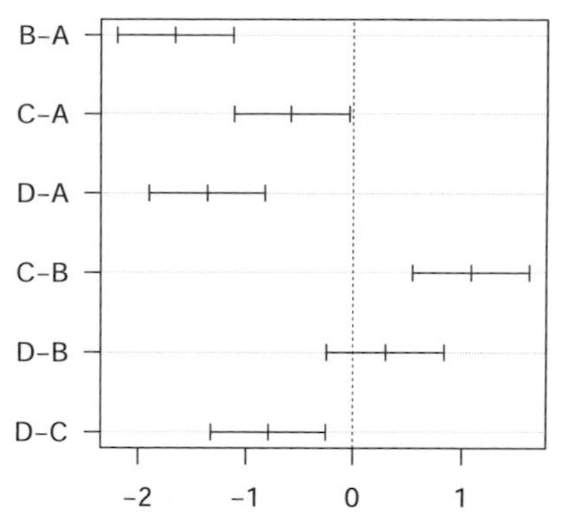

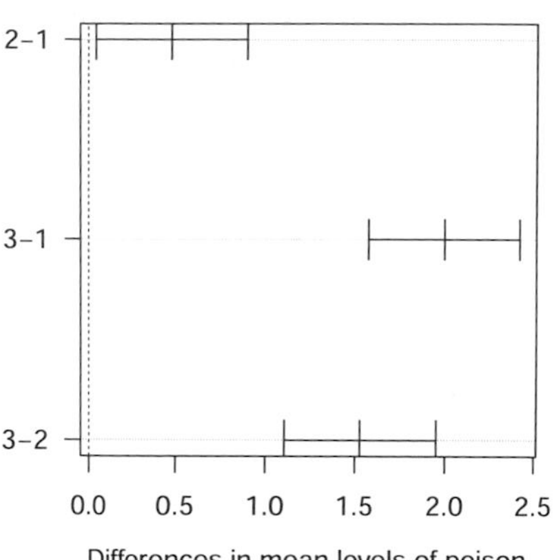

Fig. 4.9 Tukey's HSD. Mean differences and 95% CI for comparisons between treatments (left) and poisons (right).

The first questionable practice is to conduct an all-versus-all comparison between the 12 factor-level combinations. This results in 66 pairwise tests, most of which are uninteresting, but which are easily obtainable from statistics software. For example, what is the point of comparing the treatment A/poison 1 group to the treatment B/poison 2 group? These two groups have different treatments and different poisons, so if a difference exists, is it because of the treatments or the poisons? Since it is customary to correct for multiple testing, the interesting comparisons will be penalised more heavily because all of the uninteresting comparisons have been computed as well. Thus, the power to detect true and interesting effects is decreased.

The second questionable practice is to conduct the same all-versus-all comparisons but not correct for multiple testing. With so many comparisons conducted, the probability of false positives is much higher than 0.05, even if comparisons are restricted to the interesting ones. As was mentioned in Section 4.1.3 on multiple comparisons, Fisher's LSD method does not correct for multiple testing, although most software allows this as an option for such an experiment.

When there is an overall effect of treatment, the next question is which treatments differ from each other, averaging over all three poisons?[8] Similarly, when there is an overall effect of poison, the next question is which poisons differ from each other, averaging over all four treatments. *Tukey's honestly significant difference (HSD)* method can address these questions, but averaging over levels of a factor only makes sense if the treatment by poison interaction is not significant. If there is an interaction, the effect of a treatment depends on the poison used, and so averaging over the poisons can be misleading. The code below uses the `TukeyHSD()` function to print the results and to create the graphs in Figure 4.9. This function takes a statistical model created by `aov()` as the first argument

[8] This is called the *marginal effect* of treatment.

```
> # F-statistic with pooled MS residual
> 1.191/0.24
[1] 4.9625
>
> # p-value for simple effect (with pooling)
> pf(4.9625, # F-statistic calculate above
+    3,
+    36,   # residual df from the full ANOVA
+    lower.tail=FALSE)
[1] 0.00552028
```

The same approach can be used to calculate the simple effect of treatment for the other two poisons, but the `testInteractions()` function in the `phia` package makes the calculations easier. The function takes the full model as input, the `across` argument specifies the factor that is to be tested, and the `fixed` argument defines the other factor that will be held constant for each analysis. Setting `adjustment="none"` in the code below specifies that no corrections for multiple testing are done, which makes the results comparable to the manual calculations in the code above, but should be set to another option for a real experiment. For example, `"bonf"` uses the Bonferroni correction for the three tests, which controls the familywise error rate. The results are all significant, and are not surprising because the overall effect of treatment was significant and the interaction was not, implying that the effect of treatment at each level of poison is similar.

```
> phia::testInteractions(mod.2way, across="treat", fixed="poison",
+                        adjustment="none")
F Test:
P-value adjustment method: none
          treat1  treat2 treat3 Df Sum of Sq     F   Pr(>F)
1         0.7972 -0.5262  0.173  3     3.572  4.96  0.00554
2         1.5669 -0.3081  1.012  3     9.142 12.69 8.20e-06
3         1.7109 -0.0628  1.173  3     9.270 12.87 7.23e-06
Residuals                       36     8.643
```

In this analysis, the residual degrees of freedom (36) and sum of squares (8.643) are the same as in the full ANOVA, and that the degrees of freedom (3) and sum of squares (3.572) for the first poison are the same as the simple effect calculated above (slight differences are due to rounding error). Also, the *p*-value is the same as our calculation by hand ($p = 0.0055$). A similar procedure in the below code tests whether poisons differ across the treatments.

```
> phia::testInteractions(mod.2way, across="poison", fixed="treat",
+                        adjustment="none")
```

```
F Test:
P-value adjustment method: none
           poison1 poison2 Df Sum of Sq      F   Pr(>F)
A           -2.316  -1.534  2    11.104 23.12 3.48e-07
B           -1.865  -1.636  2     8.277 17.24 5.60e-06
C           -2.402  -1.551  2    11.868 24.72 1.75e-07
D           -1.402  -1.390  2     5.199 10.83 0.000208
Residuals                  36     8.643
```

This simple experiment has been sliced and diced in many ways, and we have not exhausted the possibilities. It should be apparent how easy it is to try multiple analyses and choose those that support one's hypothesis (confirmation bias) and only report them (a form of publication bias). Even though corrections for multiple testing were often used in this example, this does not take into account all of the different analyses.

4.3.4 One factor with subsamples (pseudoreplication)

Suppose we are interested in testing the effect of three treatments on the glycogen content of rats' livers and only six rats are available. The rats are randomised to the three treatments so that two rats are in each condition and the treatments, which could be different compounds, are applied to the rats. The rats' livers are then extracted and divided into three pieces, and two measurements are taken on each piece for a total of $6 \times 3 \times 2 = 36$ observations. The rats are the experimental units and there are two levels of subsampling, the liver pieces within rats and the measurements within pieces. The data are in the `glycogen` data set in the `labstats` package.

Design summary

Data:	`glycogen` data set in the `labstats` package
N:	6 (36 observations)
Outcome:	Glycogen levels
Treatment effects:	Treatment (fixed): levels = {1, 2, 3}
Biological effects:	Liver piece (fixed or random): levels = {1, 2, 3}
	Measurement (fixed or random): levels = {1, 2}
Notes:	Measurements are nested under liver pieces which are nested under rats

$$\underset{(6-1)}{\text{Outcome}} = \underset{(2)}{\text{Treatment}} + \underset{(3)}{\text{Error}}$$

The variables treatment, rat, and liver are numeric values and they need to be converted into factors because they are categories.

```
> head(glycogen)
  Glycogen Treatment Rat Liver
1      131         1   1     1
2      130         1   1     1
3      131         1   1     2
4      125         1   1     2
5      136         1   1     3
6      142         1   1     3
>
> sapply(glycogen, class) # check whether variables are factors
 Glycogen Treatment       Rat     Liver
"integer" "integer" "integer" "integer"
>
> # make numeric variables into factors
> glycogen$Treatment <- factor(glycogen$Treatment)
> glycogen$Rat <- factor(glycogen$Rat)
> glycogen$Liver <- factor(glycogen$Liver)
>
> summary(glycogen)
    Glycogen    Treatment Rat    Liver
 Min.   :125   1:12       1:18   1:12
 1st Qu.:136   2:12       2:18   2:12
 Median :141   3:12              3:12
 Mean   :142
 3rd Qu.:150
 Max.   :162
```

This data set is a good example of how analyses can go wrong, especially if the data were given to you by someone else. The first place an error can occur is by not confirming that the factors are indeed categorical variables. Without converting the variables from numbers to factors, R will try to fit regression lines through the data, but this is inappropriate because the treatments (1, 2, 3) and pieces of liver (1, 2, 3) do not have an inherent order, even though they have been assigned numbers. A second way that the analysis can go wrong is by not taking the nested structure into account, and the way these data are labelled is ambiguous. If the variables treatment and rat are cross-tabulated the following result is obtained, which indicates the number of observations at all factor level combinations.

```
> xtabs(~ Treatment + Rat, data=glycogen)
         Rat
Treatment 1 2
        1 6 6
        2 6 6
        3 6 6
```

Do you see anything suspicious? There are six rats but the output only shows values for Rat 1 and 2. This occurred because rats were not given a unique identifier but instead a unique number *within* each treatment group. Thus there is a Rat 1 in Treatment 1, a Rat 1 in Treatment 2, and a Rat 1 in Treatment 3, but these are different rats. Unless we have information about the experimental design, it is unclear whether the three treatments were applied to all rats (and there are two rats) or whether each rat received only one treatment (and there are six rats). *Experimental units should be given unique identifiers to avoid any confusion about the factor arrangement.* The same problem arises with the liver variable, and although it might be clear to us that liver pieces are nested within livers from the same rat, how is the computer supposed to know?

```
> xtabs(~ Liver + Rat, data=glycogen)
     Rat
Liver 1 2
    1 6 6
    2 6 6
    3 6 6
```

We therefore need to create a unique rat identifier and a unique liver piece identifier by pasting together two or more variables using the `paste()` function. The variables are separated by a period for readability, converted to a factor, and are saved back to the `glycogen` data frame.

```
> glycogen <- within(glycogen, {
+             uniq.rat <- factor(paste(Treatment, Rat, sep="."))
+             uniq.liver <- factor(paste(Treatment, Rat, Liver, sep="."))
+                              })
>
> # examine new variables
> head(glycogen)
  Glycogen Treatment Rat Liver uniq.liver uniq.rat
1      131         1   1     1      1.1.1      1.1
2      130         1   1     1      1.1.1      1.1
3      131         1   1     2      1.1.2      1.1
4      125         1   1     2      1.1.2      1.1
5      136         1   1     3      1.1.3      1.1
6      142         1   1     3      1.1.3      1.1
```

Cross-tabulating the unique rat ID with treatment shows there are six rats (not two) and that they are nested within treatment.

```
> xtabs(~ Treatment + uniq.rat, data=glycogen)
         uniq.rat
Treatment 1.1 1.2 2.1 2.2 3.1 3.2
        1   6   6   0   0   0   0
        2   0   0   6   6   0   0
        3   0   0   0   0   6   6
```

The same is true if the unique liver ID is cross-tabulated with the unique rat ID. As we will see below, even if the correct model syntax is used, incorrect results can be produced if the IDs are not unique.

```
> xtabs(~ uniq.liver + uniq.rat, data=glycogen)
          uniq.rat
uniq.liver 1.1 1.2 2.1 2.2 3.1 3.2
     1.1.1   2   0   0   0   0   0
     1.1.2   2   0   0   0   0   0
     1.1.3   2   0   0   0   0   0
     1.2.1   0   2   0   0   0   0
     1.2.2   0   2   0   0   0   0
     1.2.3   0   2   0   0   0   0
     2.1.1   0   0   2   0   0   0
     2.1.2   0   0   2   0   0   0
     2.1.3   0   0   2   0   0   0
     2.2.1   0   0   0   2   0   0
     2.2.2   0   0   0   2   0   0
     2.2.3   0   0   0   2   0   0
     3.1.1   0   0   0   0   2   0
     3.1.2   0   0   0   0   2   0
     3.1.3   0   0   0   0   2   0
     3.2.1   0   0   0   0   0   2
     3.2.2   0   0   0   0   0   2
     3.2.3   0   0   0   0   0   2
```

The data are plotted in Figure 4.10 using the original (non-unique) variables and the code is shown below. There appear to be differences between treatment groups, especially between Treatment 2 and Treatment 3. Treatment 1 is odd because one rat has high values – similar to the rats in Treatment 2 – while the other rat has low values, which are similar to the rats in Treatment 3. It is also apparent that the two measurements on each piece of liver tend to be more similar than measurements on different pieces within the same animal (points with the same symbols are closer to each other).

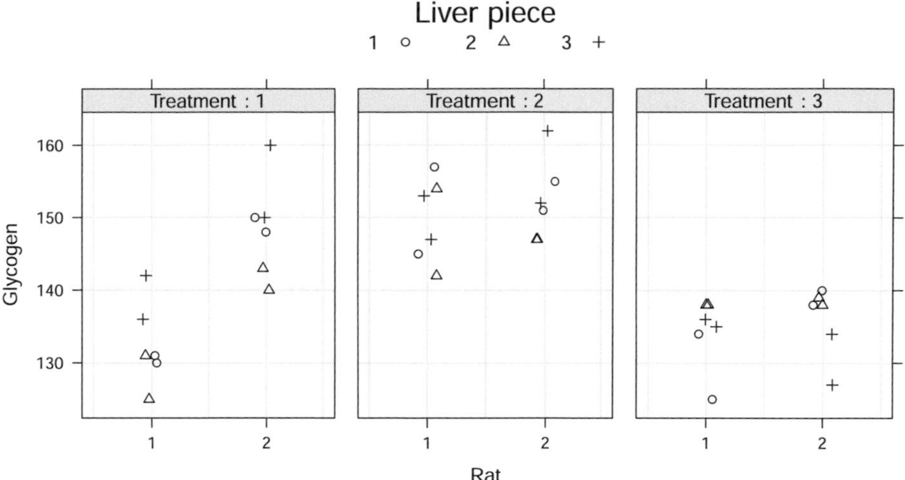

Fig. 4.10 Example of subsampling. Glycogen levels are shown from two measurements taken on three pieces of liver from six rats.

```
> library(lattice)
> trellis.par.set(superpose.symbol=list(col="black", pch=1:3))
>
> xyplot(Glycogen ~ Rat|Treatment, data=glycogen, groups=Liver,
+        type=c("g","p"), jitter.x=TRUE, layout=c(3,1),
+        scales=list(alternating=FALSE), between=list(x=1),
+        auto.key=list(columns=3, title="Liver piece"),
+        strip = strip.custom(var.name="Treatment",
+            strip.names = TRUE))
```

There are several appropriate and inappropriate ways to analyse the data. The first inappropriate analysis is to mistake each observation as an experimental unit; that is, to use a sample size of 36 instead of 6. The code below ignores the pseudoreplication when testing for differences between treatment groups.

```
> # incorrect analysis
> summary(aov(Glycogen ~ Treatment, data=glycogen))
            Df Sum Sq Mean Sq F value Pr(>F)
Treatment    2   1558     779    14.5  3e-05
Residuals   33   1773      54
```

The analysis is inappropriate because the residual degrees of freedom (equal to 33) is greater than the number of experimental units (the six rats). The correct residual df is three (as calculated in the experimental design equation at the beginning of this section), and

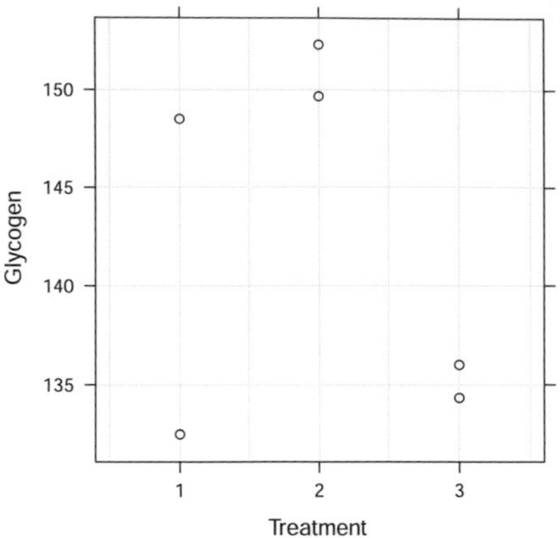

Fig. 4.11 Summary measure analysis. Points represent the means of the subsamples.

therefore this analysis artificially inflates the sample size by a factor of 10, leading to a significant but meaningless *p*-value.

One way to appropriately analyse the data is to average the subsamples. This is called a *summary measure* or *derived variable* analysis and results in a simple analysis. The code below is one of several ways to calculate the mean glycogen level for each rat. The `ddply()` function from the `plyr` package takes a data frame as an argument and returns a reduced data frame (`gly.red`), where we indicate that the mean of the glycogen values for each treatment and each rat should be calculated.

```
> library(plyr)
> glyc.red <- ddply(glycogen, .(Treatment, uniq.rat), summarize,
+                    Glycogen = mean(Glycogen))
>
> glyc.red
  Treatment uniq.rat Glycogen
1         1      1.1  132.500
2         1      1.2  148.500
3         2      2.1  149.667
4         2      2.2  152.333
5         3      3.1  134.333
6         3      3.2  136.000
```

The summarised data are plotted in Figure 4.11 and the difference in values for the two rats in Group 1 is even more striking. There are three lessons to be learnt here. First, it is impossible to determine which rat is the outlier with only two genuine replicates per group. A third rat in each group could help resolve the issue. Second, two genuine replicates per group is not enough for many biological experiments. Methods for determining the appropriate sample size are discussed in Sections 5.2 and 5.3.11 in Chapter 5. Third, the only information we have on the animals is their treatment group. What about their sex, age, litter, and other factors that could influence glycogen levels or their measurement? For all we know, the three rats with high glycogen levels could be from one litter and the other three from another litter, and what appears to be a treatment effect between Treatment 2 and 3 is instead a litter effect coupled with an imbalance between litter and treatment condition.

```
> xyplot(Glycogen ~ Treatment, data=glyc.red,  type=c("g","p"),
+        col="black")
```

The model for the reduced data is below, and the pseudoreplication has been taken care of by averaging. The ANOVA table shows that the residual df is three, which is less than the sample size, and the p-value is no longer significant.

```
> # summary measure
> summary(aov(Glycogen ~ Treatment, data=glyc.red))
            Df Sum Sq Mean Sq F value Pr(>F)
Treatment    2    260   129.8    2.93    0.2
Residuals    3    133    44.3
```

Another appropriate analysis uses the original data and specifies in the model that the rats are the experimental units. This is done in the code below with the `Error()` argument in the `aov()` function. This analysis treats rats as a fixed factor, and in later analyses rats will be treated as a random factor (Section 2.6 discussed the distinction between fixed and random factors).

```
> # indicate that the EU is the rat
> summary(aov(Glycogen ~ Treatment + Error(uniq.rat), data=glycogen))

Error: uniq.rat
          Df Sum Sq Mean Sq F value Pr(>F)
Treatment  2   1558     779    2.93    0.2
Residuals  3    798     266

Error: Within
          Df Sum Sq Mean Sq F value Pr(>F)
Residuals 30    975    32.5
```

The output is more complex because there are two ANOVA tables. The first ANOVA table uses the rat at the error term (`Error: uniq.rat`). The degrees of freedom, F-value, and p-value are identical to the summary measure analysis. These values will not always be identical between these two analyses but are here because the design was balanced – each rat had the same number of liver pieces and measurements. The residual degrees of freedom for the `Error: uniq.rat` ANOVA table is three. The second ANOVA table (`Error: Within`) is for the variation within the subsamples and has 30 df. A key point is that the residual df used to calculate the *p*-value for predictor variables is always the df in the same table as the predictor variable. In the above output the predictor is Treatment and the residual df in the line below it is used.

If the original rat indicator is used instead of the unique rat ID, the results will be incorrect because R assumes that rat and treatment are crossed instead of nested. This is shown in the analysis below; once again there are two ANOVA tables, but now the treatment effect is in the `Error: Within` table and the associated residual df is 32. We know the analysis is incorrect because the residual df associated with the treatment variable should not be greater than six.

```
> # incorrect, Rat ID is not unique
> summary(aov(Glycogen ~ Treatment + Error(Rat), data=glycogen))

Error: Rat
          Df Sum Sq Mean Sq F value Pr(>F)
Residuals  1    413     413

Error: Within
          Df Sum Sq Mean Sq F value  Pr(>F)
Treatment  2   1558     779    18.3 4.9e-06
Residuals 32   1359      42
```

The final analysis treats rats as a random effect instead of a fixed effect and is a better choice because these six rats can be thought of as samples from a larger population of rats. The necessary functions are in the `nlme` package (the `lme4` package is another popular alternative). Once again, if the original Rat and Liver variables are used the incorrect results will be obtained (not shown). The `lme()` function (for linear mixed effect) is used and the first part of the model formula is the same as the previous analyses. A `random` argument is now included, which requires the unique rat ID. The results are the same as before; three residual degrees of freedom (`denDF`) and the same F-value and p-value.

```
> library(nlme)
> lme.mod1 <- lme(Glycogen ~ Treatment, random=~1|uniq.rat, data=glycogen)
> anova(lme.mod1)
            numDF denDF  F-value p-value
(Intercept)     1    30 2738.655  <.0001
Treatment       2     3    2.929  0.1971
```

The glycogen data were analysed in several ways and the main points of this section are as follows. First, ensure that identifiers are unique, especially for the experimental units. This provides information to R about the factor arrangement, making it less likely that an incorrect analysis will be conducted. Second, in a nested design the level at which randomisation occurred and thus where the experimental error is needs to be indicated. This can be done with the `Error()` argument in the `aov()` function, with the `random` argument in the `lme()` function, or by averaging the subsamples to remove the pseudoreplication. Because of the balance in this data set, all of the methods gave the same results. This will not always be the case but differences should not be large. In Chapter 3, we mentioned the phrase *the sample size is where you randomise* and that randomisation can occur at different levels. When randomisation occurs high in the hierarchy *averaging multiple values from each experimental unit* allows a summary measure analysis to be used – a simpler analysis that is easier to interpret. A mixed-effects model may be better and some would argue that the summary measure approach is not ideal because an average ignores both the variability and the number of subsamples. Thus the averages are estimated with different precision, but are not made use of in the final analysis. However, a summary measure analysis does partition the sum of squares correctly, uses the correct number of degrees of freedom, and uses the correct error term, and so should be considered an option. It is better to use a method that you can apply and interpret correctly instead of one that is better by some standard but is more complex and has a greater chance of being misapplied.

Mixed-effects models (also known as hierarchical or multi-level models) are more complex and have more assumptions, such as the distribution of random effects being Gaussian. The random effects can be extracted from the model using the `ranef()` function for plotting.

```
> ranef(lme.mod1)
    (Intercept)
1.1   -7.022148
1.2    7.022148
2.1   -1.170358
2.2    1.170358
3.1   -0.731474
3.2    0.731474
```

The book *Mixed-Effects Models in S and S-Plus* by Pinheiro and Bates accompanies the `nlme` package and is a standard reference, but it is an advanced text [310].[9] A gentler introduction can be found in Crawley [86], and a more thorough treatment is by Gelman and Hill, although the examples are from the social sciences [129].

[9] S and S-Plus are commercial versions of R but the code in the book still works because of the similarities between the two languages.

4.3.5 One factor with a covariate

Suppose we are interested in whether the heart weight of male and female cats differs.[10] How can this experiment be conducted? This experiment has no randomisation but one approach is to collect some cats, determine their sex, and then measure their heart weights. Differences between sexes can then be tested. However, males tend to be larger than females, and since there is a relationship between body weight and heart weight, we expect that males should have heavier hearts. The simple comparison of heart weight between sexes will mainly be a test of body weight differences – most body parts are heavier in males. A more interesting question is whether hearts are *disproportionately* heavier in one sex, after controlling for the differences in body weight. Below we describe two methods of removing the effect of body weight when comparing heart weight. The data for this example are from Fisher [120] and can be found in the `MASS` package.

Design summary

Data:	`cats` data set in the `MASS` package
***N*:**	144 (cats)
Outcome:	Heart weight (g)
Biological effects:	Sex (fixed): levels = {M, F}
	Body weight (kg)

Outcome	=	Sex	+	Body weight	+	Sex:Body weight	+	Error
(144 – 1)		(1)	+	(1)	+	(1)		(140)

Dependency of the primary outcome on body weight can be accounted for by dividing heart weight by body weight, and is shown in the code below. In the `cats` data set heart weight is measured in grams and body weight in kilograms, but if they were in the same units the ratio would represent the proportion of total body weight that the heart contributes.

```
> data(cats, package="MASS")
>
> # ratio of heart weight to body weight
> cats$ratio <- cats$Hwt/cats$Bwt
>
> summary(cats)
 Sex          Bwt              Hwt               ratio
 F:47    Min.   :2.00    Min.   : 6.30    Min.   :2.62
 M:97    1st Qu.:2.30    1st Qu.: 8.95    1st Qu.:3.52
```

[10] Not a scientifically interesting question but it was hard to find a good data set! Assume there is some biological theory that predicts a sex difference.

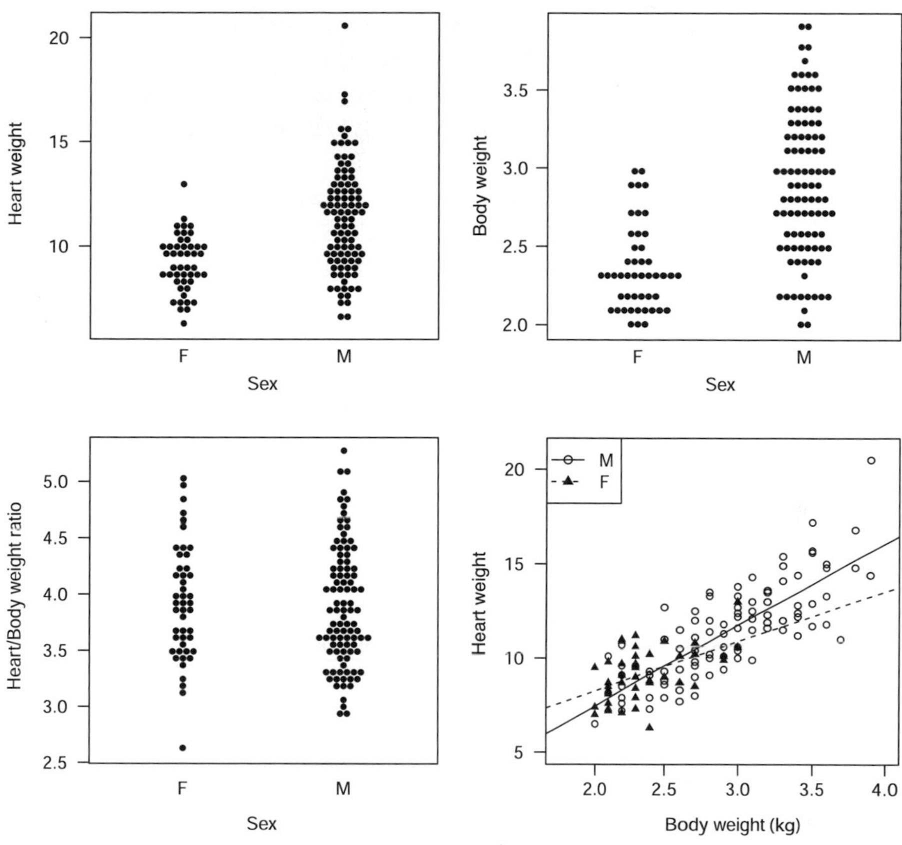

Fig. 4.12 Both heart weight and body weight differs between sexes (top graphs), but the ratio of heart/body weight is similar (bottom left). There is a strong correlation between heart and body weight (bottom right).

```
Median :2.70   Median :10.10   Median :3.87
Mean   :2.72   Mean   :10.63   Mean   :3.90
3rd Qu.:3.02   3rd Qu.:12.12   3rd Qu.:4.25
Max.   :3.90   Max.   :20.50   Max.   :5.26
```

Figure 4.12 shows the heart weight, body weight, and ratio for both sexes. Males have, on average, heavier hearts and bodies, but the ratio appears the same between the sexes.

```
> par(mfrow=c(2,2),
+     mar=c(4,4,2,1),
+     las=1)
> beeswarm(Hwt ~ Sex, data=cats, method="center", pch=16,
+          cex=0.8, ylab="Heart weight")
```

```
> beeswarm(Bwt ~ Sex, data=cats, method="center", pch=16,
+          cex=0.8, ylab="Body weight")
> beeswarm(ratio ~ Sex, data=cats, method="center", pch=16,
+          cex=0.8, ylab="Heart/Body weight ratio")
>
> plot(Hwt ~ Bwt, data=cats, subset=Sex=="M",
+      ylim=c(5,21), xlim=c(1.75,4),
+      cex=0.8, ylab="Heart weight", xlab="Body weight")
> points(Hwt ~ Bwt, data=cats, subset=Sex=="F", pch=17, cex=0.8)
>
> # add regression lines
> abline(lm(Hwt ~ Bwt, data=cats, subset=Sex=="M"))
> abline(lm(Hwt ~ Bwt, data=cats, subset=Sex=="F"), lty=2)
>
> legend("topleft", legend=c("M","F"), pch=c(1,17), lty=1:2)
```

The analysis of heart weight and the ratio is shown below. As expected, there is a large difference in heart weights between sexes ($p < 0.001$), but not for the ratio data ($p = 0.83$), that is, when controlling for body weight.

```
> summary(aov(Hwt ~ Sex, data=cats))
           Df Sum Sq Mean Sq F value  Pr(>F)
Sex         1    142     142    28.7 3.4e-07
Residuals 142    705       5
>
> summary(aov(ratio ~ Sex, data=cats))
           Df Sum Sq Mean Sq F value Pr(>F)
Sex         1    0.0  0.0134    0.05   0.83
Residuals 142   39.5  0.2785
```

Calculating a ratio to control for body weight worked well enough in this example, but it is often a poor choice and sometimes impossible. For example, suppose we had information on the age of the cats instead of their body weight. Younger cats are expected to have lighter hearts than adult cats, but a ratio of heart weight over age is not easy to interpret. The same is true if a technical variable like order of sample collection needs to be accounted for in an analysis.

A second problem with ratios is that even if both the numerator and denominator variables are normally distributed their ratio often is not. In addition, if the denominator is small (close to zero) division by a small number results in a larger number, which can be an extreme outlier (see Section 6.2.7, p. 300, for more problems with ratios). Another more general method of adjustment is to include the variable you want to adjust for as a predictor in the model. This is shown below where body weight and its interaction with sex is included in the model. A model with one or more categorical factors and one or more continuous variables is called an analysis of covariance (ANCOVA).

```
> summary(aov(Hwt ~ Bwt * Sex, data=cats))
             Df Sum Sq Mean Sq F value Pr(>F)
Bwt           1    548     548  263.64 <2e-16
Sex           1      0       0    0.07  0.785
Bwt:Sex       1      8       8    4.01  0.047
Residuals   140    291       2
```

The p-value for the effect of sex is large, similar to the ratio analysis.[11] However, the interaction effect is significant and so we have to be careful with interpreting the main effect of sex. The interaction tests whether the two lines in the bottom right panel of Figure 4.12 have the same slopes, and the small p-value suggests that the slopes are unequal. This means that there is no simple answer for 'what is the effect of sex?' because it depends on the body weight of the cats. At a body weight of 2.5 kg, the sex difference is almost zero, at lower body weights females have proportionally heavier hearts, and at higher body weights males have proportionally heavier hearts.[12] This relationship was completely missed by the ratio analysis and is another benefit of using the ANCOVA model.

Suppose that the interaction is believed to be unlikely *a priori* – based on prior physiological knowledge – and the barely significant p-value is unconvincing, especially when we consider the range of data where the observations of both sexes overlap (between 2–3 kg). The interaction can be removed from the model to obtain a simpler interpretation of the effect of sex and is shown in the code below.

```
> summary(aov(Hwt ~ Bwt + Sex, data=cats))
             Df Sum Sq Mean Sq F value Pr(>F)
Bwt           1    548     548  258.14 <2e-16
Sex           1      0       0    0.07   0.79
Residuals   141    299       2
```

The p-value for the effect of sex is still large and so the interpretation is the same as the ratio analysis. With no interaction in the model the slopes of the two lines are constrained to be equal. If the lines were plotted in Figure 4.12 they would be parallel, with little difference between them because there is almost no difference between the sexes. Since

[11] The sum of squares and mean squares for sex is zero in the above output because it has been rounded up from 0.2; sex does account for a small amount of variation.

[12] A common follow-up question is 'at what body weights do the sex differences appear?' This can be determined with the Johnson–Neyman procedure [90, 393] using the `jn()` function `probemod` package.

the distance between two parallel lines is constant, the effect of sex (if present) is the same at all body weights.

⚠ A final point about adjustment with ANCOVA is that *order matters!* Suppose we enter sex as the first predictor, followed by body weight. This model does not include the interaction but either model could be used to illustrate the point.

```
> summary(aov(Hwt ~  Sex + Bwt, data=cats))
             Df Sum Sq Mean Sq F value  Pr(>F)
Sex           1    142     142      67 1.4e-13
Bwt           1    406     406     191 < 2e-16
Residuals   141    299       2
```

Now sex has an extremely small p-value and could be misinterpreted as a sex effect. Recall the discussion in Section 4.1.1 on partitioning the sum of squares with multiple predictor variables (Figure 4.2 on page 129 and Table 4.1 on page 130). ANCOVA designs are almost always nonorthogonal and so the order that the predictor variables enter the model matters if the default Type I SS is used. Recall that a Type I (sequential) SS tests each predictor in the order that it appears in the model. If the point of including body weight in the model is to remove its effect before testing for the effect of sex, then body weight should be included first. Alternatively, a Type II or III SS can be used where order does not matter. The `Anova()` function in the `car` package gives a large (correct) p-value for sex in the code below.

```
> car::Anova(aov(Hwt ~  Sex + Bwt, data=cats))
Anova Table (Type II tests)

Response: Hwt
          Sum Sq  Df F value Pr(>F)
Sex          0.2   1   0.073  0.788
Bwt        405.9   1 191.160 <2e-16
Residuals  299.4 141
```

4.4 Randomised block designs

In a randomised block design the experimental units are randomised to the treatment groups within each block (Section 2.4). This restricts all possible randomisations, but in such a way that unfavourable randomisations do not occur [166]. For example, suppose there are eight animals and we flip a coin for each animal to decide whether it is assigned to the control or treated group. The number of possible assignments is $2^8 = 256$, which includes the case where all animals are assigned to the treated group (coin lands heads for all eight tosses), all to the control group, and also all cases with a large imbalance in the sample size between groups. These randomisations are unsuitable and if they occurred we would do another randomisation to obtain a better balance. It is simpler though to restrict the randomisations to those assignments that have four animals in each group. This is a completely randomised design (CRD) and there are $\binom{8}{4} = \frac{4!}{2!4!} = 70$ such randomisations.[13] Suppose further that there are four males and four females, and we would like to ensure that the control and treated condition has exactly two animals of each sex. Here, the sex of the animal is a blocking variable and imposes a further restriction on the allowable randomisations. There are now $\binom{8/2}{8/4}^2 = 36$ ways to assign four males to two groups and four females to two groups. Finally, instead of sex as a blocking variable suppose that the eight animals come from four litters, and that we would like one animal from each litter in the control condition and the other in the treated condition. With such a paired design, once one member of the pair has been assigned, the other member must be in the remaining condition. This places even more restrictions on the allowable randomisations, such that there are only $2^{(8/2)} = 16$ assignments.

Why does any of this matter for the analysis? Recall from the section on statistical inference (Section 1.4) that the calculation of a p-value depends on the space of possible outcomes. There we noted that the space of possible outcomes is different if a coin is tossed for a fixed number of times versus tossed until a fixed number of heads is reached, and that different p-values would be calculated from two experiments that had the same results (e.g. 7 heads out of 10 tosses) but used different tossing procedures. In the present example, if the randomisation procedure disallows some assignments, then these assignments cannot be used to form the reference distribution, from which the p-values are calculated. This is why (frequentist) statisticians insist that if blocking was used in the design then the blocking factor should be included in the analysis, even if it is not significant [67, 274]. The method of randomisation therefore determines and justifies the use of the statistical procedure.

4.4.1 With no replication

Festing describes an experiment to test whether diallyl sulfide (DS) affects the activity of the liver enzyme glutathione-S-transferase (Gst) [115]. Four strains of mice were used and for logistical reasons the experiment was conducted in two batches. Each batch was an independent 'mini-experiment' and the housing conditions differed between batches. The data are in the `festing` data fame from the `labstats` package and only data from the first batch will be used to illustrate a simple randomised block design. The full data set is analysed in Section 4.4.2.

[13] The $\binom{N}{n}$ notation indicates the number of ways that n items (e.g. animals) can be chosen from a total of N. The exclamation mark is the notation for a factorial and is short hand for writing the product of all whole numbers equal to or smaller than the number indicated. For example $4! = 4 \times 3 \times 2 \times 1 = 24$.

Design summary

Data:	`festing` data set in the `labstats` package
***N*:**	8
Outcome:	Glutathione-S-transferase (Gst) levels
Treatment effects:	Treatment (fixed): levels = {Control, DS}
Biological effects:	Strain (fixed): levels = {129/Ola, A/J, BALB/c, NIH}
Notes:	Only data from batch 1 is used

$$\begin{array}{ccccccc} \text{Outcome} & = & \text{Treatment} & + & \text{Strain} & + & \text{Error} \\ (8-1) & & (1) & + & (3) & + & (3) \end{array}$$

The first step is to make a new data frame (`f2`) that has only the values for the first batch.

```
> # select data from the first batch
> f2 <- subset(festing, batch==1)
> f2
    strain treatment batch value
1      NIH   Control     1   444
3      NIH        DS     1   614
5   BALB/c   Control     1   423
7   BALB/c        DS     1   625
9      A/J   Control     1   408
11     A/J        DS     1   856
13 129/Ola   Control     1   447
15 129/Ola        DS     1   719
```

In this smaller data set, there are two mice from each strain, which form a natural pair. Since DS activity might differ by strain, we do not want both animals from the same strain in the same treatment condition. Therefore one mouse from each strain is randomly assigned to either the control or DS condition, and the other mouse is assigned to the remaining condition. Thus, randomisation to treatment group occurs within each pair of animals. The pairs (strains) are the blocks and are connected with a line in Figure 4.13.

The treatment has a large effect and it appears consistent across all strains, but the A/J mice might be more responsive than the others. The analysis below fits a model with strain, treatment, and the interaction. The interaction tests whether the effect of DS is constant across strains, that is, whether the lines are parallel in Figure 4.13.

```
> summary(aov(value ~ strain * treatment, data=f2))
                 Df Sum Sq Mean Sq
strain            3  15548    5183
treatment         1 149058  149058
strain:treatment  3  23138    7713
```

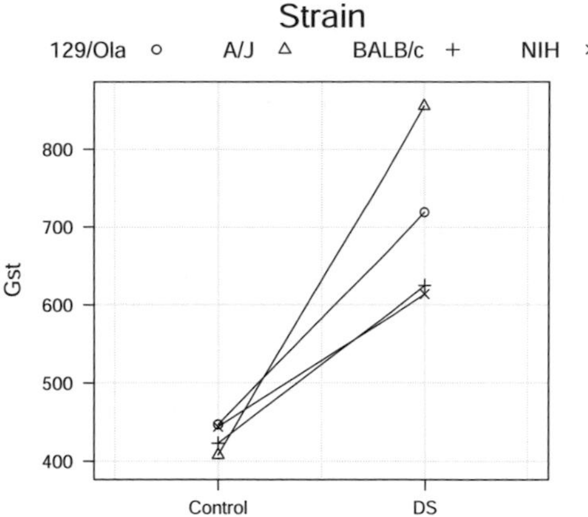

Fig. 4.13 A randomised block design. The strains are blocks and randomisation to treatment groups occurs within strains.

There are no p-values in the output and no residual sum of squares or df. What happened? A randomised block design without replication cannot test for an interaction because there are no df remaining for the error. This can be confirmed by counting the df.

$$\begin{array}{ccccccccc} \text{Outcome} & = & \text{Strain} & + & \text{Treatment} & + & \text{Strain:Treatment} & + & \text{Error} \\ 8-1 & = & 3 & + & 1 & + & 3 & + & \text{Error} \\ 0 & = & & & & & & & \text{Error.} \end{array} \tag{4.6}$$

For a randomised block design with no genuine replication, p-values can only be calculated when the model does not include the interaction. The numbers in the last line of the output below (residuals) are identical to the last line of the previous output (strain by treatment interaction). In a randomised block design, the interaction and the error are equivalent, so an interaction cannot be tested.

```
> summary(aov(value ~ strain + treatment, data=f2))
            Df Sum Sq Mean Sq F value Pr(>F)
strain       3  15548    5183    0.67  0.624
treatment    1 149058  149058   19.33  0.022
Residuals    3  23138    7713
```

4.4.2 With genuine replication

The experiment by Festing was conducted in two separate batches, 2 months apart, and the previous analysis used only data from the first batch. Now the second batch is included. There are two types of blocks in this experiment. The first are the strains of mice and the second are the batches (which were called blocks in the original paper but are called

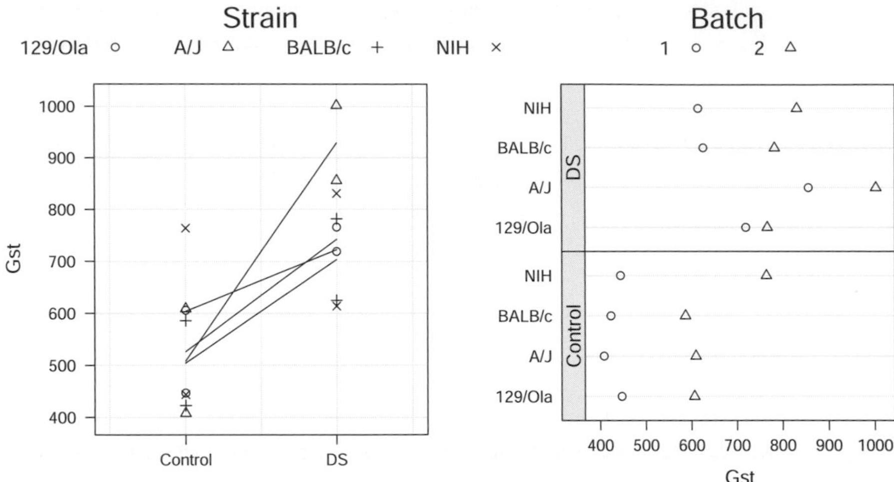

Fig. 4.14 A randomised block design with strain and batch as blocks. There is genuine replication of treatments within strains.

batches here to avoid ambiguity).Thus there are eight factor level combinations: 4 strains × 2 treatments × 2 batches. The left graph of Figure 4.14 shows that there are now two mice from each strain in each factor level combination, thereby providing genuine replication.[14] The right graph plots the same data with the batch effects highlighted. In all cases, the values for the second batch are higher than the first. The batch effect cannot be seen from the graph on the left, nor would a standard mean and error bar plot show the batch effects. Many experiments are divided into more manageable batches but manuscripts rarely mention if this was done, how the samples were divided across batches to avoid confounding, whether batch effects are present, and how they were removed.

Design summary

Data:	`festing` data set in the `labstats` package
***N*:**	16
Outcome:	Glutathione-S-transferase (Gst) levels
Treatment effects:	Treatment (fixed): levels = {Control, DS}
Biological effects:	Strain (fixed): levels = {129/Ola, A/J, BALB/c, NIH}
Technical effects:	Batch (fixed): levels = {1, 2}

$$\begin{array}{ccccccccc} \text{Outcome} & = & \text{Treatment} & + & \text{Strain} & + & \text{Batch} & + & \text{Error} \\ (16-1) & & (1) & + & (3) & + & (1) & & (10) \end{array}$$

The code below shows the analysis for the full data, where batch and the strain by treatment interaction are included in the model. As expected from the graphs, there is an effect

[14] A randomised block design with genuine replication is called a *generalised randomised block design*, although this term is rarely used in the biological literature.

of batch ($p < 0.001$) and a large effect of treatment ($p < 0.0001$). There is also some evidence that DS affects the strains differently (interaction: $p = 0.028$).

```
> summary(aov(value ~ batch + strain * treatment, data=festing))
                 Df Sum Sq Mean Sq F value  Pr(>F)
batch             1 124256  124256   42.02 0.00034
strain            3  28613    9538    3.23 0.09144
treatment         1 227529  227529   76.94   5e-05
strain:treatment  3  49591   16530    5.59 0.02832
Residuals         7  20701    2957
```

There are two lessons here. First, planning ahead ensured that the strains and treatments were balanced across the two batches so that these effects could be estimated unambiguously. Second, it is a good idea to plot the data in several ways to understand all of the relationships and all the factors that might affect the outcome. Do not look only at the treatment effects!

4.4.3 With pseudoreplication

Suppose that in the above example multiple measurements of enzyme activity were taken on each animal. These measurements are subsamples and do not contribute to the error degrees of freedom. The appropriate way to analyse the data is the same as in Section 4.3.4. The easiest option is to average the subsamples so that the number of data points corresponds to the number of experimental units. Alternatively, the `Error()` argument in the `aov()` function or a mixed-effects model can be used (e.g. `lme()`). If subsamples are present, a treatment by strain interaction still cannot be tested, although R will provide p-values for the interaction unless the pseudoreplication is dealt with appropriately.

4.5 Split-unit designs

Split-unit or split-plot designs have randomisation at multiple levels of a biological or technical hierarchy and thus have multiple types of experimental units. The example in this section is from Mehta *et al.* [275] and was also analysed by Lazic and Essioux [222], where the full data can be obtained. A subset of the data is used for this example and is in the `VPA` data frame in the `labstats` package. The full data contained 14 litters and here 6 were selected so that there is an equal number of samples across all conditions. Removing data to obtain a balanced design is not a good idea, and is only used here to make the analysis and important points easier to explain.

Design summary

Data:	`VPA` data set in the `labstats` package
***N*:**	6 females (higher level unit)
	24 offspring (lower level unit)
Outcome:	Locomotor activity (measured on the offspring)
Treatment effects:	Group (fixed): levels = {Saline, VPA}
	Drug (fixed): levels = {Saline, MPEP}
Biological effects:	Litter (fixed or random): levels = {C–J}
	Sex (fixed): levels = {Male, Female}
Notes:	VPA was applied to the pregnant females and MPEP to the offspring. The sex of the offspring is not considered in this example but is balanced with all other groups and is not an important predictor.

Higher level units (females):

$$\begin{array}{ccccc} \text{Outcome} & = & \text{Group} & + & \text{Error} \\ (6-1) & & (1) & + & (4) \end{array}$$

Lower level units (offspring):

$$\begin{array}{ccccccccc} \text{Outcome} & = & \text{Litter} & + & \text{Drug} & + & \text{Drug:Group} & + & \text{Error} \\ (24-1) & & (5) & + & (1) & + & (1) & & (16) \end{array}$$

In this experiment six pregnant female mice were randomly assigned to receive an injection of valproic acid (VPA, $n = 3$) or saline ($n = 3$). The offspring of these mice ($n = 24$) were then randomly assigned to receive an injection of the glutamate receptor antagonist MPEP ($n = 12$) or saline ($n = 12$). There are two levels of randomisation: the pregnant females to the VPA or control condition, and their offspring to the MPEP or control condition. The design is similar to the example in Figure 3.17 on page 118.

A summary of the data is shown below and the `relevel()` function sets the saline control condition (SAL) as the baseline so that it appears first in the graphs (the default order is alphabetical). The cross-tabulation shows that litters are nested under groups (saline and VPA).

```
> summary(VPA)
 litter group     drug        sex         activity
 C:4    SAL:12   MPEP:12   Female:12   Min.    :45258
 D:4    VPA:12   SAL :12   Male  :12   1st Qu.:54557
 E:4                                   Median :63500
 H:4                                   Mean   :63643
 I:4                                   3rd Qu.:70549
 J:4                                   Max.   :84131
>
```

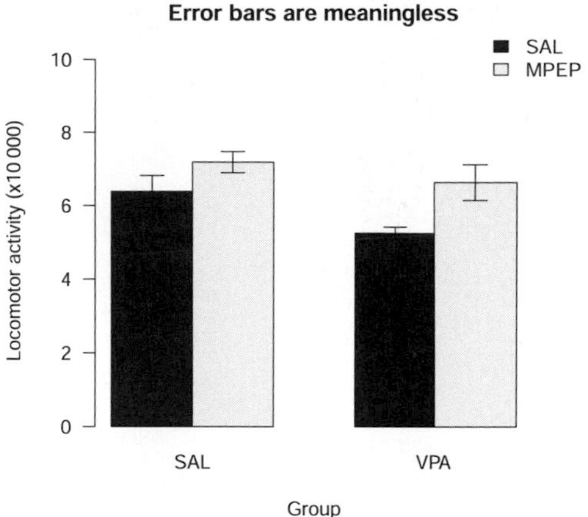

Fig. 4.15 A mean and error bar plot. Error bars in a split-unit design do not convey any meaningful information.

```
> # set SAL as the baseline group (for graphs)
> VPA$drug <- relevel(VPA$drug, "SAL")
>
> xtabs(~litter+group, VPA)
      group
litter SAL VPA
     C   4   0
     D   4   0
     E   4   0
     H   0   4
     I   0   4
     J   0   4
```

Plotting a split-unit design in a compact way to communicate the results to others is hard. Figure 4.15 is a standard mean ± SEM plot, and although the means are correct, the error bars are meaningless because different sources of variation and sample sizes are jumbled together. Error bars are calculated from the sample size, which is 6 for some comparisons and 24 for others. Also, the variation between litters is unaccounted for, which inflates the size of the error bars. Unfortunately, most split-unit experiments in publications use these graphs. Researchers often estimate the magnitude of the effects by looking at the difference between groups relative to the size of the error bars, but with split-unit designs nothing can be deduced from such graphs.

A better graph is Figure 4.16, because error bars are absent, but the variation in the points is a mixture of variation between litters and between mice within litters. It is a useful plot for quality control but offers little insight about the size of the effects relative to the variability in the data.

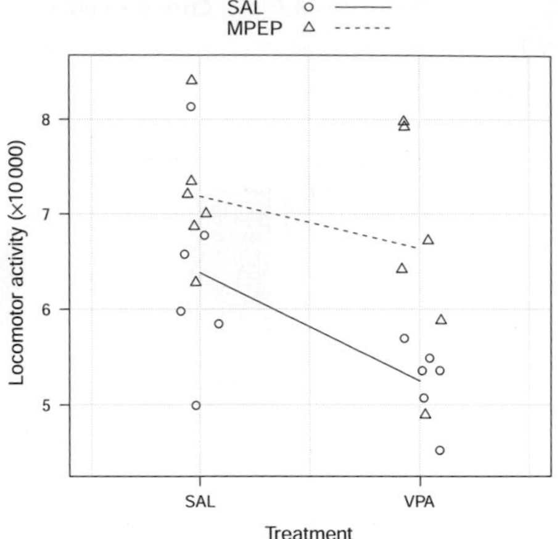

Fig. 4.16 Raw data for a split-unit design. The variability in the data is due to both variation between litters and between mice within litters.

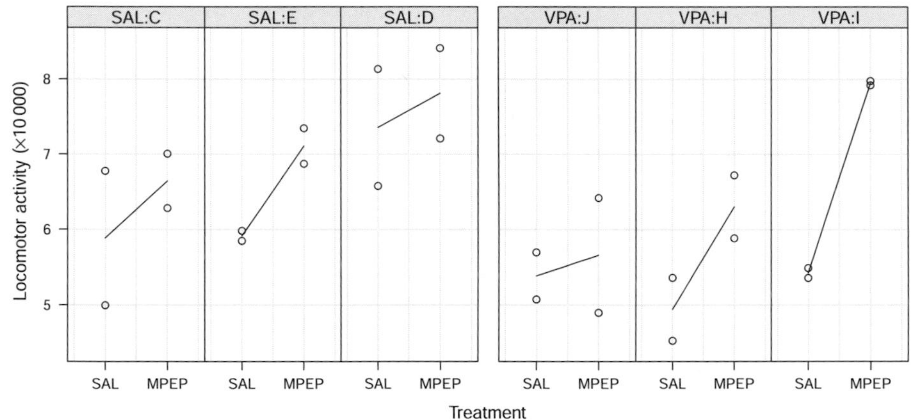

Fig. 4.17 A graph that partitions all sources of variability and makes it easy to understand the split-unit design of the experiment.

Figure 4.17 separately and appropriately displays all sources of variation, but the answers to the main research questions are not conveyed succinctly. The six panels are the experimental units at the top of the hierarchy (the pregnant females or litters) that were randomised to either the VPA or saline groups. Litters C, E, and D were assigned to the saline group while J, H, and I were assigned to the VPA group. The four points within each panel are the offspring, which were randomly assigned to either the MPEP or saline conditions. Some general patterns are: (1) in all panels the mean of the two MPEP mice is higher than the SAL mice (all lines have a positive slope), (2) the effect of MPEP varies across litters (the slopes of the lines vary), (3) the values are, on average, higher in the saline condition compared with the VPA condition, and (4) animals in the same drug group (SAL or MPEP) within a litter are sometimes similar (litter I) and sometimes dissimilar (litter D). The three litters within each group (SAL and VPA) have been ordered (using the `reorder()` function) by mean activity.

```
> xyplot(activity/10000 ~ drug|group:reorder(litter,activity,mean),
+      data=VPA, type=c("g","p","a"), col="black", layout=c(6,1),
+      xlab="Treatment", ylab="Locomotor activity (x10000)",
+      scales=list(alternating=FALSE), between=list(x=c(0,0,1,0,0)))
```

Group and Drug are fixed effects and in the analysis below litter is also treated as fixed. The ANOVA table has two sources of error. The first indicates that the error term is litter and there are four residual degrees of freedom. This makes sense because there are six litters and the effect of group (VPA) is being tested. The effect of VPA is not significant ($p = 0.2$), but with only six litters, the power to detect an effect is low.

The second table has 16 residual degrees of freedom and tests the effect of MPEP (drug) and the interaction between MPEP and VPA. The offspring are the experimental units for both the main and interaction effect of MPEP. There are 24 mice in total, so 16 residual degrees of freedom is expected.

```
> summary(aov(activity ~ group*drug + Error(litter), data=VPA))

Error: litter
          Df   Sum Sq  Mean Sq F value Pr(>F)
group      1 4.27e+08 4.27e+08    2.35    0.2
Residuals  4 7.27e+08 1.82e+08

Error: Within
           Df   Sum Sq  Mean Sq F value Pr(>F)
drug        1 7.18e+08 7.18e+08   13.09 0.0023
group:drug  1 5.11e+07 5.11e+07    0.93 0.3489
Residuals  16 8.78e+08 5.49e+07
```

Additional analyses are conducted below to get some insight into the above analysis and split-unit designs. First, the values for mice within litters are averaged and saved in the `VPA.red` data frame. Since litters are the experimental units when testing the effect of VPA, averaging the multiple values for each experimental unit allows a summary measure analysis to be used (same approach as Section 4.3.4, p. 157). Since averaging combines the MPEP and saline mice within a litter, an effect of MPEP cannot be tested, only an effect of VPA. In the analysis below, the df, F-value, and p-value are the same as the first ANOVA table in the previous analysis (`Error: litter`). This reinforces the idea that no matter how many offspring there are, the sample size is still six when testing for the effect of VPA.

```
> VPA.red <- ddply(VPA, .(litter), summarise,
+                  group=unique(group),
+                  activity=mean(activity))
>
> VPA.red
  litter group activity
1      C   SAL  62638.8
2      D   SAL  75833.8
3      E   SAL  65108.5
4      H   VPA  56217.5
5      I   VPA  66853.0
6      J   VPA  55204.8
>
> summary(aov(activity ~ group, data=VPA.red))
            Df   Sum Sq  Mean Sq F value Pr(>F)
group        1 1.07e+08 1.07e+08    2.35    0.2
Residuals    4 1.82e+08 4.54e+07
```

In the next analysis the effect of litter is first removed by including it as the only variable in the model. The `resid()` function extracts the residuals, which are the activity values with litter effects removed. These values are stored as a new column (`adj.act`) in the `VPA` data frame. A second analysis is then run using the adjusted activity variable as the outcome and only group and drug as factors.

```
> VPA$adj.act <- resid(aov(activity ~ litter, data=VPA))
>
> summary(aov(adj.act ~ group*drug , data=VPA))
            Df   Sum Sq  Mean Sq F value  Pr(>F)
group        1 0.00e+00 0.00e+00    0.00 1.00000
drug         1 7.18e+08 7.18e+08   16.36 0.00063
group:drug   1 5.11e+07 5.11e+07    1.16 0.29345
Residuals   20 8.78e+08 4.39e+07
```

The above output shows that the variation due to group (VPA) is zero, seen in the `Sum Sq` and `Mean Sq` columns. This occurred because the effect of VPA was completely removed when we adjusted for differences between litters. Since VPA was applied to the females (litters), removing the litter effects made the mean of each litter identical, and thus there is no variation between the VPA and SAL groups. Of greater interest is the drug and group by drug interaction. The residual sum of squares (`8.78e+08`) is the same as in the `Error: Within` table of the split-unit analysis above, but the df, F-value, and p-value are different – the p-value is smaller in this analysis. Both the previous split-unit and this two-step analysis account for differences between litters when testing for drug effects, but the two-step analysis does not account for the parameters estimated in the first step (the litter effects) when computing the results in the second step, and so the degrees of freedom differ.[15] This is why the two-step analysis has 20 residual degrees of freedom while the split-unit analysis has 16. On the one hand, this could be considered 'cheating' because we are not accounting for all parameters estimated from the data, making the residual degrees of freedom larger and thus the p-values smaller. On the other hand, this is done all the time and called *preprocessing*, which refers to all of the data manipulation that occurs before formal inference and includes transformation, normalisation, correction, and summarising/data reduction. There is a grey area between what should be considered preprocessing and what should be considered part of the model. The point is revisited in Section 6.2.7 and Figure 6.7 (p. 305).

The final model in this section treats litter as a random effect, which is appropriate because litters are sampled from a population of litters and there is little interest in differences between litters (see Section 2.6, p. 65 for the difference between fixed and random effects). The `lme()` function in the `nlme` package can once again be used for modelling random effects (it was also used in Section 4.3.4). The results are the same as the split-unit analysis above, which is once again the result of a balanced design.

```
> anova(lme(activity ~ group*drug, random=~1|litter, data=VPA))
            numDF denDF F-value p-value
(Intercept)     1    16 535.039  <.0001
group           1     4   2.350  0.2001
drug            1    16  13.088  0.0023
group:drug      1    16   0.931  0.3489
```

4.6 Repeated measures designs

The final design that we consider is a longitudinal or repeated measures design, where the defining feature is multiple measurements on the same experimental units over time. In these designs the experimental units are randomly assigned to treatment conditions, and there may be one or more biological or technical factors that are constant for each experimental unit across time. The interest is whether there are (1) changes over time on the outcome variable, (2) overall differences between treatment groups, and (3) the groups have a different profile over time, which represents the group by time interaction. Such designs are usually analysed with a *repeated measures ANOVA (RM-ANOVA)*, but this is a statistical

[15] Recall that the degrees of freedom depends on the number of estimated parameters; whenever a parameter is estimated a df is removed.

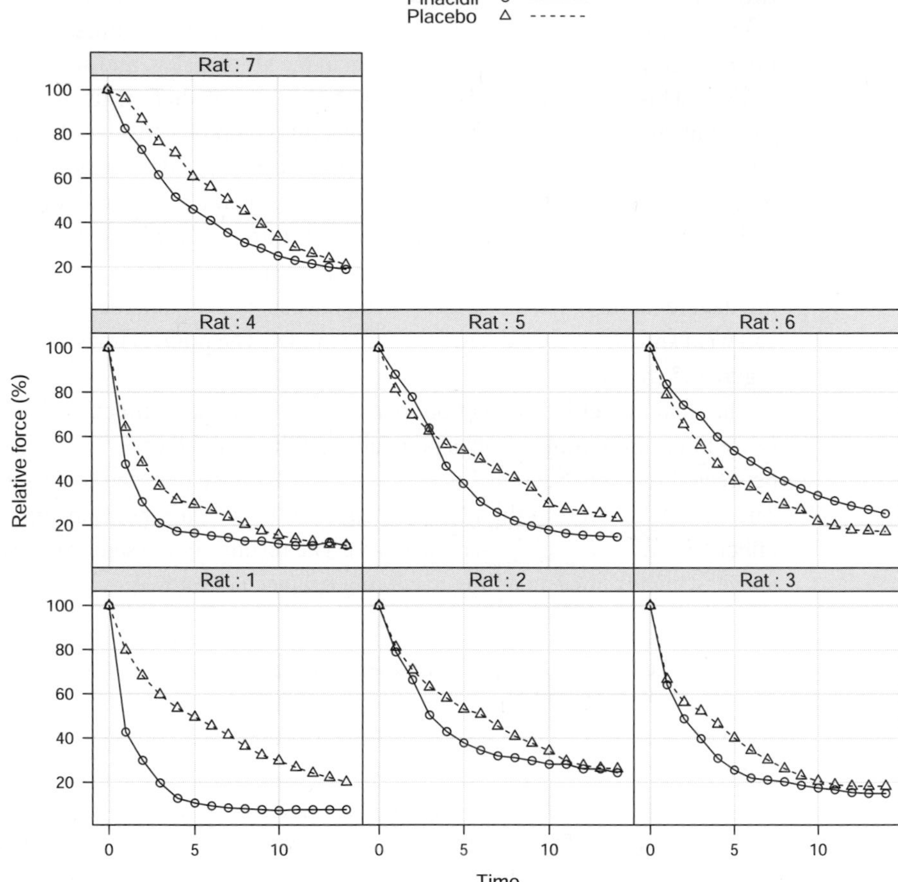

Fig. 4.18 Repeated measures design. The force of muscle contraction over time is shown for two treatment conditions. The pinacidil condition has lower values compared with the control, except for Rat 6 where the relationship is reversed.

method that is best consigned to the history of statistics [145, 199, 387]. RM-ANOVA has been superseded by mixed-effects models, which we used earlier for the analysis of split-unit designs (Section 4.5). One advantage of a RM-ANOVA is that it can be calculated with a pencil and paper, but this is irrelevant nowadays. A RM-ANOVA is simpler than a mixed-effects model, but only because it lacks flexibility and relies on assumptions that are rarely met in practice.

Data from Kristensen and Hansen are used to illustrate the limitations of the RM-ANOVA [199], and can be found in the `KH2004` data set from the `labstats` package. In this experiment seven rats were euthanised and two soleus muscles from the lower legs were extracted from each rat. One muscle from each rat was randomised to a pinacidil (a vasodialator) condition and the other to the control condition. Fifteen measurements of the force of muscle contraction were taken every 30 s on each muscle and a summary of the data is shown below. The rat identification number is numeric and we convert it into a factor. The data are plotted in Figure 4.18.

```
> summary(KH2004)
      time              cond              rat           values
 Min.    : 0   Pinacidil:105   Min.    :1   Min.    :  7.3
 1st Qu.: 3   Placebo   :105   1st Qu.:2   1st Qu.: 20.4
 Median : 7                    Median :4   Median : 31.1
 Mean    : 7                    Mean    :4   Mean    : 39.9
 3rd Qu.:11                    3rd Qu.:6   3rd Qu.: 53.4
 Max.    :14                    Max.    :7   Max.    :100.0
>
> KH2004$rat <- factor(KH2004$rat)
```

The first limitation of a RM-ANOVA is that it cannot deal with missing values. These data does not contain any missing values but many do, and by default most statistics software will remove those samples (experimental units) with incomplete data. This is called a *complete case analysis* and can dramatically reduce the sample size if many samples have a missing value. Mixed-effects models can analyse data with missing values and so samples do not need to be removed.

A second limitation of a RM-ANOVA is that the observations must be taken at the same time points for all subjects. If observations are taken at 0, 2, 4, and 6 weeks for most subjects, then including data from a subject with observations at 0, 3, 5, and 6 weeks is not possible. This is less of a problem for laboratory experiments because the observation times are under experimenter control. Different observation times are a special case of missing data; we could think of the experiment as having observation times at 0, 2, 3, 4, 5, and 6 weeks, with most subjects having missing values at 3 and 5 weeks and one subject with missing values at 2 and 4 weeks. Mixed-effects models do not require the same observation times, but it may make the analysis simpler.

A third limitation of a RM-ANOVA is that variances are assumed constant at all time points and between conditions. This is the usual homogeneity of variance assumption, and is not satisfied for this data set. Figure 4.19 shows the variances at each time point for both treatment groups. These data were normalised by Kristensen and Hansen so that all values equal 100% at the first time point, and explains why the variance is zero at $t = 0$.[16] Even if this time point is ignored, the variances differ between groups and over time. If the variance was constant across groups this graph would have two superimposed horizontal lines. It may be possible to transform the data to make the variances more alike, but homogeneity of variance is not required with mixed-effects models because more complex variance structures are allowed.

A fourth limitation of a RM-ANOVA is that correlations (or covariances) between all time points are assumed to be constant. Figure 4.20 shows the correlation of all time points with each other for the placebo group, and the strength of the correlation is depicted by the narrowness of the ellipses. Starting from the top left of the graph, the correlation between

[16] This is one reason to avoid unnecessary normalisations and is discussed in Section 6.2.

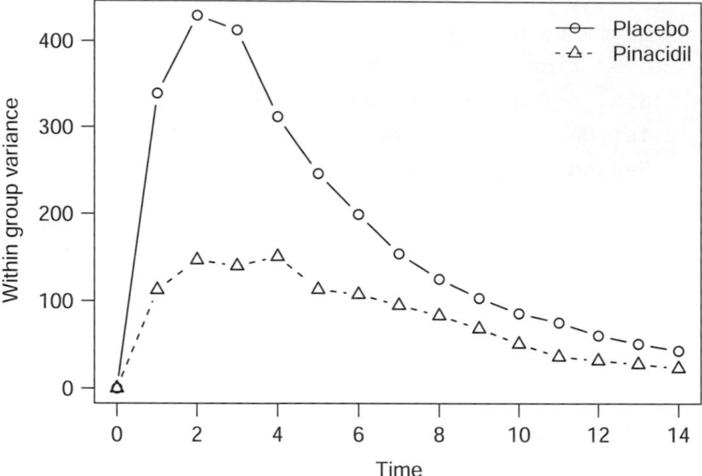

Fig. 4.19 A RM-ANOVA assumes that the variances are constant between groups and across time points, which is not the case for these data.

the first time point with itself (row 1, column 1) is perfect, indicated by a diagonal line. As we move along the first row, the correlation between successive time points with the first becomes weaker, as indicated by the ellipses becoming rounder. A RM-ANOVA assumes that all of the correlations in the figure are the same, and along with the previous equal variance assumption is the *compound symmetry* assumption that this method requires. Although corrections for a lack of compound symmetry such as the Greenhouse–Geisser and Huynd–Feldt have been developed, they are *ad hoc* adjustments to the degrees of freedom and do not model the covariance structure directly. Constant correlations across time rarely occur, especially over long periods. Time points close in time tend to have a higher correlation than time points further apart. For example, the weight of several people tomorrow will be similar to their weight today, but 1 year from now some people will gain weight and some will lose weight, so the correlation becomes weaker. A lack of compound symmetry is not a problem for mixed-effects models because they can directly model different correlation structures.

A fifth limitation of a RM-ANOVA is that the results are hard to interpret and communicate. In this example, a p-value is obtained for the main effect of condition, time, and for the interaction. The change over time is expected because muscles fatigue, and so a significant p-value is uninformative. The data were normalised to be the same at $t = 0$ and the groups are similar at the final time points, but they diverge at the intermediate time points (Figure 4.18). The main effect of pinacidil is therefore uninteresting because the size of the effect varies across time. This means that the condition by time interaction tests the biological hypothesis of interest. A RM-ANOVA provides a p-value for the interaction, significant in this case ($p < 0.001$, calculations not shown), which tells us ‘the lines do something different over time’. Despite all the calculations, this is a qualitative conclusion bereft of any biological meaning. How are the lines different? One has to look at the graph to provide a verbal description, or many might be tempted to conduct multiple *post hoc* tests to show that the groups are different at the intermediate time points but not at the

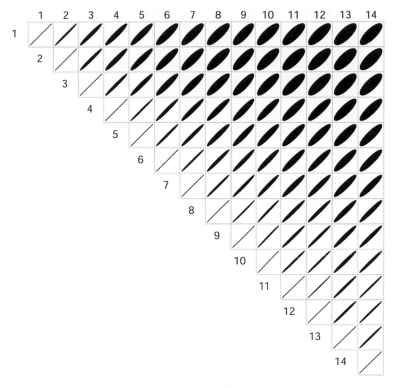

Fig. 4.20 A plot to visualise the correlation matrix of all time points versus all other time points. The greater the narrowness of the ellipses, the greater the correlation between time points. Time points closer to each other have higher correlations than time points further apart.

early or late ones. How can these results be compared to other similar studies? Should we conclude that the results are reproducible if another group also found that the lines do something different over time?

Kristensen and Hansen analyse these data in several ways, including a nonlinear mixed-effects model [199]. The change in force over time can be described by an exponential function, and the parameters of this model have a straightforward biological interpretation. The slope parameter is the *rate of decrease* and indicates how fast the muscles are fatiguing. It is in units of force per second and the difference in the rate of decrease between the two groups is also biologically meaningful. The rate of decrease can also be meaningfully compared across studies. The paper by Kristensen and Hansen is a tutorial on mixed-effects models and can be consulted for further details.

A final limitation of a RM-ANOVA is that the models are often overly complex. Time is always treated as a categorical factor and so the mean of each group at each time point is estimated. If more time points are included, the model becomes even more complex because more parameters are estimated. Mixed-effects models enable time to be treated as a continuous variable (like in the analysis by Kristensen and Hansen), which provides a more parsimonious description of the data and will often lead to more powerful statistical tests [214].

In summary, classic RM-ANOVA is an obsolete method that will provide similar results to a mixed-effects model in those rare cases when no data are missing and all assumptions hold. Below, a simpler data set originally from Levey *et al.* [230] but taken from Casella [67] is used to show how to analyse repeated measures data. The RM-ANOVA is included mainly to compare it with a summary measure analysis and a mixed-effects model, but it is also useful to see how to partition the sources of variance and count the degrees of freedom as we have been doing in the other examples.

In this experiment, 10 patients were randomly assigned to a high or low dietary calcium condition, and their blood pressure was measured at three time points. The data can be found in the `hypertension` data set in the `labstats` package. A summary of the data is below and the values are plotted in Figure 4.21.

Design summary

Data:	`hypertension` data set in the `labstats` package
***N*:**	10 (30 observations)
Outcome:	Blood pressure
Treatment effects:	Diet (fixed): levels = {LowCa, HighCa}
	Time (fixed): levels = {1, 2, 3}

Higher level units (patients):

Outcome	=	Diet	+	Error
(10 – 1)		(1)	+	(8)

Lower level units (time points):

Outcome	=	Subject	+	Time	+	Diet	+	Time:Diet	+	Error
(30 – 1)		(9)	+	(2)	+	(1)	+	(2)		(16)

```
> summary(hypertension)
    Subject           Diet          Time            Y
 Min.   : 1.0   HighCa:15   Min.   :1   Min.   :100
 1st Qu.: 3.0   LowCa :15   1st Qu.:1   1st Qu.:129
 Median : 5.5               Median :2   Median :142
 Mean   : 5.5               Mean   :2   Mean   :141
 3rd Qu.: 8.0               3rd Qu.:3   3rd Qu.:153
 Max.   :10.0               Max.   :3   Max.   :190
>
> # convert Subject and Time into factors
> hypertension$Subject <- factor(hypertension$Subject)
> hypertension$fac.time <- factor(hypertension$Time)
>
> xyplot(Y~fac.time|Diet, data=hypertension, groups=Subject,
+        type=c("g","b"), scales=list(alternating=FALSE),
+        ylab="Blood pressure", xlab="Time", col="black",
+        lty=1, pch=1)
```

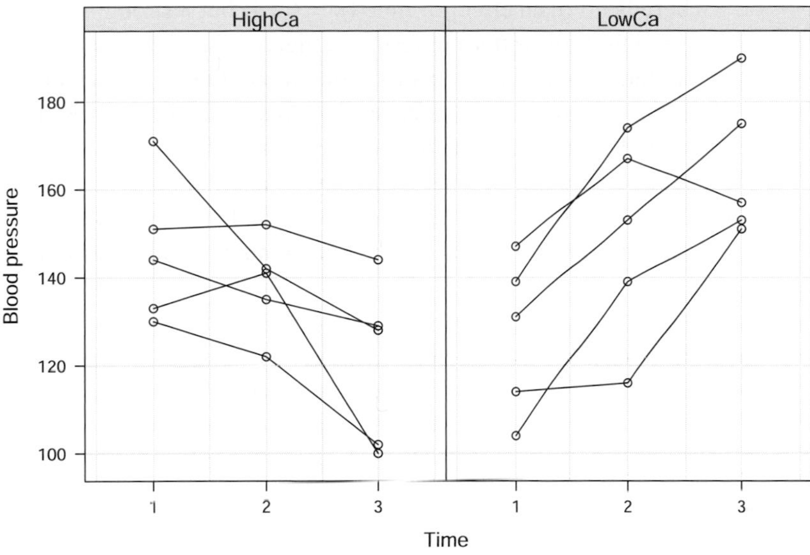

Fig. 4.21 Hypertension repeated measures design.

The analysis below is a classic RM-ANOVA, which uses the `Error()` argument to define the experimental units. Note the similarities with the split-unit analysis conducted in Section 4.5. A classic RM-ANOVA is in fact a split-unit model where subjects are the higher level experimental units that are randomly assigned to diets, and time points are the lower level units, although there is no randomisation to the time points.

```
> summary(aov(Y ~ fac.time*Diet + Error(Subject), data=hypertension))

Error: Subject
          Df Sum Sq Mean Sq F value Pr(>F)
Diet       1   1153    1153     1.6   0.24
Residuals  8   5773     722

Error: Within
              Df Sum Sq Mean Sq F value  Pr(>F)
fac.time       2    343     172    1.55    0.24
fac.time:Diet  2   5028    2514   22.70 2.1e-05
Residuals     16   1772     111
```

In this analysis time, diet, and subject are all treated as fixed effects and the ANOVA table has two sources of error. The first indicates that the error term is subject and there are eight residual df. This makes sense because there are 10 subjects and the effect of the treatment is tested. There is no main effect of diet ($p = 0.24$). The second table shows the results for time and the time by treatment interaction. The residual df is 16, which is correct.

There is no main effect of time ($p = 0.24$) but a strong interaction ($p < 0.001$), and is expected from the pattern of results in Figure 4.21 (the values decrease in the high calcium group and increase in the low calcium group). One drawback of the above analysis is that checking assumptions is hard, and is partly a limitation of R. For example, the `plot()` function lacks a method defined for `aov()` models that use the `Error()` argument, and so the residuals cannot be checked easily. In addition, checking the correlation structure of the data also requires writing additional code. Functions have not been developed because, although the above analysis is valid (assuming assumptions hold), it is not the preferred method.

The next analysis is a two-step procedure. First, the data are summarised to one value for each subject (experimental unit). A summary statistic could be the average blood pressure for each subject, but there are clear time trends and a better summary statistic is the slope of the lines. The biological question determines what summary statistic is suitable. If time trends are expected, the average value will miss this effect. In the code below the `lmList()` function from the `nlme` package calculates the slopes for each subject. The model is specified in the usual way with `Y` as the outcome and `Time` as the predictor (the continuous variable `Time` is used, not the categorical `fac.time`), and `|Subject` indicates that the model is to be fit separately for each subject. The `coef()` function then extracts the coefficients (intercepts and slopes for each subject) as a matrix with two columns. The slopes are then extracted from the `Time` column and stored in `slopes`.

```
> fits <- coef(lmList(Y ~ Time|Subject, data=hypertension))
> head(fits)
  (Intercept)  Time
1     157.667 -16.5
2     146.000 -14.0
3     156.000  -3.5
4     151.000  -7.5
5     190.000 -21.5
6      83.000  24.5
>
> slopes <- fits[,"Time"]
```

A new factor to indicate the treatment groups for the values in `slopes` is needed. The `gl()` function (generate levels) creates this factor with five HighCa and five LowCA values. The results are then plotted in Figure 4.22.

```
> # make new treatment factor
> treatment <- gl(2, 5, labels=c("HighCa","LowCA"))
>
> par(las=1)
> beeswarm(slopes ~ treatment, pch=16)
```

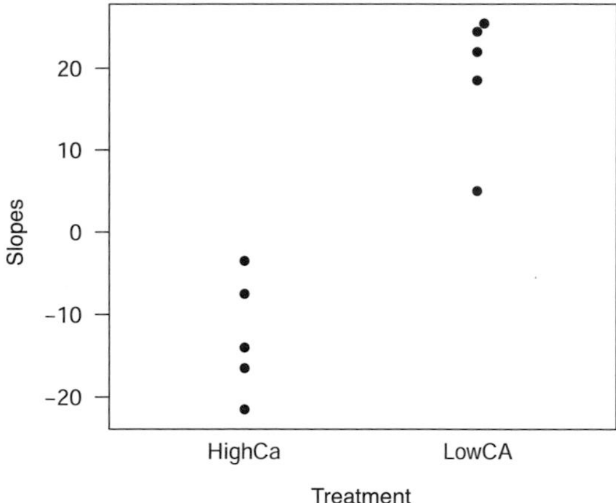

Fig. 4.22 Summary measure analysis. The slope for each person is used as a new outcome variable.

The second step of this two-step procedure is to analyse the summary statistics, that is, the slopes. The analysis has been reduced to an independent samples t-test, but we use the `aov()` function to make the outputs comparable to the other analyses. The degrees of freedom are the same as the split-unit analysis and the treatment effect is significant ($p < 0.001$).

```
> summary(aov(slopes ~ treatment))
            Df Sum Sq Mean Sq F value Pr(>F)
treatment    1   2512    2512    41.6  2e-04
Residuals    8    483      60
```

This two-step approach is not the preferred analysis, but it is a simple and valid analysis that may be good enough. The analysis is straightforward because there are 10 subjects and 10 outcome values. Both the subject and time variables have been eliminated from the analysis and the dependencies in the data from multiple observations on each subject have been removed. Also, the research hypothesis is now based on the effect of the treatment instead of the treatment by time interaction. Thus, the results are easier to interpret and communicate. One drawback of the above analysis is that there are only three data points available to estimate the slopes (and intercepts) for each subject. The estimated slopes are therefore uncertain and one unusual value can have a large effect. In addition, some subjects may have more observations than others. The slopes for these subjects will be estimated with greater certainty but this information is not used in the second stage of the analysis.

The mixed-effect analyses below are the preferred methods, but they are more complex and therefore require greater knowledge to use appropriately. The trade-off is that greater complexity means greater flexibility to model all of the relationships in the data. In these analyses Subject is treated as a random effect. The first mixed-effects analysis uses the categorical time variable (`fac.time`) and the df, F-statistics, and p-values are the same as the split-unit analysis conducted above (differences are due to rounding error). A plot of the residuals indicates no problem with the model fit (Figure 4.23), and recall that this

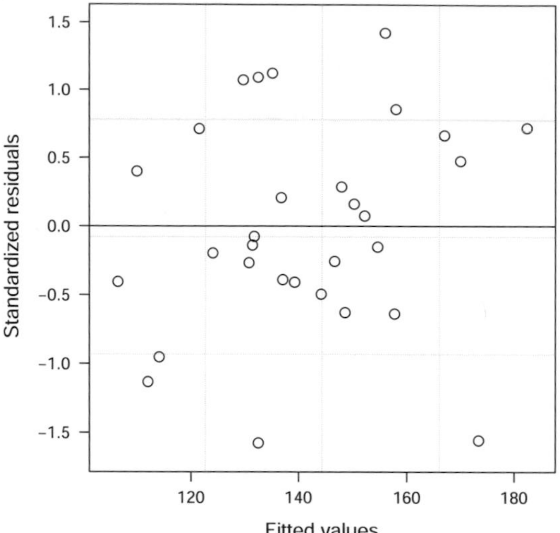

Fig. 4.23 Diagnostic plot from the mixed-effects model.

diagnostic graph could not be easily obtained with the aov() model (see Figure A.6 on page 376 and the corresponding text on how to interpret diagnostic plots).

```
> lme.mod1 <- lme(Y ~ fac.time * Diet, random=~1|Subject, data=hypertension)
> anova(lme.mod1)
              numDF denDF F-value p-value
(Intercept)       1    16 828.082  <.0001
fac.time          2    16   1.550  0.2425
Diet              1     8   1.598  0.2418
fac.time:Diet     2    16  22.702  <.0001
>
> plot(lme.mod1, col="black")
```

Similar to the two-step procedure, Time can be treated as a continuous variable in the analysis, and is shown below. The degrees of freedom for Time and the Time by Diet interaction are equal to one instead of two, and the residual df (denDF) is equal to 18 for these effects. Treating time as a continuous variable results in a simpler model with fewer estimated parameters and thus more residual degrees of freedom, leading to more powerful tests – although is makes no difference for the interpretation of these results. Much like the two-step procedure, this model is only reasonable if the change over time is linear. With more complex dynamics nonlinear models would be required, or Time could be treated as a categorical variable.[17]

[17] The nlme() function (nonlinear mixed-effects) in the nlme package can be used for nonlinear models.

```
> lme.mod2 <- lme(Y ~ Time*Diet, random=~1|Subject, data=hypertension)
> anova(lme.mod2)
            numDF denDF F-value p-value
(Intercept)     1    18 828.083  <.0001
Time            1    18   1.993  0.1750
Diet            1     8   1.598  0.2418
Time:Diet       1    18  47.410  <.0001
```

Whole books are devoted to describing mixed-effects models and we have barely scratched the surface. Two important arguments of the `lme()` function have not yet been discussed. They are the `weights` argument, which models unequal variances and the `correlation` argument, which models covariance structures other than compound symmetry. The help page for `lme()` provides further information and the book by Pinheiro and Bates provides all the details for the `nlme` package [310].

Further reading

There are well over a hundred books on analysis with R and it is impossible to make recommendations for all. The R Project website contains a list of R books that might be useful to browse.[18]

General analysis with R: *The R Book* by Crawley is comprehensive and covers many models and analyses [86]. An earlier book by Crawley is based on S-Plus but most of the code works with R [85].

Designed experiments: There are few R books exclusively about designed experiments but Lawson is an exception [213].

Mixed-effects models: The book by Pinheiro and Bates is the standard reference for the `nlme` package [310]. The book by West *et al.* is a gentler introduction and describes how to fit mixed-effects models using several statistical packages [392]. Gelman and Hill's book is a (not so old) classic, but examples are from the social sciences [129]. Zuur *et al.* provide a readable introduction to mixed-effects models with examples from ecology. They also describe more complex methods such as generalised additive models [416].

Nonlinear regression: Pinheiro and Bates [310] discuss nonlinear models and nonlinear mixed-effects models (e.g. Figure 4.18) and Ritz and Streibig provide a shorter and more introductory treatment [326].

[18] `https://www.r-project.org/doc/bib/R-books.html`

5 Planning for Success

I have not failed. I've just found 10 000 ways that won't work.

Thomas Edison

If Edison had a needle to find in a haystack, he would proceed at once with the diligence of the bee to examine straw after straw until he found the object of his search . . . I was a sorry witness of such doings, knowing that a little theory and calculation would have saved him ninety per cent of his labor.

Nikola Tesla

Edison's quote is often used to exemplify perseverance, but when set beside Tesla's, Edison's approach seems inefficient, not virtuous. In this chapter we use 'a little theory and calculation' to improve experiments.

Many decisions need to be made when designing an experiment and the fundamental experimental design equation (Section 2.2) can guide the discussion:

$$\text{Outcome} = \text{Treatment effects} + \text{Biological effects} + \text{Technical Effects} + \text{Error.} \quad (5.1)$$

How do we decide on a good outcome variable? Even if we know which treatments to test, how do we decide the doses and time points, or the number of genuine replicates and subsamples? If we include another biological factor do we lose too much power to detect the treatment effect? How can sources of technical variation be removed? The choices made can have a dramatic effect on the success of the experiment.

5.1 Choosing a good outcome variable

It is becoming easier to measure more and more variables, but decisions still need to be made about what to record or measure. In addition, confirmatory studies require a primary outcome and one or more secondary outcomes to be defined before the experiment is started. Exploratory studies do not require, but may benefit from, the selection of a primary outcome.

The primary outcome is the variable considered the best for testing the experimental hypothesis; it is where you place your bet. Selecting it after the experiment is completed is like placing your bet after the roulette wheel has stopped – you will win every time, but it's unimpressive.

What criteria can be used to select a good primary outcome or to decide between variables that cannot all be measured? Several are discussed below, and like many other aspects of experimental design, trade-offs and compromises are required. Some of the criteria discussed below are predictions or guesses based on the literature or what is known about the experimental system, and others require data to determine.

5.1.1 Qualitative criteria

Precedence

An outcome variable should be generally accepted as a relevant readout for a biological process or function. Using such a variable puts the results into the context of previous research and makes the study comparable to others. Using a familiar outcome makes it easier to convince others that the correct phenomenon has been measured. For example, if children's growth is commonly measured by their height, then how can a new study be interpreted if it uses body weight instead, especially if previous results are not replicated [103]? Height and weight both capture an aspect of growth, but they are distinct concepts and may differ in biological significance. Precedence also helps because the validity and reliability of the outcome may be established by long use. On its own, however, precedence is no argument for continued use of a poor outcome variable.

Objectively measured

An objectively measured outcome variable is beneficial because it is less likely to be influenced by experimenter biases. This in turn will make the results more convincing to a sceptical audience, especially if the experimenter is not blinded. One reason for the large investment in biomarker studies is to objectively measure disease states and the effects of interventions to replace subjective clinical evaluations.

Measured close to the action

An outcome variable should be measured as close to the action as possible. If the interest is the brain, the brain itself should be measured. This may not be possible with living human subjects, and an alternative is to measure the variable in the cerebrospinal fluid (CSF) – the fluid surrounding the brain. This requires an invasive lumbar puncture and so one might have to resort to taking a blood sample, since the CSF drains into the bloodstream. A final option is to use a urine sample, but now we are far removed from the brain. The further the measurement is from the action, the weaker the association between the measured values and what we want to quantify. Also, readouts measured far from the action are likely influenced by other factors, and so the causal links become less certain and biases can be introduced.

Suppose we are interested in determining if a protein is phosphorylated and thereby activated. It would be preferable to measure the phosphorylation status of the protein directly –

for example, with an antibody that only recognises the phosphorylated form of the protein. If such an antibody is unavailable, another option is to measure the immediate consequence of the activated protein such as the production of a second messenger, or if the protein is a kinase, the phosphorylation of its target protein. These are better than measuring effects further downstream such as changes in gene expression. The further from the action, the weaker the relationship and the greater the chance of bias.

5.1.2 Statistical criteria

Unlikely to be missing

An outcome variable should have (or is predicted to have) few missing values. In a longitudinal human study, subjects may be more likely to provide multiple urine samples than blood samples, as collecting blood is more invasive and uncomfortable. It may be better to measure the desired biology in the urine instead of the blood, even though the measurement may be further from the action. Fewer missing values may be a suitable trade-off.

Unlikely to be censored

An outcome variable that is unlikely to be censored is preferred. A value is censored when it is known only up to a boundary value, but not beyond. For example, values beyond the upper and lower limits of detection are censored; the values are known to be at least at the limit of detection, but not how far beyond. When the outcome is a latency measurement or the time to the occurrence of an event, censoring occurs when the event (e.g. death) does not happen for some subjects before the experiment is completed. Information is therefore lost and censored data require special statistical methods such as survival or time-to-event models to obtain unbiased estimates.

Normally distributed with constant variance

Normally distributed outcome variables with a constant variance are beneficial because they can be analysed with standard statistical methods. Variables that become normally distributed after a transformation are suitable as well. For example, area under the curve (AUC) values tend to have a positive skew, but the log-AUC values are usually normally distributed. Some outcomes might be prone to outliers for biological or technical reasons, making them less suitable.

Bounded data are less likely to be normal; counts cannot be negative and proportions are between zero and one. If many values are near the boundaries then the assumption of normality is questionable. For both proportion and count data, the variance is not constant and related to the mean. Methods exist for analysing proportion and count data and this criterion is only relevant if you are unfamiliar with them. It is better to choose an outcome variable that you can analyse well instead of fitting an inappropriate model to the data [220].[1]

High information content

A good outcome variable integrates information throughout an assay and thus has a high information content. For example, suppose the locomotor activity of rodents is recorded using an automated system and an activity count is provided every 5 minutes during a 30-minute testing session. Values for the last 5 minutes can be used as the primary readout but it might be better to sum the values from all of the 5-minute bins to obtain the total activity. If all of the recorded locomotor activity is informative for the hypothesis, then using all of the data is better than using a part of it. The total activity makes full use of the available data. A caveat is that the maximal difference between groups may occur at a specific time point, which should then be used instead. In this case, summing all the data may dilute the signal.

In pharmacokinetic (PK) studies, three key variables are usually estimated: the maximum concentration of a compound in the blood or other compartment (C_{max}), when this maximal concentration occurs (T_{max}), and the area under the PK curve (AUC). Unless the hypothesis is about C_{max} or T_{max}, the AUC would be the best choice for a primary outcome because it reflects the total exposure of the animal or human to the compound. In practice C_{max}, T_{max}, and AUC tend to be highly correlated and so it may not matter which is chosen, but the general principle applies.

Many behavioural tests measure the latency until an event occurs and also the duration or the total time of the event. An example is the latency for a rodent to enter a brightly lit chamber and the total time they spend in it. The interpretation is that an animal has low anxiety if they enter the bright chamber quickly (low latency) or if they spend a lot of time in the bright chamber. The total time is a better outcome variable because every second that a rodent is in the bright chamber contributes to the value, whereas a latency is a one-off event (latencies also tend to be skewed and censored).

In general, a readout that measures more of the phenomenon is better than one that measures a small aspect of it, unless the hypothesis is specifically about that small aspect.

Good sensitivity and specificity

An outcome variable should have good sensitivity and specificity. Good sensitivity means that the outcome changes when the underlying biology changes. Good specificity means that the outcome remains constant when the underlying biology is constant, even though other biological processes may change. For example, if gene expression is used to measure the activation of a pathway, the ideal gene would be one that is consistently overexpressed

[1] The `glm()` function in R can be used for proportion and count data. See the `glm()` help page for details.

when the pathway is active (sensitivity) and never overexpressed when the pathway is inactive (specificity). Sensitivity and specificity are often traded-off, as more of one often implies less of the other. For example, a threshold for overexpression must be set; some value is chosen and everything above is considered overexpressed. The higher the threshold, the lower the sensitivity, because only large values will be considered as overexpressed and small but true effects will be missed. However, a high threshold implies high specificity because small and moderate effects that are due to chance will be less likely to pass. The choice of threshold depends on how one wants to trade-off false positives versus false negatives based on the costs associated with each type of error.

Good reliability

A good outcome variable should have high reliability or consistency of measurements. Measured values should be similar when:

- multiple measurements are taken on the same sample,
- two people measure the same samples,
- the same samples are measured on two occasions, and
- when a new method is compared with a gold standard.

Suppose we measure two outcomes, A and B, on five samples, and for each outcome we take three measurements, which are subsamples or pseudoreplicates. The data are in the `CV` data frame in the `labstats` package, and the first few lines are shown.

```
> library(labstats)
> head(CV)
  Sample    A     B
1      1  8.7 121.8
2      1  7.9 122.1
3      1 10.3 125.5
4      2 10.4 125.9
5      2 10.9 129.1
6      2 10.8 126.5
```

The variation between the three pseudoreplicates for each sample is due to measurement error. The two outcomes are highly correlated (Figure 5.1, left graph) and when the three measurements are plotted for each sample, we can get an idea of the variation between the samples and between the three measurements per sample (middle and right graphs). Which of the two outcomes is more reliable? It is hard to tell because the values are on different scales; Outcome A has a mean of 10 and Outcome B a mean of 125. Looking at the middle and right panels of Figure 5.1 does not immediately suggest an answer.

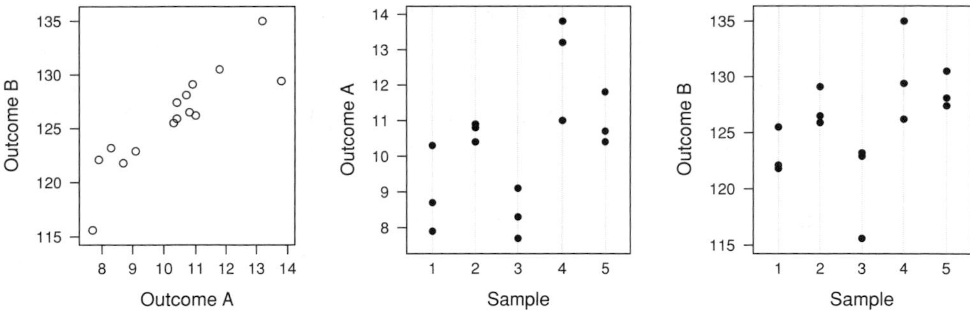

Fig. 5.1 Two outcome variables, A and B, are measured on five samples and are highly correlated. Three measurements are taken on each sample (subsamples) to estimate the measurement error and are plotted by sample number. Which variable would make a better primary outcome?

```
> # load required packages
> library(lattice)
>
> p1 <- xyplot(B ~ A, data=CV, col="black",
+              xlab="Outcome A", ylab="Outcome B")
> p2 <- dotplot(A ~ Sample, data=CV, col="black",
+               xlab="Sample", ylab="Outcome A")
> p3 <- dotplot(B ~ Sample, data=CV, col="black",
+               xlab="Sample", ylab="Outcome B")
>
> trellis.par.set(axis.components=list(right=list(tck=0),
+                                      top=list(tck=0)))
> print(p1, split=c(1,1,3,1), more=TRUE)
> print(p2, split=c(2,1,3,1), more=TRUE)
> print(p3, split=c(3,1,3,1))
```

The coefficient of variation (CV) enables outcomes measured in different units or with different means to be compared.[2] The CV is calculated for each sample, by dividing standard deviation (SD) of the subsamples divided by their mean (M):

$$\mathrm{CV} = \frac{\mathrm{SD}}{M}. \tag{5.2}$$

A drawback of the CV is that if the mean of an outcome is near zero, the CV can be large because of division by a small number, and so the CV is sensitive to small changes in the mean.

The R code below calculates the CV with the `ddply()` function in the `plyr` package. This takes a data frame as the first argument, the `.(Sample)` argument indicates that the

[2] In some fields the CV is called the *relative standard deviation* and often expressed as a percentage.

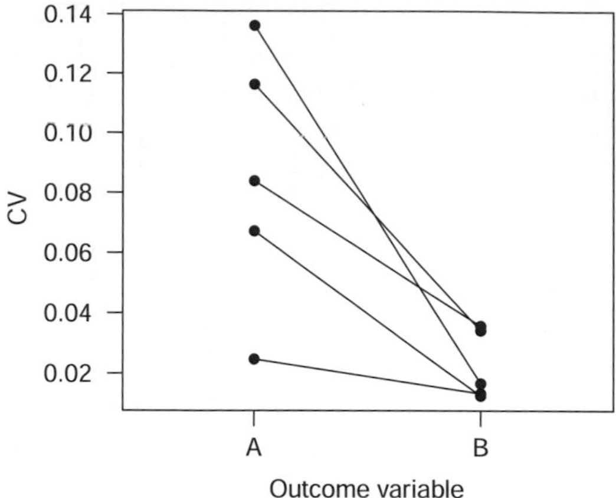

Fig. 5.2 Coefficient of variation for three measurements on five samples for two outcome variables. Outcome B is preferred because the measurements are more reliable.

variables are to be summarised separately for each sample. Then, the CV for each outcome is calculated as the standard deviation divided by the mean. The results are then saved to the `cv.red` data frame and graphed with the `matplot()` function (Figure 5.2). Outcome B is more reliable because the variation of the three measurements – relative to their mean – is much lower.

```
> library(plyr)
> # calculate the CV for both variables
> cv.red <- ddply(CV, .(Sample), summarize,
+                  CV.A = sd(A)/mean(A),
+                  CV.B = sd(B)/mean(B))
>
> cv.red
  Sample      CV.A      CV.B
1      1 0.1362848 0.0166898
2      2 0.0247266 0.0133760
3      3 0.0839494 0.0356970
4      4 0.1163860 0.0342105
5      5 0.0672138 0.0126360
>
> par(las=1)
> matplot(t(cv.red[,2:3]), xlim=c(0.5,2.5), pch=16,
+         col="black", ylab="CV", xaxt="n",
+         xlab="Outcome variable")
>
> axis(1, at=1:2, labels=c("A","B"))
> # add lines to connect samples
> segments(rep(1,5), cv.red[,2], rep(2,5), cv.red[,3])
```

A second type of reliability is the agreement between a new variable and a gold standard. The gold standard may be expensive or hard to use and an alternative is desired. The `goldstandard` data set from the `labstats` package is used for this example and the first few lines of data are shown. The data set contains simulated values for a gold standard and for four new methods that have different relationships with the gold standard.

```
> head(goldstandard)
  goldstandard perfect.cor noise location scale
1         16.3        16.3  15.5     17.5  20.4
2          4.7         4.7   6.1      8.1   7.5
3         16.5        16.5  15.3     17.3  20.2
4         10.7        10.7  10.7     12.7  13.9
5         18.6        18.6  20.3     22.3  25.9
6         11.0        11.0  10.4     12.4  13.7
```

In Figure 5.3, the gold standard is plotted on the x-axis and the new variables are plotted on the y-axes for 20 samples. The diagonal line represents perfect reliability; if the data points fall on this line then the new method gives the same value as the gold standard (Figure 5.3A). There are several ways that a new variable can depart from the gold standard. One type of departure occurs when the new variable is a noisier version of the gold standard. The new variable provides the same value as the gold standard, on average, but there is some scatter around the diagonal line (Figure 5.3B). Another type of departure is a *location shift*, where the new method either consistently over- or underestimates the value of the gold standard. In Figure 5.3C, the values for the new variable are about two units higher than the gold standard (most of the points are above the line). Another type of departure is a *scale shift*, where the two methods agree for low values, but not for higher values because the variance of the new variable is larger than the gold standard (Figure 5.3D). A location plus a scale shift is also possible, as is attenuation of the variance, where the new method overestimates low values and underestimates high values compared with the gold standard (not shown).

Although the correlation between the gold standard and the new variable quantifies the scatter around the diagonal line, it will not detect location or scale shifts. A correlation only measures the association between two variables but not the reproducibility or agreement, and so is unsuitable for comparing a new method with a gold standard. Lin developed a concordance correlation coefficient (CCC; Eq. (5.3)), which is interpreted as a regular correlation coefficient (values close to one are good) but takes scale and location shifts into account [237, 238]:

$$\mathrm{CCC} = \frac{2S_{xy}}{S_x^2 + S_y^2 + (\bar{X} - \bar{Y})^2}. \tag{5.3}$$

S_{xy} is the covariance between the two variables (X and Y) and measures the strength of association, S_x^2 and S_y^2 are the variances, and $\bar{X}$ and $\bar{Y}$ are the means. The values of the Pearson correlation and CCC are shown in Figure 5.3 and are the same when the new

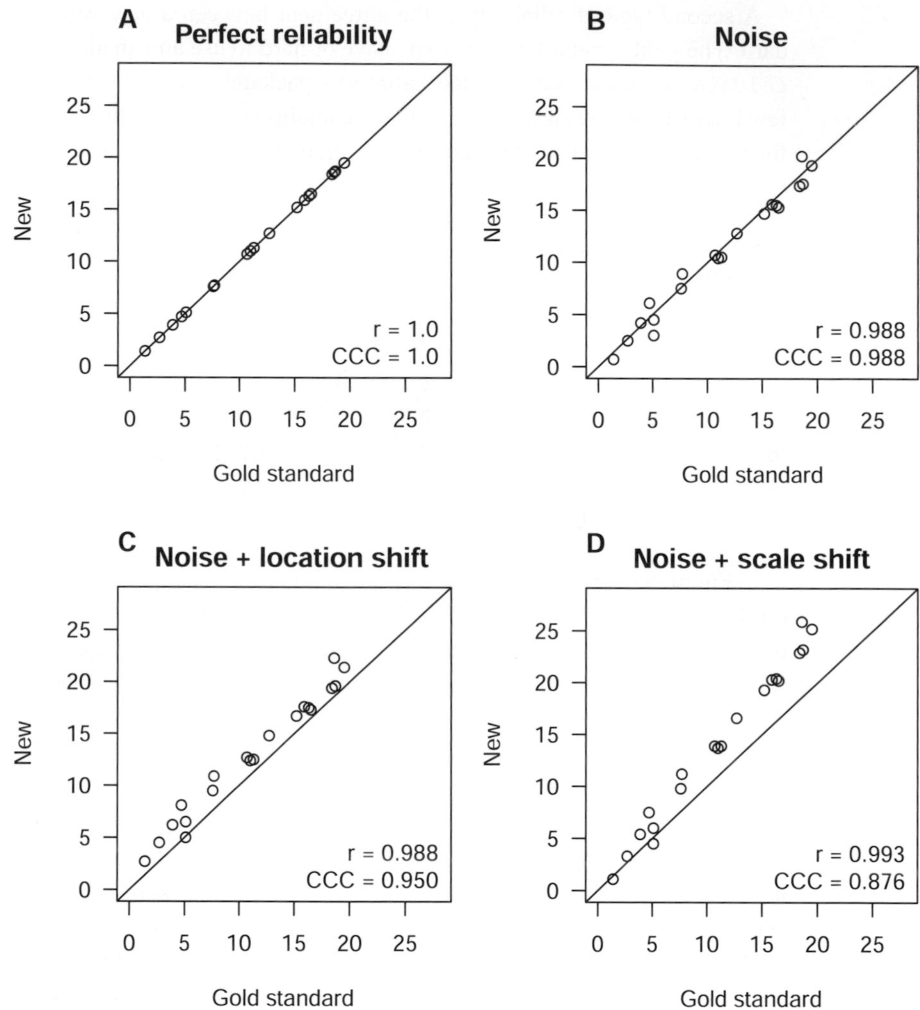

Fig. 5.3 Comparing a new variable with a gold standard. r = Pearson correlation; CCC = Lin's concordance correlation coefficient.

variable is only a noisy version of the gold standard (Figure 5.3B) but the CCC is smaller than the correlation when there is a location or scale shift (Figures 5.3C and D).

Equation (5.3) is used in the `lin.cor()` function below to calculate the CCC, which takes two vectors as arguments (`x` and `y`); one is the new variable and the other is the gold standard. The code below then calculates the Pearson correlation and CCC between the gold standard and the variables, and the values are also shown in Figure 5.3.

```
> # function to calculate CCC
> lin.cor <- function(x,y){
+     cov.xy <- cov(x,y)
```

```
+     var.x <- var(x)
+     var.y <- var(y)
+     mean.x <- mean(x)
+     mean.y <- mean(y)
+
+     2*cov.xy / (var.x + var.y + (mean.x - mean.y)^2)
+ }
>
>
> # compare Pearson correlations with CCC
> with(goldstandard, cor(goldstandard, noise))
[1] 0.988493
> with(goldstandard, cor(goldstandard, location))
[1] 0.988493
> with(goldstandard, cor(goldstandard, scale))
[1] 0.993052
>
> with(goldstandard, lin.cor(goldstandard, noise))
[1] 0.987502
> with(goldstandard, lin.cor(goldstandard, location))
[1] 0.949378
> with(goldstandard, lin.cor(goldstandard, scale))
[1] 0.875887
```

The graphs in Figure 5.3 are not ideal for visually comparing the reliability of two methods because the eye tends to join the points to the closest part of the line, but the difference between methods is the vertical distance from each point to the line. A better graph is a Tukey mean-difference plot (Figure 5.4).[3] This graph plots the difference between the new and gold-standard measurements on the *y*-axis and the average of the two measurements on the *x*-axis. These are the same data as shown in Figure 5.3C and D. The constant location (vertical) shift in the left graph is apparent, as is the greater departure at higher values in the right graph. The code for the Tukey mean-difference plot is below and requires wrapping the `xyplot()` function with the `tmd()` function, both of which are from the `lattice` package.

```
> p1 <- tmd(xyplot(location ~ goldstandard, data=goldstandard,
+                  main="Noise + location shift"),
+           ylim=c(-1,5), col="black")
> p2 <- tmd(xyplot(scale ~ goldstandard, data=goldstandard,
+                  main="Noise + scale shift"),
```

[3] Also known as a Bland–Altman plot in some fields and an MA plot in the microarray literature [43].

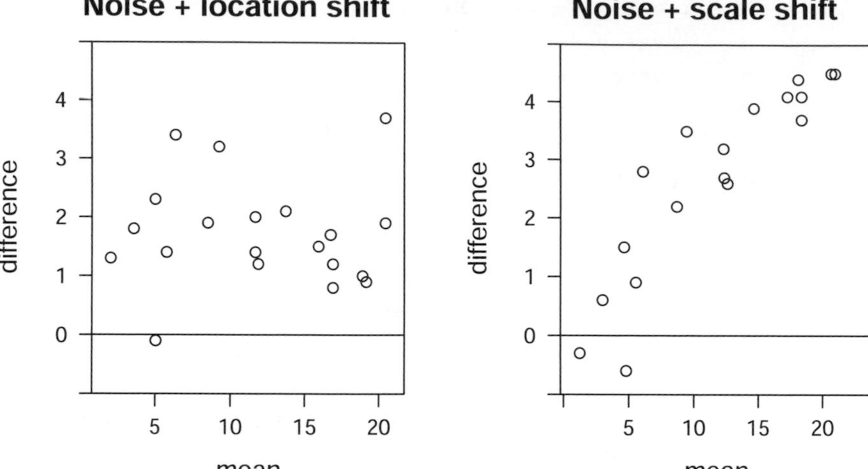

Fig. 5.4 Tukey mean-difference plot for comparing measurements with a gold standard.

```
+                ylim=c(-1,5), col="black")
>
> print(p1, split=c(1,1,2,1), more=TRUE)
> print(p2, split=c(2,1,2,1))
```

Four situations where reliability can be measured were listed at the beginning of this subsection. The first (multiple measurements on the same sample) differs from the other three in that measurements on the same sample are interchangeable. The labels 'measurement 1' and 'measurement 2' do not have any inherent meaning and can be interchanged without affecting the interpretation of the results. The CCC assumes that pairs of values cannot be interchanged because one value comes from the gold standard and the other from the new method, or one from Researcher A and the other from Researcher B. Thus, the CCC would be inappropriate to estimate the reliability of the example in Figure 5.1 (even if there were only two values instead of three).

Good assay window

A final consideration when choosing the primary outcome is the separation between the positive and negative control groups – assuming that a positive control is available. This separation is called the *assay window* or *signal window* and is a measure of how easily the two control groups can be distinguished. A small assay window is a problem because if it is hard to distinguish the positive control from the negative control, then it will likely be hard to distinguish another experimental condition from the negative control – in other words, to find significant effects. The `assay.window` data set from the `labstats` package is used for this example and the first few lines of the data are shown. There are two outcomes, A and B, and each sample is either a positive or negative control.

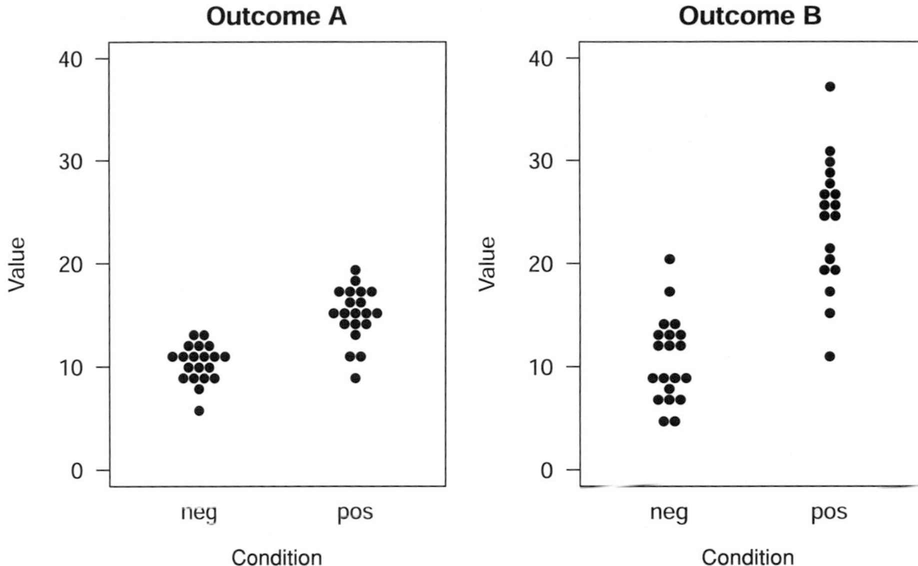

Fig. 5.5 Assay window. Outcome A has a smaller difference between means, but less variability within the two groups, compared with Outcome B. Which outcome has a better assay window?

```
> head(assay.window)
     A    B condition
1  8.7  9.2       neg
2 10.4  8.7       neg
3  8.3 13.5       neg
4 13.2 12.8       neg
5 10.7  6.6       neg
6  8.4  6.5       neg
```

In Figure 5.5, the difference in means between the positive and negative control groups is larger for Outcome B compared with Outcome A, but since Outcome B also has a larger variance, it is unclear which outcome better separates the two groups.

```
> library(beeswarm)
> par(mfrow=c(1,2),
+     mar=c(4,4,2,1),
+     las=1)
>
> beeswarm(A ~ condition, data=assay.window, ylab="Value",
+          method="center", pch=16, ylim=c(0,40), main="Outcome A")
> beeswarm(B ~ condition, data=assay.window, ylab="Value",
+          method="center", pch=16, ylim=c(0,40), main="Outcome B")
```

Many methods have been developed to quantify the separation of two groups [364, 412, 413]. Only one is mentioned here because it leads to a discussion of power analyses and sample size calculations – the topic of the next section. The separation between groups can be quantified by calculating the difference between the means relative to their variability and is called a *standardised effect size*. The most common standardised effect size for a two group comparison is Cohen's d (Eq. (5.4); [78]). It is the difference between the mean of the positive (M_p) and negative (M_n) control group, divided by the within-group standard deviation (S):

$$\text{Effect size (ES)} = \frac{M_p - M_n}{S}, \tag{5.4}$$

where S is calculated as a weighted average of the two variances,

$$S = \sqrt{\frac{(n_p - 1)S_p^2 + (n_c - 1)S_n^2}{n_p + n_c - 2}}. \tag{5.5}$$

S_p^2 and S_n^2 are the variances of the positive and negative control group, respectively. If the sample size is equal in the two groups ($n_p = n_c$), this formula reduces to

$$S = \sqrt{\frac{S_p^2 + S_n^2}{2}} \tag{5.6}$$

and is easy to compute with R. The `tapply()` function calculates the mean and variance for the positive and negative control groups for each outcome. These values are then used to calculate the standardised effect size using Eq. (5.6) for the pooled within-group standard deviation. The `abs()` function ensures that the numerator is always positive.

```
> # calculate mean and variance for Outcome A
> with(assay.window, tapply(A, condition, mean))
   neg    pos
10.390 14.985
> with(assay.window, tapply(A, condition, var))
    neg     pos
3.31253 6.86134
>
> # standardised effect size
> abs(10.390 - 14.985) / sqrt((3.31253 + 6.86134)/2)
[1] 2.03731
>
>
> # calculate mean and variance for Outcome B
> with(assay.window, tapply(B, condition, mean))
   neg    pos
10.695 25.815
```

```
> with(assay.window, tapply(B, condition, var))
    neg     pos
16.3310 70.4434
>
> # standardised effect size
> abs(10.695 - 25.815) / sqrt((16.3310 + 70.4434)/2)
[1] 2.29547
```

The two outcomes can now be compared because they are on the same standardised scale, which is in 'standard deviation units'. An effect size of 1.5 indicates that the means of the two groups are one-and-a-half standard deviations apart, so the larger the value the better the assay window. Standardised effect sizes are less intuitive than unstandardised effect sizes and are only used here to compare two outcomes. The numerator of Eq. (5.4) could be positive or negative and the sign is ignored, only the magnitude of the effect size is important. Outcome B is preferred because it has a larger effect size (2.30) than Outcome A (2.04).

An assumption of this calculation is that the values are normally distributed. If there are outliers then the median and median absolute deviation (MAD) can replace the mean and standard deviation in Eq. (5.4). Also, with few positive and negative control samples the uncertainty in the estimated mean and SD will be large. We have calculated point estimates for the two effect sizes but not the uncertainty in these estimates, such as 95% CIs. Although this is possible, what we want to know when planning an experiment is whether the difference in effect size will have any practical difference in the number of samples required. This is the topic of the next section, and Box 5.1 summarises the criteria for choosing an outcome variable.

Box 5.1 **Properties of good outcome variables**

Qualitative:

- Precedence
- Measured objectively
- Measured close to the action

Quantitative:

- Unlikely to be missing
- Unlikely to be censored
- Normally distributed
- High information content
- Good sensitivity and specificity
- Good reliability
- Good assay window

5.2 Power analysis and sample size calculations

Before conducting an experiment, it is useful to know, if only approximately, the chance that it will be successful. A successful experiment is one that finds a true effect or relationship, or that correctly concludes that no effect or relationship exists. The probability that an experiment or a statistical procedure detects a real effect is called the *power* of the experiment or procedure. Being a probability, power ranges from zero to one, but is often converted into a percentage. Thus, an experiment with 80% power has a probability of 0.8 of successfully detecting a real effect; that is, to reject the null hypothesis.

There are two types of power calculations. The first is *prospective power* and is calculated before the experiment to determine a suitable sample size. The second is *retrospective* or *observed power* and is calculated after the experiment with the data that were obtained. Since there is a one-to-one mapping from *p*-values to observed power, observed power provides no new information or insights. Hoenig and Heisey describe the use of observed power as flawed [156], and others also argue against its use [138, 229, 232, 352, 357].[4] Only prospective power is discussed below.

The design of the experiment and the analysis must be chosen before calculating the power or sample size. How to choose and compare designs is discussed in Section 5.3, and here we assume that the design and analysis have been chosen and proceed from there. Five pieces of information are required for the calculations, usually four are available, and they are used to calculate the fifth. They are:

1. **Sample size (*N*).** This is the number of experimental units. When performing a sample size calculation, this value is calculated from the others.
2. **Effect size (ES).** Depending on the experiment, the ES could be the correlation between two variables, the difference between two means, the difference between two proportions, or the ratio of the between-group to within-group variability (for an ANOVA). The values used for the ES are usually the minimum effect that one is interested in detecting or the predicted size of the effect. When the ES is calculated from the other values, the interest is in determining the smallest effect that can be detected.
3. **Variability of the outcome (σ^2).** Refers to the within-group variability (for example, Eq. (5.5)). The variability may be available from previous experiments, but is usually estimated from published studies or an educated guess. It is a prediction about the variability that will be observed in a future experiment.[5]
4. **Power.** If this is chosen by the researcher, values of 0.8 or 0.9 are often used. When performing a power analysis, this value is calculated from the others.
5. **Significance threshold (α).** This is usually set at 0.05.

[4] Gelman and Carlin discuss the use of a retrospective 'design analysis', which resembles a power analysis but focuses instead on the probability of obtaining significant results in the wrong direction and an estimate of how much the effect size is overestimated [128].

[5] In most calculations the standard deviation (σ) is used instead of the variance (σ^2).

The only equation shown in this section is

$$\text{Power} \propto \frac{ES\,\alpha\,\sqrt{n}}{\sigma^2}, \tag{5.7}$$

which shows the relationship between the five items [320]. This equation shows that power increases as (1) the ES increases, (2) α increases (that is, a less stringent threshold is used), (3) the sample size increases, and (4) the variability decreases. Power is shown as proportional to ($\propto$) the other items because the details depend on the specific analysis.

When planning an experiment there are three related questions that can be asked:

1. What sample size is required? This is a sample size calculation.
2. What is the power of the experiment? This is a power analysis.
3. What is the smallest effect that can be detected in this experiment?

The questions are related because they use the same equation (Eq. (5.7)), but solve for a different unknown in each case.

5.2.1 Calculating the sample size

The assay window data in Figure 5.5 are used for this example and recall that Outcome B had a larger standardised effect size and was therefore a better outcome, but we were unsure if this represented a real improvement over Outcome A. We can decide by calculating the sample size required for both outcomes, and if Outcome B requires fewer samples then it is better. For this calculation the power is fixed at 0.8 and the significance threshold at 0.05. The difference in means and the variability in the outcomes can be calculated from the data in `assay.window` using Eq. (5.5). This provides the four values needed to determine the sample size.

The `power.t.test()` function can answer all three of the above questions by calculating the sample size, power, or the minimum detectable effect. The function requires four of the five items in Eq. (5.7) to be specified and these are used to calculate the fifth item that was left unspecified (this argument is set to `NULL` in the function). The function has other options such as the type of *t*-test (independent or paired samples) and whether a one- or two-tailed is used. The default values are independent samples and two-tailed, which corresponds to our design and so do not need to be specified.

Using the summary statistics for Outcome A calculated above (the code below Eq. (5.5) on page 204), the mean difference is $14.985 - 10.390 = 4.595$ and the pooled within-group standard deviation is $\sqrt{(3.31253 + 6.86134)/2} = 2.25542$. In the code below, these values are provided to `power.t.test()`, the power is set to 0.8, and the significance level to 0.05. `n` is set to `NULL` because this is the value we want to calculate. The output returns five values, the four that were provided and the fifth that was calculated, which was the

⚠ sample size `n = 4.95395`. The reported sample size is the number for *each* group, so the experiment will require $5 + 5 = 10$ samples to have an 80% chance of detecting a 4.595 unit difference between the two groups.

```
> # Outcome A in assay.window data set
> power.t.test(n = NULL, delta = 4.595, sd = 2.25542,
+              sig.level = 0.05, power = 0.8)

     Two-sample t test power calculation

              n = 4.95395
          delta = 4.595
             sd = 2.25542
      sig.level = 0.05
          power = 0.8
    alternative = two.sided

NOTE: n is number in *each* group
```

The same approach is taken to calculate the sample size for Outcome B in the `assay.window` data set.

```
> # Outcome B in assay.window data set
> power.t.test(n = NULL, delta = 15.12, sd = 6.5869,
+              sig.level = 0.05, power = 0.8)

     Two-sample t test power calculation

              n = 4.19528
          delta = 15.12
             sd = 6.5869
      sig.level = 0.05
          power = 0.8
    alternative = two.sided

NOTE: n is number in *each* group
```

Outcome A requires 4.95 samples per group while Outcome B requires 4.20. Since it is impossible to have a fraction of a sample, it is customary to round these values upward to the nearest whole number because it is better to slightly overestimate than underestimate the number of samples required. For both outcomes the sample size is rounded up to five in each group, or 10 samples in total. Because the same number of samples are required for both outcomes, the size of the assay window does not distinguish between them, and other criteria must be used (although Outcome B will have slightly greater power).

A more common use for a sample size calculation is to determine the number of samples required to detect the smallest difference that is considered biologically or clinically relevant. The treatments used in an experiment will likely be less effective than the positive control, and a larger sample size than what we calculated above will be required. Suppose we decide to use Outcome A from Figure 5.5, which had a difference between groups of 4.6 units. Furthermore, suppose that we are interested in detecting a minimum difference of 3 units between groups with 80% power.

The R code below calculates the number of samples required when the minimum relevant difference is defined to be three (`delta = 3`). The values of the other arguments for Outcome A are the same, and here `n` is set to NULL because we want to solve for the sample size. The output indicates that 10 samples per group are required (`n = 9.93121`), or a total sample size of 20.

```
> # Outcome A with smallest relevant difference
> power.t.test(n = NULL, delta = 3, sd = 2.25542,
+              sig.level = 0.05, power = 0.8)

     Two-sample t test power calculation

              n = 9.93121
          delta = 3
             sd = 2.25542
      sig.level = 0.05
          power = 0.8
    alternative = two.sided

NOTE: n is number in *each* group
```

When performing sample size calculations researchers are often surprised at the large number of samples required. A common response is to question the variability and effect size values that were used. If the sample size calculation is required for a grant application, then the first calculation is often followed by some tweaking of the options until the sample size is what the researcher thinks is suitable. It is not uncommon for researchers (or statisticians acting on their behalf) to retrofit a sample size calculation to justify a predetermined sample size. This makes sample size calculations a box-ticking exercise, and if used in this way, is a waste of everyone's time. In practice, three factors determine the number of samples. The first is feasibility; there may be limits on what one experimenter can do in a fixed period of time, the number of cages that one research group can use, or the availability of patient samples. The second factor is the amount of resources investigators are willing to spend on the experiment. Finally, convention; if other labs (that is, potential peer-reviewers) are using 5–8 animals per group, then it would be hard for them to criticise a study that used a similar number of animals.

The purpose of a sample size calculation is to know if there is any point in carrying out the experiment. If the power turns out to be 40% for the number of samples that can be afforded, then there is little chance of getting a significant result – assuming that the effect exists. If so, we might decide that it is not worth conducting the experiment, or that more samples are required and we'll forgo another experiment.

5.2.2 Calculating power

Instead of fixing power and calculating the sample size, the sample size can be fixed at the maximum number feasible and the power that this provides can be calculated. Suppose that only six samples per group are available for the experiment with Outcome A in Figure 5.5, and that we want to detect an effect size of three. What is the probability of detecting this effect?

In the R code below the effect size is set to `delta = 3`, the sample size to `n = 6`, and the power left unspecified (`power = NULL`). The calculated power is approximately 0.55. In other words, there is only a 55% chance of getting a significant result for our chosen effect size and variability. Since the power is low, we need to decide if it is worth performing the experiment. If so, more resources need to be invested.

```
> # Outcome A for power
> power.t.test(n = 6, delta = 3, sd = 2.25542,
+              sig.level = 0.05, power = NULL)

     Two-sample t test power calculation

              n = 6
          delta = 3
             sd = 2.25542
      sig.level = 0.05
          power = 0.547994
    alternative = two.sided

NOTE: n is number in *each* group
```

5.2.3 Calculating the minimum detectable effect

It is often useful to calculate the smallest effect that can be detected for a given power and sample size. The values for Outcome A in the `assay.window` data set are used once again. In the code below we specify that the sample size is eight in each group (assume this is all we can use) and that power is 80%. The effect size (`delta`) is left unspecified and the output shows that the smallest mean difference between groups that can be detected is about 3.4. Based on the research question, experimental system, and background knowledge, we can conclude either that such a large effect is unlikely, and so the experiment should not be conducted with a sample size of eight, or that the effect size (or an even larger one) is likely and that the experiment should proceed.

```
> # Outcome A: calculate minimum detectable effect
> power.t.test(n = 8, delta = NULL, sd = 2.25542,
+              sig.level = 0.05, power = 0.8)

     Two-sample t test power calculation

              n = 8
          delta = 3.39812
             sd = 2.25542
      sig.level = 0.05
          power = 0.8
    alternative = two.sided

NOTE: n is number in *each* group
```

5.2.4 Power curves

In the above examples, all but one of the items that go into a power analysis were fixed at a single value, and the value for the remaining item was calculated. This provides a narrow view of how one item varies as a function of the others. When planning an experiment it is useful to know how the calculated value varies as the other items vary. For example, how quickly does the power increase as a function of the sample size, how is this affected by increases or decreases in the variability, and how does this vary across different effect sizes? These questions put the calculated values into context.

In the code below, power is calculated for five estimates of variability (`SD`), two effect sizes (`diff`), and 18 sample sizes (`N`). The `expand.grid()` function creates a matrix with all possible combinations of these values and a column of `NA` values is added to store the calculated power values. The first few rows are shown and the total number of rows is 180.

```
> # various sample sizes, SDs, and mean differences
> pow <- expand.grid(N=seq(5, 40, 2),
+                    SD=seq(1.85, 2.65, 0.2),
+                    diff=c(1.5, 2),
+                    power=NA)
>
> head(pow)
   N   SD diff power
1  5 1.85  1.5    NA
2  7 1.85  1.5    NA
3  9 1.85  1.5    NA
4 11 1.85  1.5    NA
```

```
5 13 1.85  1.5    NA
6 15 1.85  1.5    NA
>
> dim(pow)
[1] 180   4
```

Next, we loop through each row of the data frame and calculate the power using the specification for the sample size, variability, and effect size in that row, and then save the result back to the data frame. The power value from the `power.t.test()` function is extracted with `$power`.

```
> # Calculate power for each combination
> for (i in 1:nrow(pow)){
+     pow$power[i] <- power.t.test(delta = pow$diff[i],
+                                  n=pow$N[i], sd = pow$SD[i],
+                                  sig.level = 0.05)$power
+ }
```

Then, the code below plots the results in Figure 5.6.

```
> xyplot(power ~ N|factor(diff), data=pow, groups=SD, type="l",
+        ylab="Power", xlab="Sample size per group",
+        ylim=c(0,1), between=list(x=1),
+        strip = strip.custom(var.name=c("Effect size"), strip.names=TRUE),
+        scales=list(alternating=FALSE),
+        auto.key=list(columns=1, space="right",
+            points=FALSE, lines=TRUE, title="SD"))
```

The nonlinear relationship between the sample size and power can be seen. Increasing the sample size from 10 to 20 results in a large increase in power, but a similar increase from 30 to 40 results in a much smaller increase in power. There are diminishing returns to increasing the sample size. By drawing a horizontal line at the desired power, say 0.8, one can determine when experimental objectives will be achieved by finding where the horizontal line intersects with the curves and dropping a vertical line down to find the corresponding sample size. For example, when the effect size is 1.5 (left panel) 25 samples are required if the standard deviation is 1.85 and 40 samples if the variability is 2.25.

5.2.5 Simulation-based power analysis

Standard power and sample size calculations only provide a single estimate and the power curves in Figure 5.6 ignore that some effect size and variability values are more likely than others. The power tells us that *if* the planned experiment has a given difference between the

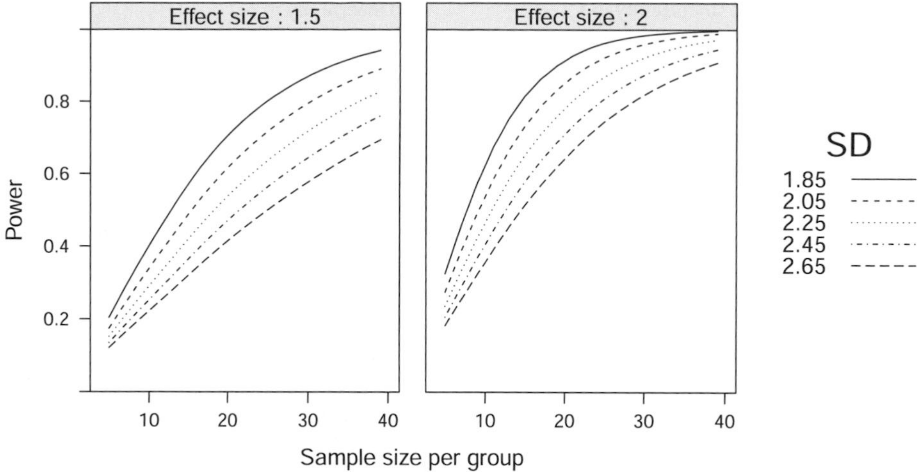

Fig. 5.6 Power as a function of the sample size, effect size, and within-group variability (SD).

groups and variability, then there is fixed probability of getting a significant result. But it is unlikely that the effect size and variability will be *exactly* the values used in the calculation, so the actual power will be different. If we are unlucky and get a smaller effect size and larger variability, then the power will be much lower.

Power analyses and sample size calculations are predictions about future experiments based on background information, prior data, and some educated guesses. The inputs (variability and effect size) are uncertain and therefore so are the outputs (power and sample size). There is little value in reporting a prediction without also reporting a confidence in that prediction. Yet, this is standard practice – and what we did in the above calculations.

A standard sample size calculation answers the question, 'What sample size do I need to have 80% power?' A better question to ask is 'What sample size do I need to be 90% certain that the experiment will have 80% power?' By representing the effect size, variability, or both as a distribution instead of a single value, this second question can be addressed [359]. Using the results for Outcome A in the `assay.window` data set once again, suppose an effect size of 4.6 is the most likely value – one that we would have used in a standard calculation. We need to choose a distribution to represent our uncertainty in this value and a normal distribution is suitable because it has a peak at 4.6 and then drops off symmetrically. The standard deviation for the normal distribution reflects the uncertainly around the value of 4.6. Since it is hard to think in standard deviations, we can choose a 95% confidence interval and then calculate the required standard deviation. Suppose we are 95% certain that the effect size will be between 4.5 and 4.7, which is 0.1 units above and below the mean. The standard deviation can then be approximated by taking half the distance from the mean to the upper or lower 95% interval ($0.1/2 = 0.05$) and this distribution is the left histogram in Figure 5.7. Where does the 95% interval come from? It can come from existing data, just like the effect size used in the calculations, but more often it reflects our uncertainty in the value. Representing uncertainty as a probability distribution may be an unfamiliar procedure and some may be uncomfortable with introducing a subjective element into the

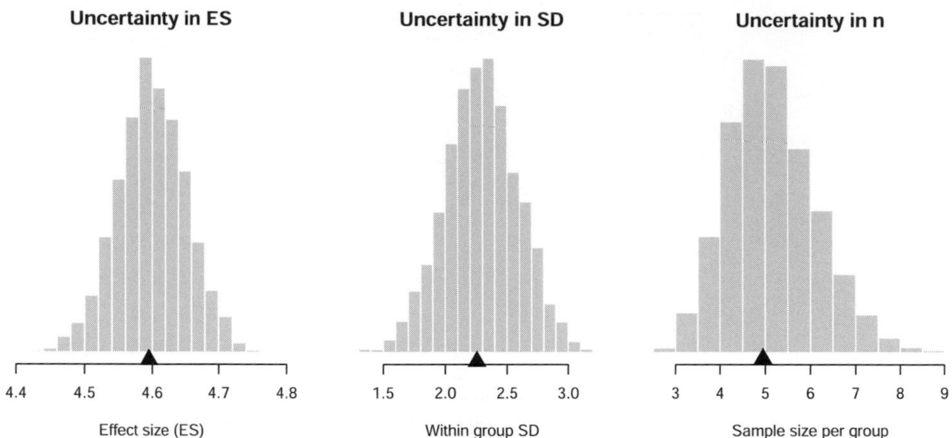

Fig. 5.7 Simulation-based sample size calculations. The uncertainty in the effect size and variability is represented with a normal distribution. The number of samples required also has a distribution from which we can calculate useful summaries. Black triangles are the values from the standard sample size calculation.

calculations. But choosing a value of 4.6 for the effect size is just as subjective, and is identical to using a normal distribution with a standard deviation of zero; in other words, that one is 100% certain that the effect size will be 4.6 – a highly unrealistic assumption.

A similar approach is taken with the within-group standard deviation. The uncertainty is represented by a normal distribution with a mean of 2.3 (our estimate of the most likely value) and a standard deviation of 0.3, to give a 95% interval from about 1.7 to 2.9 (middle histogram in Figure 5.7). Since standard deviations can only be positive numbers and it is important to check that the distribution includes no negative values.

To perform a power analysis via simulation a value for the effect size and within-group variability are generated from their respective distributions and then used to calculate the sample size in the usual manner. This is repeated many times giving the distribution of sample sizes. In the code below, 5000 values for the effect size (`delta`) and within-group variability (`sigma`) are generated from normal distributions with the parameters specified above. These values are then combined into a data frame and the first few lines are shown.

```
> set.seed(1)
> # generate values for mean difference and within group SD
> delta <- rnorm(5000, 4.6, 0.05)
> sigma <- rnorm(5000,  2.3, 0.3)
>
> # combine into a data frame
> vals <- data.frame(delta=delta, sd=sigma)
>
> head(vals)
    delta      sd
```

```
1 4.56868 1.84509
2 4.60918 2.48874
3 4.55822 1.79654
4 4.67976 2.65393
5 4.61648 2.63530
6 4.55898 1.92868
```

The sample size is calculated for each of the 5000 pairs of values, but instead of using a `for()` loop like the previous example, the more efficient `apply()` function is used. The `vals` data frame is given as the first argument to the `apply()` function, the `1` indicates that the processing will be done on the rows (2 means columns), and then we supply the values to the `power.t.test()` function, and also extract the sample size with `$n`.

```
> # calculate samp size for each combination of effect size
> # and within group SD
> res <- apply(vals, 1, function (x){
+                   power.t.test(delta = x[1], sd = x[2],
+                                power=0.8)$n })
```

The code below plots the distributions and the distribution of calculated sample sizes is the right histogram in Figure 5.7.

```
> par(mfrow=c(1,3),
+     mar=c(4.5,1.5,3,0.5))
> hist(delta, breaks=20, col="grey", border="white",
+      main="Uncertainty in ES", xlab="Effect size (ES)",
+      ylab="", yaxt="n")
> points(x=4.595, y=-20, pch=17, cex=2)
>
> hist(sigma, breaks=20, col="grey", border="white",
+      main="Uncertainty in SD", xlab="Within group SD",
+      ylab="", yaxt="n")
> points(x=2.255, y=-20, pch=17, cex=2)
>
> hist(res, breaks=20, col="grey", border="white",
+      main="Uncertainty in n", xlab="Sample size per group",
+      ylab="", yaxt="n", xlim=c(3,9))
> points(x=4.95, y=-20, pch=17, cex=2)
```

Since a distribution of sample sizes is available, other information can be calculated. The most relevant summary addresses a question posed earlier: if we want to be 90% certain that we have at least 80% power, how many samples are required? The code below uses the quantile() function to answer this question. The 0.9 quantile is the value that divides the sample size distribution into the lower 90% and the upper 10%. This tells us the sample size that ensures that we have at least 80% power in 90% of the simulations.

```
> # how many samples to ensure 90% prob of 80% power?
> quantile(res, 0.9)
    90%
6.47136
```

The sample size is 7 per group (rounding up from 6.47), which is greater than the 5 per group originally calculated, but ensures that the power will be at least 80% even if we are unlucky and have a smaller effect size or larger variability.

The above examples relied on the power.t.test() function, but if we are simulating data then we can dispense with built-in functions altogether. The idea is to simulate *data* from a hypothesised model with a chosen sample size, effect size, and within group SD. The simulated data are then analysed with the desired test and we note whether the *p*-value is less than 0.05. This procedure is repeated many times, say 10 000, and the proportion of significant results out of the total number of simulations is the power of the test. This approach offers complete flexibility to specify the model and parameters. The code below creates a function called sim.reg() that we use to calculate the power of a linear regression analysis. Suppose we are testing a compound at doses of 0, 5, 10, and 20 mg/kg and we want to know the power to detect a linear trend. The function takes as input the sample size at each dose (n), the intercept (the value of the outcome when dose equals zero), the slope, which is the main parameter of interest, and the within group SD (sigma). The values for the predictor variable (i.e. design points) are hard-coded in this example in the vector x, but they could be provided as arguments as well. The second line of code in the function simulates the errors based on the value of sigma. These are the deviations from the mean of each dose and provide the within group variation in the data. The values are generated from a normal distribution with a mean of zero and we need one value for each data point; length(x) automatically calculates the number of values required based on the number of elements in the predictor variable x. The third line of code generates the data, and you may recognise this as the equation for a straight line, plus the errors (e). The final line uses aov() to analyse the simulated data and the brackets at the end extract the *p*-value for the slope, which is returned as the output of the function.

```
> sim.reg <- function(n, intercept, slope, sigma){
+     # values for x
+     x <- rep(c(0, 5, 10, 20), each=n)
+
+     # use within group SD to calculate errors
+     e <- rnorm(length(x), 0, sigma)
+
+     # generate data
```

```
+     y <- intercept + slope * x + e
+
+     # calculate and return p-value
+     summary(aov(y ~ x))[[1]]["x", "Pr(>F)"]
+ }
```

The code below calculates the p-value for one simulated data set with a slope of 10 and 5 observations at each of the four doses, and the result is significant. To determine the power, we repeat this procedure 10 000 times using the `replicate()` function and calculate the proportion of significant p-values, which is about 74%.

```
> # run one simulation
> set.seed(1)
> sim.reg(n=5, intercept=10, slope=0.25, sigma=3)
[1] 0.00230296
>
> # run 10000 simulations and save p-values
> set.seed(1)
> pvals <- replicate(10000, sim.reg(n=5, intercept=10, slope=0.25, sigma=3))
>
> # power (proportion of significant p-values)
> sum(pvals < 0.05) / 10000
[1] 0.7416
```

The above function can be modified in many ways. For example, we could allow the sample size to vary at each dose to see the effect on power (see the discussion of Figure 5.8, p. 221). We could allow the within-group SD to vary by dose to see what happens to the power when the variances are unequal. We could calculate a second p-value from an analysis that treats dose as a categorical factor instead of a continuous variable, and the function can return both. Or, we could incorporate uncertainty in the slope and within-group SD by allowing them to vary from run to run by drawing values from a distribution. Finally, more complex models with multiple effects can be simulated.

Most of the above examples were for a simple two group design that would be analysed with an independent samples t-test. The `power.t.test()` function used for those examples can also be used for a paired design or for testing if a single mean differs from a specified value. The functions `power.anova.test()` and `power.prop.test()` in the base R installation are used in a similar way for one-way ANOVA designs or comparing proportions. Functions for other tests and designs can be found in the `pwr` and `powerAnalysis` packages. One useful function from the `pwr` package is `pwr.t2n.test()`, which can handle two groups with unequal sample sizes. This is useful if the sample size is fixed for one group (e.g. number of clinical samples available), but the other group can be increased to reach the desired power. The `pwr` package also has a function to calculate power and

Sample size calculations are essential for maximising the chance of a successful *confirmatory* experiment and simulations are recommended because the uncertainty in the variation and effect size is incorporated. Traditional sample size calculations, as shown above, are for hypothesis testing (Section 1.4, p. 38). But for studies where parameter estimation (Section 1.4, p. 42) is more relevant a better objective is to calculate the sample size required to obtain a given precision for an estimate (e.g. a difference between groups); in other words, calculate the sample size required to have confidence intervals of a given width. Maxwell, Kelly, and Rausch describe these *accuracy in parameter estimation* (AIPE) methods [182, 266], and provide some R code in their 2003 paper [182].

The low power of many published studies has been discussed for nearly half a century. The first edition of Cohen's classic book on the topic was published in 1969 and focused on the behavioural sciences [78], but a recent review of the neuroscience literature found that not much has changed over the years [65]. Maxwell points out a paradox: scientists continue to conduct underpowered studies, yet they want significant effects so that they can publish, which high power would enable them to do [265]. Maxwell argues that low powered studies persist because experiments have multiple analyses or hypotheses, and although the power for any individual analysis is low, taken together, there is a good chance that some results will be significant.

5.3 Optimal experimental designs (rules of thumb)

The goal of optimal experimental design is to maximise the amount of information obtained given fixed resources by obtaining precise estimates and thus greater power to detect true effects. Optimal designs can reduce the number of samples required, thereby saving time and resources. When we calculated the power and sample size above, the experimental design was taken as given. But how do we decide on the design itself? There is a large literature on optimal experimental designs, and much of it highly technical. The aim of this section is to provide some rules of thumb that can be applied to improve many biological experiments.

To say that a design is optimal implies that it is optimal with respect to some criterion, and optimising one criterion often means being less optimal for another. When the optimisation reflects the goals of the experiment, the likelihood of a successful experiment is increased.

Suppose we are interested in testing a compound. Figure 5.8 shows several designs that we will use in this section to discuss options for designing an experiment. The figure shows 9 designs with 20 samples (experimental units) and depicts several ways of distributing these samples across doses of a compound. Assume that assigning samples to the doses is under the experimenter's control.

The code below shows how the designs were generated and can be referred to later in the chapter to remember what the variables `x1`, `x2`, and so on mean. The graphs in

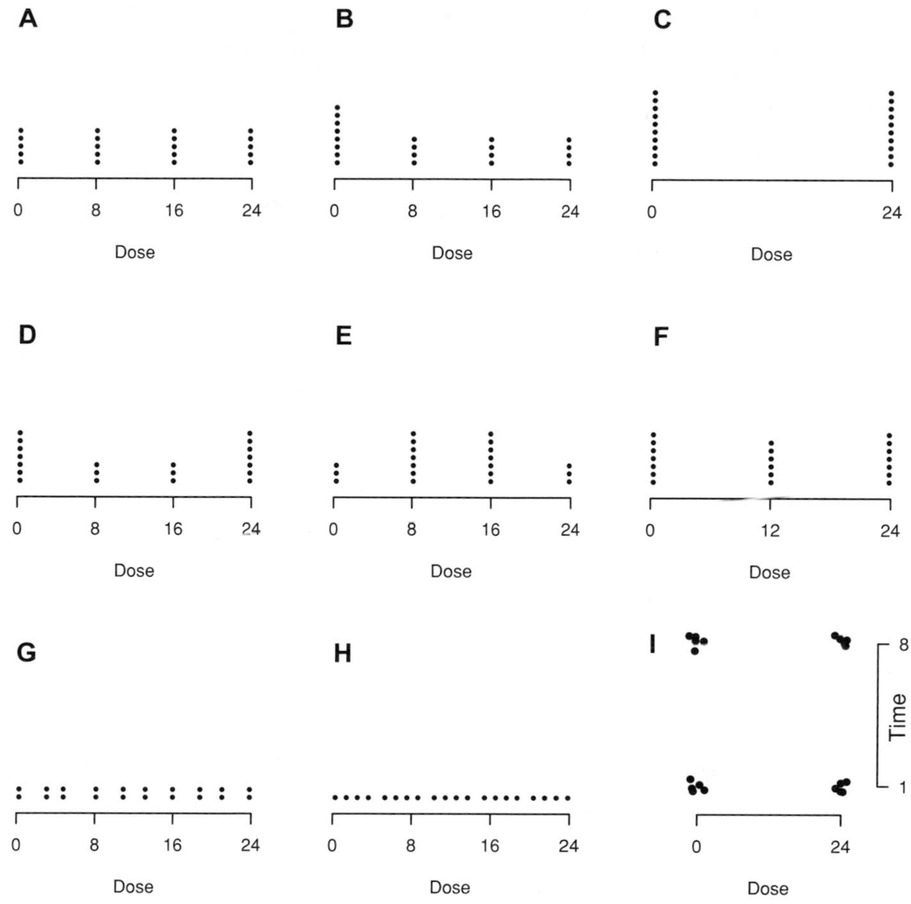

Fig. 5.8 Nine designs with 20 samples (black dots). All designs have the same design space for Dose (0–24 mg/kg) but different design points and number of samples per-design point. Design (I) has Time as an additional variable.

Figure 5.8 were created with the `dotPlot()` function in the `BHH2` package and the code for the first plot is shown.

```
>                                                          # Panel in graph
> x1 <- rep(c(0,8,16,24), each=5)                          # A
> x2 <- rep(c(0,8,16,24), times=c(8,4,4,4))                # B
> x3 <- rep(c(0,24), each=10)                              # C
> x4 <- rep(c(0,8,16,24), times=c(7,3,3,7))                # D
> x5 <- rep(c(0,8,16,24), times=c(3,7,7,3))                # E
> x6 <- rep(c(0,12,24), times=c(7,6,7))                    # F
> x7 <- rep(round(seq(0,24, length.out=10),0), each=2)     # G
> x8 <- round(seq(0,24, length.out=20),1)                  # H
> z1 <- rep(c(1,8,1,8), each=5) # time variable            # I
```

```
> library(BHH2)
> dotPlot(x1, pch=16, xlab="Dose", base=FALSE, axes = FALSE)
> axis(1, at=c(0,8,16,24))
```

The first thing to consider is the range of values for continuous predictor variables; for example, the minimum and maximum dose, concentration, time, age, pH, or cell density. A minimum value of zero often makes sense and the highest level is based on biological or technological considerations. The range that a predictor variable takes is called the *design region* or *design space*. In Figure 5.8, the main predictor variable is the dose of a drug and in all examples the minimum is 0 and the maximum is 24 mg/kg.

Once the minimum and maximum values have been selected, one also has to decide if intermediate values will be used, and if so, which ones. The values of the predictor where observations are made are called the *design points* or *support points* and include the minimum, maximum, and all intermediate points. In Figure 5.8, the options range from no intermediate design points (C) to having 20 design points (H). The spacing between the design points is the same in all the examples, but this need not be the case and in Section 5.3.7 we discuss when unequal spacing is beneficial.

Once the design points and total sample size have been decided, there is still the question of how many samples to allocate to each design point. An equal number of samples at each design point is often the default, but it may not always be the best option.

A final point to consider is whether to include other variables. If so, how much precision is lost in estimating the main effect of interest. Figure 5.8I includes Time as an another variable, which enables another effect to be estimated with the same number of samples.

How do we choose between these designs (plus others not shown in the figure)? The short answer is that the goals of the experiment along with background knowledge will determine the best design. Some designs are excellent for some goals and poor for others, while other designs are not especially good or bad for any goal but are reasonably good for many. Goals that we might have are:

1. Determine if the compound is active at all.
2. Determine if the compound is active at a given dose.
3. Verify that the dose–response is linear within a given range of doses.
4. Estimate a full dose–response curve.
5. Determine the minimum effective dose (MED) or the dose that gives half of the maximum response (ED50).

A good design estimates effect sizes and other parameters with high precision, meaning that the variance of the estimate is small (precision is the reciprocal of variance). Such a design is *efficient* and has greater power to reject a null hypothesis. By making the estimates that address the goal of the experiment as precise as possible, the chance of finding true effects is increased.

Relative efficiency (RE) is the efficiency of the optimal (or better) design over the efficiency of another less efficient design:

$$\mathrm{RE} = \frac{\text{Efficiency of better design}}{\text{Efficiency of worse design}} \tag{5.8}$$

and will always be less than one because the efficiency values are variances, and the variance in the numerator will be smaller than the variance in the denominator. Relative efficiency can be used to compare the efficiencies of two designs and to calculate the number of additional samples required with the less efficient design to achieve the same power as the more efficient design. For example, suppose the variance for an efficient design is 12 and for another less efficient design is 15.5. The relative efficiency is therefore $RE = 12/15.5 = 0.77$ and we would need approximately $1/0.77 = 1.3$ times as many samples with the less efficient design.

In the examples below we assume that the variance is constant in all groups and the data are normally distributed. The analyses do not tell us what sample size to use because that would require an estimate of the within-group standard deviation. We only find the design that has the highest precision, but even the optimal or most efficient design can be underpowered, so one would first choose an efficient design, and then use that for the power calculations.

5.3.1 Use equal n with two groups

Suppose we have an experiment with two groups and the total sample size is $N = 20$ (Figure 5.8C). n_1 samples are allocated to Group 1, $n_2 = N - n_1$ samples are allocated to Group 2, and we have to decide how many samples to allocate to each group. Intuition suggests that an equal number of samples in each group is best such that $n_1 = n_2 = N/2$ (assuming that N is an even number), and this does indeed provide the most power for testing differences between the means of the groups. Suppose that the outcome is a continuous variable and the means of the two groups will be compared with an independent samples t-test. The variance of the difference between means (that is, the uncertainty in the size of the effect) is equal to

$$\sigma^2 \sqrt{\frac{1}{n_1} + \frac{1}{n_2}}, \tag{5.9}$$

where σ^2 is the within-group variance. The value of σ^2 is not required for comparing efficiencies and we can ignore it. In the R code below, a vector of sample sizes is generated for `n1` from 10 to 18, and another for `n2` from 10 to 2, such that the sum of the sample sizes for the two groups always equals 20.

```
> # sample sizes for two groups
> n1 <- 10:18
> n2 <- 10:2
>
```

```
> # confirm that total is 20
> n1 + n2
[1] 20 20 20 20 20 20 20 20 20
```

Next, we calculate the variance of the estimator using Eq. (5.9), store it in the vector v, and plot it against the sample size of n1. Setting xaxt=''n'' suppresses the x-axis labels so that we can draw our own using the axis() function. The result is in Figure 5.9, which shows how the variance of the mean difference (y-axis) increases as the sample size imbalance increases.

```
> # variance of the estimator
> v <- sqrt(1/n1 + 1/n2)
>
> par(las=1,
+     mar=c(5.1,7,1,1))
> plot(v ~ n1, type="b", xaxt="n", xlab="",
+      ylab="")
> axis(1, at=n1)
> axis(1, at=n1, labels=n2, line=1.5, tick=FALSE)
> axis(1, at=9, labels=~n[1], xpd=TRUE,
+      tick=FALSE, font=2)
> axis(1, at=9, labels=~n[2], xpd=TRUE,
+      tick=FALSE, font=2, line=1.5)
>
> mtext(expression(sqrt(frac(1,n[1]) + frac(1,n[2]))), side=2, line=4)
> mtext("Balance of samples", side=1, line=4)
```

Suppose we want to calculate the relative efficiency of a balanced design with one that has a 18:2 allocation. The code below shows that we need to divide the variance of the estimator for the balanced design (stored in the first element of v) by the variance of the design with an 18:2 sample allocation (stored in v[9]). Compared with a balanced design, having 18 samples in one group and 2 in the other has a RE of $(0.45/0.75) \times 100 = 60\%$. Or, the 18:2 design requires 1.7 times more samples to have the same power as the 10:10 design. Efficiencies for the other allocation ratios can be calculated in a similar way.

```
> # Relative efficiency
> v[1]/v[9]
[1] 0.6
>
> # number of additional samples
> v[9]/v[1]
[1] 1.66667
```

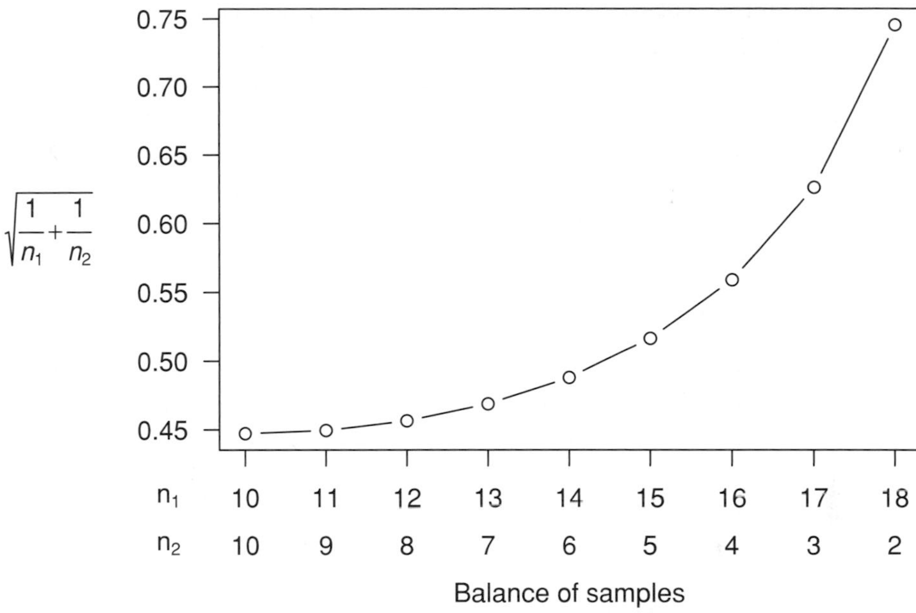

Fig. 5.9 Efficiency of estimating a mean difference. The *y*-axis is the variance of the estimate and lower values are better. An 18:2 sample allocation requires 1.7 times more samples compared with a 10:10 allocation.

5.3.2 Use more controls when comparing multiple groups to the control

The objective of some experiments is to compare several treatment groups to a common control group, and comparing treatment groups to each other is less relevant; for example, determining if three compounds are active in a biochemical or cellular assay. Here, the interest is in determining whether each compound is active, and there is less interest in determining if one compound is better than another because all active compounds will be progressed further along the drug discovery pipeline; the activities relative to each other are unimportant at this stage. The research question is only 'is a compound active?'.

If all possible comparisons are equally important, then an equal sample size in all groups has the most power for all comparisons. If, however, the goal of the experiment is to compare each treatment group with the control group, then an unequal allocation of samples has greater power. Let N represent the total sample size and t the number of treatment groups (excluding the control group). Assume that all comparisons with the control group are equally important and therefore the sample size in each treatment group will be the same, denoted as n_t. The number of samples in the control group is n_C. Then, the optimal design allocates $\sqrt{t}$ more samples to the control group than to the treated groups [23]. In the example with three compounds, whatever we choose for n_t we need $\sqrt{t} = \sqrt{3} = 1.73$ times more for the control group. The result will be a decimal number, and so we round to the nearest whole number (or up to the next whole number). This experiment is represented by the arrangement in Figure 5.8B, but assume that the 8, 16, and 24 dose groups are different compounds instead of different doses of the same compound.

The calculation can be done in R as follows. First, determine the number of treated groups, `t` (excluding the control group). Then, determine the number of additional samples required in the control group by calculating the scaling factor as `sqrt(t)`. If the number of samples in the treated groups is `n.t`, the number of samples in the control group will be `n.c = n.t * sqrt(t)`, and rounded to the nearest whole number. Finally, calculate the number of control samples and total sample size for different values of `n.t`. The output shows how `N` total samples should be divided between the control and treated group.

```
> t <- 3 # number of treated groups
> k <- sqrt(t) # scaling factor
> n.t <- 2:10  # various sample sizes for treated groups
> n.c <- round(k*n.t) # number in control group
> N <- n.c + t*n.t # total sample size
>
> # combine into data frame
> (data.frame(n.t, n.c, N))
  n.t n.c  N
1   2   3  9
2   3   5 14
3   4   7 19
4   5   9 24
5   6  10 28
6   7  12 33
7   8  14 38
8   9  16 43
9  10  17 47
```

Suppose that the maximum sample size we can afford for our experiment with three compounds is $N = 24$. The above output table shows that we need three treated groups of $n_t = 5$ and one control group of $n_c = 9$ giving a total of $3 \times 5 + 9 = 24$ samples. What is the improvement in efficiency compared with a balanced design, which has $n = 6$ in all treated and control conditions (the total sample size is the same: $4 \times 6 = 24$)? We can use Eq. (5.9) and assume that $\sigma^2 = 1$, so it drops out from the calculations below.

$$
\begin{array}{ccc}
\textbf{Optimal Design} & & \textbf{Equal } n \textbf{ Design} \\
\sqrt{\frac{1}{n_c} + \frac{1}{n_t}} & < & \sqrt{\frac{1}{n_c} + \frac{1}{n_t}} \\
\sqrt{\frac{1}{9} + \frac{1}{5}} & < & \sqrt{\frac{1}{6} + \frac{1}{6}} \\
0.558 & < & 0.577.
\end{array}
\tag{5.10}
$$

The reduction in variance for the optimal design is small (0.558 compared with 0.577) giving a relative efficiency of $0.558/0.577 = 0.97$. However, the 'optimal' design is worse than the balanced design for *treated versus treated* comparisons, but this is the trade-off that has been made. By increasing the precision of the comparisons with the control, we have decreased the precision of comparing the drug groups with each other. But by how much? The variance when comparing any two treated groups with the optimal design is $\sqrt{1/5 + 1/5} = 0.632$ and with the balanced design is $\sqrt{1/6 + 1/6} = 0.577$. The RE for comparing two treated groups for the optimal design is $0.577/0.632 = 0.91$. The loss in efficiency with the optimal design for treated versus treated comparisons (0.91) is greater than the gain in efficiency for the treated versus control group comparison ($1/0.97 = 1.03$). This may or may not be a good trade-off, depending on the objectives of the experiment. This illustrates that 'optimal' is always relative to a specific comparison or set of comparisons. A balanced design may be preferred because of the desire to 'not miss anything' (Section 1.2.2); a balanced design hedges one's bets to find true effects between any comparison. Balance is also advantageous if the groups have unequal variances.

⚠ It follows that having *fewer samples* in the control group is worse than the equal *n* design if the goal is to test for differences from the control. However, sometimes there is little interest in testing the treated groups against the control group because all of the treated groups are known to be different. In the example with three compounds, the control group might only be used to ensure that the experiment is working properly and the comparisons of interest are between the three compounds. In this case it would make sense to have fewer samples in the control group and more in the treated groups.

5.3.3 Use fewer factor levels

Suppose that the goal of an experiment is to determine if a compound has an effect. This is an exploratory study; we are uncertain about the size of the effect, if it exists, and at what doses the effect might be seen. We do not know the form of the dose–response relationship but believe that it is linear within the range of doses we plan to use.

Consider the three designs in Figure 5.8A, C, and F. They all have 20 samples and the same design space, but differ in the number of design points; C has only two, F has three, and A has four. When the underlying variable is continuous the most efficient design to detect an effect is to place all of the samples at the extremes of the design space (Figure 5.8C). This is appropriate if the relationship between dose and the outcome is linear. But what if the relationship is quadratic – a 'U' or inverted 'U' shape – where the compound becomes less effective at high doses? Such a relationship would be impossible to detect with only two design points. A design with two groups maximises the efficiency of detecting a linear effect but has zero efficiency of detecting a quadratic effect. The good news is that only one additional design point is required to detect a quadratic effect (Figure 5.8F), but at the cost of a less efficient estimate for the main goal of the experiment. Adding two additional design points (Figure 5.8A) further reduces the efficiency of testing for an overall linear effect but it does allow a more complicated dose–response relationship to be detected; for example, the outcome first increases, then decreases, then increases again with increasing dose. Such a relationship is biologically unlikely, and so it is probably not a useful design, especially when the cost is a further reduction in efficiency to detect if any effect exists. Given the background to the problem, the design in Figure 5.8F is a good compromise between finding an effect and also verifying that the relationship is linear between 0 and 24 mg/kg.

What is the reduction in efficiency when using a three or four group design compared with a two group design? First, we need to decide on the analysis. Recall from Section 4.3.2 (p. 145) that we can treat the predictor as continuous or categorical, leading to a regression or ANOVA analysis. Dose is treated as continuous here because it is easier to explain the key point, but the same principle applies when dose is categorical. If dose is continuous the main interest is testing if the slope of the line is zero. The efficiency of the design is therefore determined by uncertainty or variance in the estimate of the slope, calculated as

$$\text{var(slope)} = \frac{\sigma^2}{N\,\text{var}(x)}, \tag{5.11}$$

where N is the sample size, σ^2 is the within-group variance (same as in Eq. (5.9)), and var(x) is the variance of the predictor (dose). A small value for var(slope) is desired because it means the estimate of the slope is precise, that is, the confidence intervals are narrow. From Eq. (5.11) we see that var(slope) can be made smaller by

1. **Reducing σ^2.** Reducing noise in the measurements (e.g. choosing a more reliable outcome) makes the estimate of the slope more precise.
2. **Increasing N.** Increasing the sample size is the first and sometimes only option considered, but it costs more and sometimes samples are hard to get.
3. **Increasing var(x).** Increasing the variance of the predictor is rarely considered but can increase the efficiency of a design without additional cost.

Both σ^2 and N are constant in the designs that we are comparing so they cancel out when calculating the relative efficiencies. Thus, the relevant part of Eq. (5.11) for comparing designs is

$$\text{var(slope)} = \frac{1}{\text{var}(x)}. \tag{5.12}$$

The relative efficiency can then be calculated as before by taking the ratio of the optimal or better design (with the *opt* subscript) to the less efficient design:

$$RE = \frac{\text{var(slope}_{\text{opt}})}{\text{var(slope)}} = \frac{\frac{1}{\text{var}(x_{opt})}}{\frac{1}{\text{var}(x)}} = \frac{\text{var}(x)}{\text{var}(x_{opt})}. \tag{5.13}$$

The equation simplifies to comparing the variance of the predictor variables and the code below calculates the variance of dose for each design and the REs.

```
> # calculate variance of predictor
> var(x1) # A
[1] 84.2105
> var(x3) # C
[1] 151.579
> var(x6) # F
```

```
[1] 106.105
>
> # RE
> var(x1)/var(x3) # four vs. two group
[1] 0.555556
>
> var(x6)/var(x3) # three vs. two group
[1] 0.7
```

The variance of x3 for the two group design is the largest and is therefore the most efficient. The four group design (Figure 5.8A) is only 56% as efficient as the two group design (Figure 5.8C), requiring 1.8 times the number of samples (36 instead of 20) to have the same power as the two group design for detecting a linear effect of the compound. This is a substantial reduction in power for what might appear to be a trivial change in the design of the experiment.

The three group design (Figure 5.8F) is only 70% as efficient as the two group design and requires 1.4 times as many samples (28 instead of 20). Although the two group design can only detect a linear relationship, it does so with good efficiency.

The rule of thumb is to use as few factor levels or design points as necessary for the goal of the experiment, and if little is known about the experimental system, only one additional design point is required to check that assumptions hold. For example, if linearity is assumed, only one additional design point is required to verify this assumption. Thus, the more you know about the experimental system the better the experiment that can be designed.

5.3.4 Increase the variance of predictor variables

In the previous section, we saw that by using fewer factor levels the variance of the predictor increases, thereby making the design more efficient. Here we consider other ways of increasing the variance of the predictor. Consider the designs in Figure 5.8A, D, and E. All have 20 samples and the same 4 design points, but they differ in how the samples are distributed at the design points. Figure 5.8A has an equal number of samples at each design point, D has more samples at the highest and lowest doses, and E has more samples at the two middle doses. Suppose once again that there is little background knowledge about the compound and so multiple design points are used. The goal is to determine if an effect exists, and we take it as given that there are four design points. Which design is better? The equal N design is appealing, but we can increase the efficiency of detecting a linear trend by allocating more samples to the extremes as in Figure 5.8D. Allocating more samples to the middle two design points reduces the efficiency of detecting a linear effect.

Placing more samples at the extremes increases the variance of the predictor (dose), which leads to more precise estimates. The rule of thumb is therefore to maximise the variance of the predictor variables. The design in Figure 5.8C has the maximum possible variance, which is why it is the most efficient design for detecting a linear effect. In all three designs the mean dose is 12 and the variances are A = 84, D = 111, and E = 57. The code below calculates the variances and relative efficiencies.

```
> var(x1) # A
[1] 84.2105
> var(x4) # D
[1] 111.158
> var(x5) # E
[1] 57.2632
>
> # RE
> var(x1)/var(x4)
[1] 0.757576
>
> var(x5)/var(x4)
[1] 0.515152
```

Since the design in Figure 5.8D has more points at the extremes, it has the largest variance of the three designs. The relative efficiency of the equal N design (Figure 5.8A) is only 0.75 compared with the design with more samples at the extremes (Figure 5.8D). The REs for the designs in Figure 5.8D versus A is 0.76 and for D versus E is 0.52. McClelland explains in more detail why increasing the variance of the predictor is beneficial and discusses optimal designs for detecting both linear and quadratic effects [268].

Often a predictor variable is a property of the experimental units, such as their age, weight, or disease severity, and is not a treatment to which the subjects are assigned. Figure 5.10 shows an example where an arbitrary outcome for 100 people is plotted against age. The graph on the left has an age range from 20–80 and shows a clear relationship between the variables. The graph on the right has a narrower age range from 40–60 and the relationship looks weak. The same equation was used to generate both data sets and they both have a slope of one. A wide age range is better both visually and statistically. The relative efficiency of the narrow age range design is only 33% – a dramatic loss in power. Therefore, ensure that the predictor variables cover a wide range when selecting subjects and creating inclusion and exclusion criteria. It is the variance of the predictor and not the range per se that matters, but by increasing the range the variance increases as well.

There are two main disadvantages to the unequal N designs (Figure 5.8D and E). The first is that pairwise comparisons between groups with the smallest sample sizes can have lower power. Second, when the variance is not constant across the levels of the predictor unequal N designs can be more problematic.[7] Nevertheless, unequal N designs can provide more power, and at the very least, this rule of thumb applies when the number of samples cannot be divided evenly by the number of groups; the extra samples can be placed either in the control condition or at the extremes.

[7] Unequal variances can sometimes be addressed by data transformations or can be modelled directly; for example, using the `gls` function in the `nlme` package.

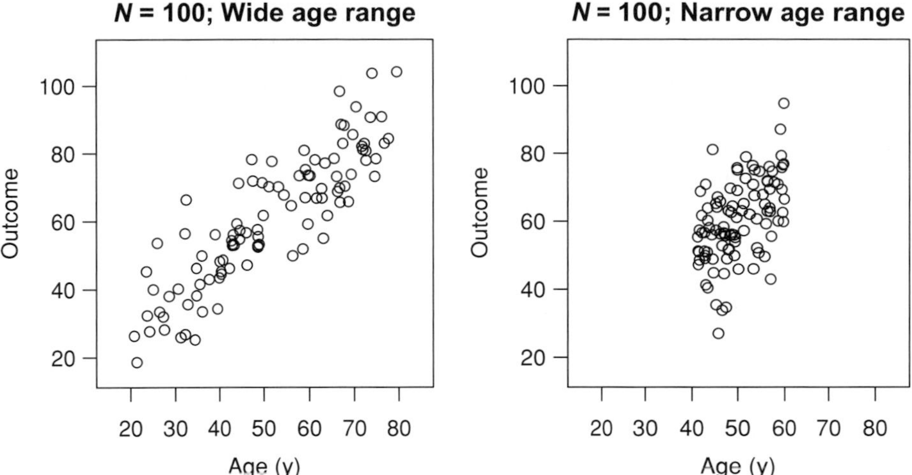

Fig. 5.10 How the range of a predictor variable (age) affects the efficiency. Both graphs have the same number of samples and the same underlying relationship between the outcome and age (slope = 1). With a narrow age range, three times as many samples are required to have the same power as with a wide age range.

A digression on dichotomising continuous variables

It might seem that by dichotomising or binning a continuous variable such as age (Figure 5.10) into a young and old group that the efficiency of the design can be increased. This, however, makes the analysis *less efficient* because information has been removed. It is common to see continuous variables made into categorical variables, despite the many papers that argue against this practice [12, 22, 33, 71, 77, 111, 118, 174, 184, 214, 250, 264, 289, 302, 335, 350, 363, 365, 371, 374, 385, 404, 407]. Even if you do not read these references, their titles are informative:

- *The cost of dichotomization*
- *Breaking up is hard to do: the heartbreak of dichotomizing continuous data*
- *Leave 'em alone: why continuous variables should be analyzed as such*
- *Why carve up your continuous data?*
- *Dichotomizing continuous predictors in multiple regression: a bad idea*
- *Negative consequences of dichotomizing continuous predictor variables*
- *Bivariate median splits and spurious statistical significance*
- *Analysis by categorizing or dichotomizing continuous variables is inadvisable*
- *Disappointing dichotomies*
- *Bias and efficiency loss due to categorizing an explanatory variable*
- *Against quantiles: categorization of continuous variables in epidemiologic research, and its discontents*

Binning often takes the form of a median split – dividing the data into two equal sizes – or sometimes a cut-off is based on an arbitrary value to divide the data into high and low groups. Occasionally, data are split into more groups such as high, medium, and low.

There are several (poor) reasons for binning a predictor variable. The first is to get the predictor into a form so that the data can be analysed with a preferred or familiar test, such as a t-test or ANOVA. This is a bad reason because the analysis should fit the data; the data should not be forced into a form to fit the analysis. Second, there may be a nonlinear relationship between the predictor and the outcome variable and a simple regression would be unsuitable. This is also a bad reason because a quadratic term or nonlinear regression can model the nonlinear relationship. Third, binning creates more homogeneous groups. The assumption is that the samples within the newly formed groups are homogeneous enough, such that any variation within the groups can be ignored. This is usually a false assumption, and it is the heterogeneity – that is, the variance in the predictor – that gives us power to find effects. Removing heterogeneity in a predictor variable only throws away information. *There is a consensus regarding the practice of binning continuous variables: just don't do it.*

The arguments against binning have to do with biased estimates and loss of statistical power, and the above references describe these in detail. Regardless of these statistical concerns, binning should be offensive to biologists; if the phenomenon is continuous, forcing the values into a few categories is not being true to the biological reality. People are not either obese or anorexic; body mass is a continuous variable (most people are somewhere in the middle) and should be treated as such in an analysis. Labels can be assigned to ranges (e.g. normal, overweight, obese, and so on) to make discussion and communication easier, but these artificial categories should not become the reality. Standard regression methods can easily deal with continuous predictor variables.

The example below illustrates some problems with binning. Suppose we want to determine if a biomarker, such as the expression of a gene, predicts disease severity. We measure the biomarker in 50 patients and the distribution of values is plotted in Figure 5.11A. The distribution is skewed and clearly non-normal. We divide the patients into a high and low biomarker group based on a median split (vertical dashed line in the figure; it is easier to see in panel C). Patients with a biomarker value below 0.9 are placed into the low group and the rest of the patients are placed in the high group. We then test if disease severity differs between the two groups (panel B), but despite trying (1) a t-test assuming equal variances, (2) a t-test assuming unequal variances, (3) a t-test on the log-transformed severity scores, and (4) a Wilcoxon test, all p-values are > 0.1. We conclude that the biomarker does not predict disease severity, and as is common in our field of research, we present only the bar graph in panel B to support our claim.

If we treat the biomarker as a continuous variable and plot it against the disease severity score (panel C) there is a clear relationship between the two variables, although three patients seem to be influential. The vertical dashed line is once again the median that separates the high and the low groups. The two variables have a Spearman correlation of $r = 0.75$ and a p-value of 3.7×10^{-10}. The Spearman correlation is based on the ranks of the data and so we do not have to worry about the excess influence of the three patients. Even if these three patients are excluded, there is still an overall correlation ($r = 0.32$, $p = 0.028$). What a difference in interpretation compared with binning the biomarker and analysing the data with a t-test!

A further problem with using a median split to bin the biomarker variable is that the low and high biomarker groups may not be the same across studies, making it impossible to

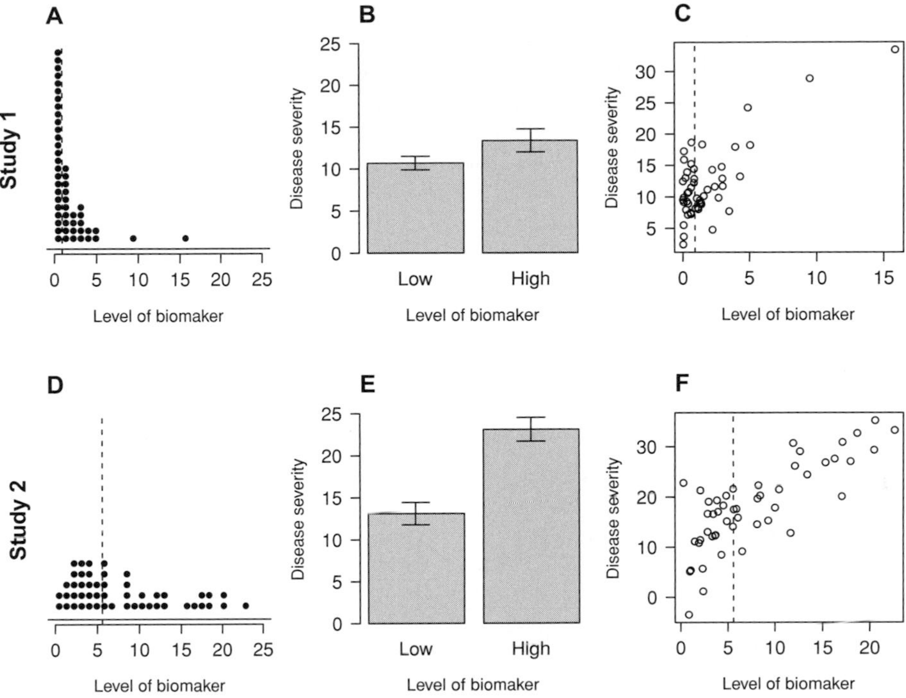

Fig. 5.11 Binning a continuous variable. Two studies (panels A–C and D–F) perform a median split (vertical dashed bar) of the biomarker to define two groups. The groups are tested if they differ on disease severity. The groups are not comparable between studies because the cut-off for the median is different. The relationship between the biomarker and disease severity is the same in both studies, they only differ in the distribution of the biomarker variable.

compare the results from several experiments. Suppose another research group conducts the same experiment and the only difference between studies is the distribution of the biomarker; the second study has more patients with greater disease severity and thus higher levels of the biomarker (Figure 5.11D). They also perform a median split (vertical dashed line) and analyse the data with a t-test, and they find a significant difference between groups (panel E). The two studies come to different conclusions (based on a t-test), but how can we compare them when the value used to define the high and low groups differs between studies? Twenty-three patients that were placed into the high group in the first study would be classified as having low biomarker levels using the criteria from the second study. *Data-dependent cut-offs create groups that do not exist in nature.* The relationship between the biomarker and disease severity is the same in the two studies; the data were generated from the following equation:

$$\text{Disease severity} = 10 + 1.1 \times \text{Biomarker value} + \text{noise}. \tag{5.14}$$

The three 'outliers' in Study 1 only appear unusual because we did not sample enough patients with high levels of the biomarker.

A final problem is that binning creates multiple groups, and then one is tempted to perform comparisons between them all, leading to problems of multiplicities. In the above

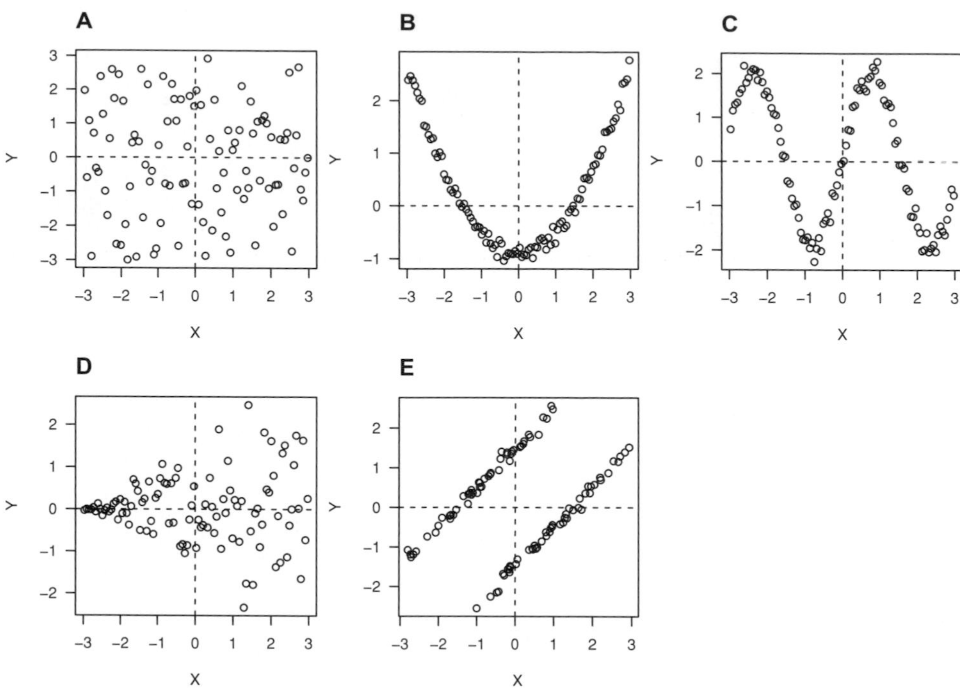

Fig. 5.12 When X and Y are dichotomised at zero these five graphs all produce an identical 2×2 table with $n = 25$ in each cell. This example is from Kuss [208].

example, the data were binned into two groups, but with three or more groups the chance of obtaining false positive results increases.

⚠ The phrase to remember is that *binning is sinning*. But like all sins, some can occasionally be forgiven. There are some situations where binning is useful. The first is displaying data with histograms (as in Figure 5.7). The data are placed into many bins, but this is only for visualisation and not for analysis. Second, when the underlying variable is discrete, binning can be useful even though the measured variable is continuous. For example, gene expression is measured as fluorescence intensity on a microarray, but some genes are either expressed or not, such as XIST, which is only expressed in females. If the sex of the samples is unknown, XIST can classify the samples by sex. It would make sense to use a binary sex variable in an analysis instead of the expression level of XIST. Finally, when a variable is used for a diagnostic test, a dichotomous decision will usually be required, such as being positive or negative for a disease. In this case the choice of cut-off is critical, and extensive validation will be required, along with estimates of the sensitivity, specificity, and other metrics.

Before leaving this topic, Figure 5.12 shows a nice example from Kuss [208]. There are 100 data points in each panel, with different relationships between X and Y. If both variables are dichotomised at zero the number of observations in each category (each of the four quadrants in the figure) is equal to 25. Testing if a relationship exists from the number of counts in each quadrant (e.g. using a Chi-squared test), we would incorrectly conclude that there is no relationship between X and Y in panels B to E.

5.3.5 Ensure predictor variables are uncorrelated

Unlike the previous examples this rule of thumb is only relevant when there are two or more predictor variables (Figure 5.8I). When predictors – either categorical or continuous – are correlated, the power to detect effects is reduced. In designed experiments, the number of samples allocated to the groups is under the control of the experimenter, and experiments can be designed such that the predictor variables are uncorrelated or orthogonal. When a categorical predictor is a property of the experimental units (a biological factor), it may not be possible to have a balanced design, especially if this factor is unknown before randomisation.

The layout below reflects the design in Figure 5.8I. It is a '2 × 2 design' (two factors with two levels each) with an equal number of samples in each group, and is commonly analysed with a two-way ANOVA. The equal N allocation of samples in the layout below is the optimal design.

	1 h	**8 h**
0 mg/kg	5	5
24 mg/kg	5	5

The next layout also has 20 samples, and the rows and columns also sum to 10. The only difference is how the samples are distributed across the four cells. There is now a correlation between dose and time (Pearson $r = -0.4$; $p = 0.080$). The p-value is not significant but that is irrelevant, any non-zero correlation will reduce the power to detect effects.

	1 h	**8 h**
0 mg/kg	3	7
24 mg/kg	7	3

Before calculating the RE we create another variable for time (`z2`) that is correlated dose and check the allocation of samples with `xtabs()`.

```
> # create another variable
> z2 <- rep(c(1,8,1,8), times=c(3,7,7,3))
>
> xtabs(~ x3 + z2)
    z2
x3   1 8
  0  3 7
  24 7 3
```

In the code below, the Pearson correlation is calculated between the two variables. As expected, the correlation is zero with the balanced design and −0.4 with the unbalanced design.

```
> # correlation between predictors with equal n
> cor.test(x3 , z1)

Pearson's product-moment correlation

data:  x3 and z1
t = 0, df = 18, p-value = 1
alternative hypothesis: true correlation is not equal to 0
95 percent confidence interval:
 -0.442521  0.442521
sample estimates:
cor
  0
>
> # correlation between predictors with unequal n
> cor.test(x3 , z2)

Pearson's product-moment correlation

data:  x3 and z2
t = -1.852, df = 18, p-value = 0.0806
alternative hypothesis: true correlation is not equal to 0
95 percent confidence interval:
 -0.7158155  0.0516661
sample estimates:
 cor
-0.4
```

How does the correlation affect the efficiency? A design like this one with two variables would usually be analysed with a two-way ANOVA. Unlike the previous examples with only one effect, we now have an effect of dose, time, and a dose by time interaction. Since there are several effects of equal interest, another method is required to calculate the efficiency. The details are beyond the scope of this book but the brief answer is that the unbalanced design has a relative efficiency of 0.84 compared with the balanced design. The rest of this section describes how the value of 0.84 was calculated, but it can be skipped. Just remember that the rule of thumb is to ensure the predictors are as little correlated as possible, and for a factorial design this means an equal number of samples in each cell.

The methods below require knowledge of topics that are not discussed such as design matrices and contrasts, and details can be found in Berger and Wong [36]. The variance of the estimates for all three effects can be calculated from the design matrix. A design matrix is the representation of a model's predictor variables in a matrix form. In the code below the `model.matrix()` function generates the design matrices. `model.matrix()` takes the right hand side of a model formula, just like the `aov()` function. We indicate that `x3`, `z1`, and `z2` are factors and the interaction is included in the model. The default contrasts are also changed to the sum-to-zero constraints (which is standard for most software, but not R).

```
> # change default contrasts
> options(contrasts=c("contr.sum","contr.poly"))
>
> # design matrix for main and interaction effects
> des1 <- model.matrix(~ factor(x3) * factor(z1)) # balanced
> des2 <- model.matrix(~ factor(x3) * factor(z2)) # unbalanced
```

The design matrices are then used to calculate the variance of each of the three effect estimates. The `solve()` function in the code below calculates the covariance matrix of the predictors. These lines of code calculate the same thing as var(x) in the previous section when there was only one predictor. The row and column names are removed by setting `dimnames()` to `NULL` to make the output nicer.

```
> # covariance matrix
> cov.des1 <- solve(t(des1) %*% des1)
> cov.des2 <- solve(t(des2) %*% des2)
>
> # remove row and column names to save space
> dimnames(cov.des1) <- NULL
> dimnames(cov.des2) <- NULL
```

The code below displays the covariances for both designs rounded to two decimal places. The balanced design (`cov.des1`) has all zeros except the top left to bottom right diagonal entries. The non-diagonal entries reflect the covariance or correlation between the predictors, which we know are zero with a balanced design. The entries on the diagonal are the variances of the predictors (which include the intercept and the interaction, and is the reason that the matrix has four rows and columns). The unbalanced design (`cov.des2`) has non-zero values for some non-diagonal entries, reflecting the correlation between predictors.

```
> # examine covariances
> round(cov.des1,2)
     [,1] [,2] [,3] [,4]
[1,] 0.05 0.00 0.00 0.00
```

```
[2,] 0.00 0.05 0.00 0.00
[3,] 0.00 0.00 0.05 0.00
[4,] 0.00 0.00 0.00 0.05
>
> round(cov.des2,2)
     [,1] [,2] [,3] [,4]
[1,] 0.06 0.00 0.00 0.02
[2,] 0.00 0.06 0.02 0.00
[3,] 0.00 0.02 0.06 0.00
[4,] 0.02 0.00 0.00 0.06
```

The final step is to combine the variances to give one value for the efficiency of each design. There are however several methods for combining the variances and we use the 'A-optimal' criterion because it is easiest to explain.[8] It is the sum of the diagonal entries of the covariance matrices, in other words, we just add the variances of all of the predictors. In the code below, the `diag()` function extracts the diagonal entries which are then summed. The last line of code calculates the relative efficiency, and the unbalanced design has a RE of 0.84. This is a large reduction in efficiency given that the sample size is the same.

```
> # Calculate A-optimality for both designs
> sum(diag(cov.des1)) # balanced
[1] 0.2
>
> sum(diag(cov.des2)) # unbalanced
[1] 0.238095
>
> # calculate RE
> 0.2 / 0.238095
[1] 0.840001
```

5.3.6 Space observations out temporally and spatially

If the body weight of 10 rats is measured today, and again tomorrow, the correlation between the two days will be high, likely greater than $r = 0.95$. This means that little has been learnt from the second set of measurements, but twice the effort has been expended. If the second measurements are taken a week later, the correlation will be weaker, and after a month, weaker still. Since the second measurements are not as easy to predict from the first when taken far apart, some new information is obtained.

Experiments that have multiple measurements taken over time on the same experimental units are called `longitudinal` or *repeated measures designs*. An initial and final time

[8] The D-optimal criterion is the most common.

defines the design space for the time variable, and the number of intermediate time points needs to be decided. This example differs from the previous ones because the same experimental units are followed over time and so all samples are observed at all time points. It is impossible therefore to place more samples at the ends of the design space. Also, additional observations between the initial and final time often costs little; for example, weighing animals more often only requires the experimenter's time. Here, the aim is to avoid wasting effort for little or no gain in useful data. If different experimental units are observed at different time points, as in Figure 5.8I, then the previous rules of thumb apply.

⚠ The rule of thumb is that *the time between observations should be long enough so that the correlation between successive time points is not very large*. 'Very large' could be anything greater than a correlation of 0.9, but this will depend on the experiment. If observations are automatically recorded then there is almost no cost to having more, regardless of the diminishing returns in information. If taking more observations is expensive, such as repeated blood samples that need to be processed, then fewer time points is better (possibly allowing more experimental units).

If the correlation between body weight measurements taken 1 week apart is 0.85, then a weekly measurement is likely enough. If the experiment will last for 4 weeks, then in addition to the initial and final measurements, only three further time points are required (measurements at weeks 0, 1, 2, 3, and 4).

Calculating the correlation between successive time points requires previous experimental data and an example was shown in Figure 4.20 (p. 185). Recall that the experiment measured the force of muscle contraction from 7 rats at 14 time points (30 s apart) [199]. The figure shows the correlation of all time points with each other and the narrowness of the ellipses represents the strength of the correlation.

This graph is good for visualising the correlation structure in the data, but the correlation matrix will need to be examined to obtain the values. Figure 5.13 plots the correlations versus the distance between time points, known as the lag. For all adjacent time points (Lag = 1) all correlations are above 0.95 and as the lag increases the correlations gradually get smaller.

Even at a lag of four all correlation are above 0.9 (horizontal line). Thus, if every fourth time point was taken the amount of data could be reduced by 75% with little loss of information. Vickers calculated the marginal benefit of including additional time points depending on the strength of the correlations [380]. For highly correlated observations (defined as $r > 0.85$), there was little benefit to using more than three time points when using a repeated measures design. Guo and colleagues also discuss sample size calculations with repeated measures designs [146].

When the outcome variable changes smoothly over time (e.g. learning or growth curves), the observations should be spaced out equally across time because the distance between time points is maximised, thereby minimising the correlations. Most experimenters already use equally spaced time points and so this will not be discussed further.

The above discussion also applies to space; for example, adjacent tissue sections and adjacent fields of view in microscope images will tend to be more alike than those further apart. Once the total number of samples or subsamples has been decided, it is best to space them out as far as possible, which implies equal spacing.

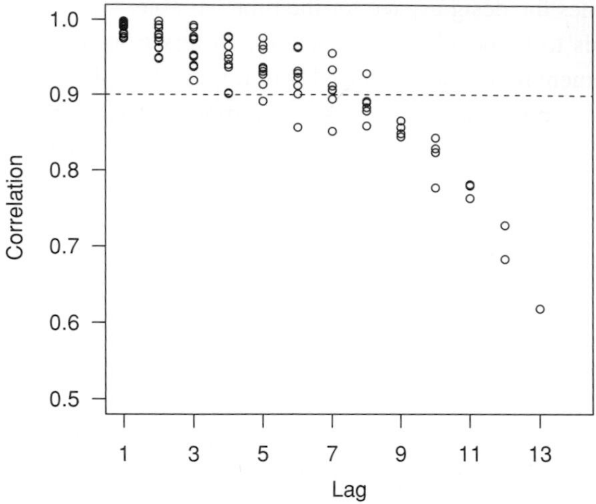

Fig. 5.13 Correlation between time points of different lags. As the distance between time points increases the correlation gets weaker.

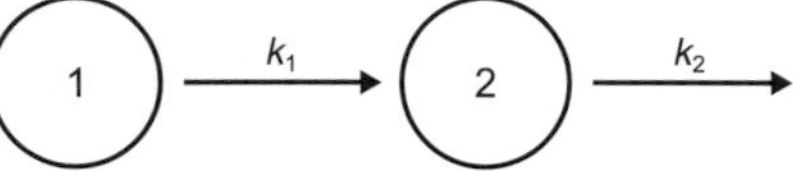

Fig. 5.14 A two compartment model. A drug is taken orally and introduced into the GI tract (compartment 1). The drug leaves the GI tract and enters the blood (compartment 2) at a rate of k_1 and leaves the blood at a rate of k_2. The concentration of the drug in the blood is measured.

One assumption in the above discussion was that the measured variable changes gradually and smoothly over time. There are situations where change is faster at some times and slower at others. It is then better to sample more intensively where change is faster, and is the subject of the next section.

5.3.7 Sample more intensively where change is faster

Consider a PK experiment with an orally administered drug and the drug's concentration in the blood is measured at several time points. The schematic diagram in Figure 5.14 is called a *compartment model* because the gastrointestinal (GI) tract and the blood are considered compartments of the body and the drug moves from one compartment to another. In Figure 5.14, the two circles represent the compartments; compartment one is the GI tract and compartment two is the blood. The drug moves from the GI tract to the blood at a rate of k_1 and leaves the blood at a rate of k_2 as it is eliminated from the body.

The concentration of the drug is measured in the blood and the purpose of the experiment is to determine the values of k_1 and k_2. These describe how quickly the drug enters and leaves the blood and are therefore used to select safe and effective doses. The relationships

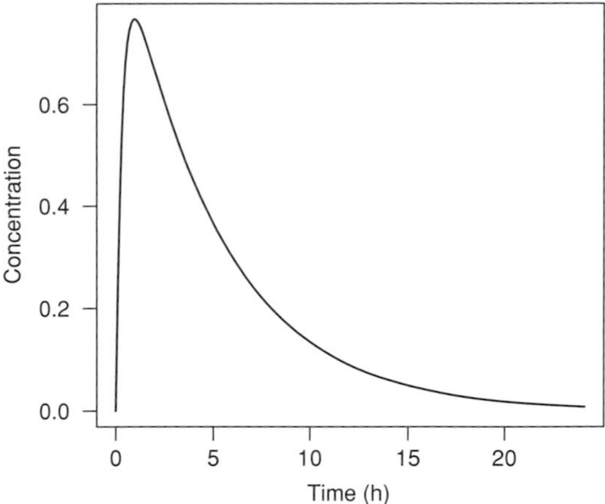

Fig. 5.15 Concentration of a compound in the blood over time.

in Figure 5.14 can be expressed as

$$\text{conc} = e^{(-k_1 \times t)} - e^{(-k_2 \times t)}, \tag{5.15}$$

where conc is the concentration of the drug in compartment two and t is time. This example is a simplified version of Lawson's [213]. A physiologically relevant model has more parameters but here they are assumed to be a convenient value such as zero or one so they can be dropped from the model.[9]

The concentration of the drug over time will resemble the curve in Figure 5.15. The blood initially contains no drug, the concentration rises over time to some maximal value, and then declines back to zero as the drug is eliminated from the blood. But the exact shape of the curve depends on the values of k_1 and k_2, which are unknown, and the purpose of the experiment is to estimate them.

Suppose that a maximum of four time points can be examined; the first will be at baseline at $t = 0$, the last will be at 24 h, at what times should the remaining two observations be taken? Spacing them apart at equal distances would put the observations at $t = 8$ and 16, but this is inefficient because most of the change happens early. Obtaining a good estimate of the peak concentration and the time of the peak is hard if there are no observations in that vicinity.

The discussion below contains some advanced topics so do not worry if some concepts are unfamiliar. The rule of thumb to sample more intensively where change is faster applies even without the formal mathematical treatment. The process below only enables a better selection of time points compared with selecting them by an educated guess.

In the code below values for time are generated between 0 and 24 h. Values for the rate constants `k1` and `k2` are chosen and are just made up for this example. These are then used

[9] Bonate discusses PK models in detail [52], Fedorov and Leonov provide a comprehensive (but mathematical) discussion on optimal designs for nonlinear models [112], and Bates and Watts is a classic book on nonlinear regression that contains some PK models [24].

to calculate the concentration of the compound in compartment 2 (y) to produce the curve shown in Figure 5.15.

```
> # make sequence of observations
> t <- seq(0, 24, 0.1)
>
> # define values for the rates
> k1 <- 0.2 # /hour
> k2 <- 3   # /hour
>
> # two compartment model with first-order kinetics
> y <- exp(-k1 * t) - exp(-k2 * t)
>
> par(las=1)
> plot(y ~ t, type="l", ylab="Concentration", xlab="Time (h)",
+       lwd=1.5)
```

Although time is a continuous variable, we need to define a discrete set of points that could be used to collect blood samples, and we space them 1 h apart. Some of these time points will be chosen as the observation times, and if the spacing is too far apart the selected times may be far from the optimal times.

```
> # make time values in 1 hour increments
> t.vals <- 0:24
```

The next step is to linearise the PK model, that is, to find a linear approximation to the curve at a given point. This is done by taking the partial derivative with respect to each parameter in the model (k_1 and k_2). If it has been a while since you differentiated an equation, R's `D()` function can perform symbolical differentiation. We define the PK model in Eq. (5.15) as an expression, and then use the `D()` function to calculate the partial derivative with respect to k_1 and then k_2.

```
> # Define the PK model
> pk.mod <- expression(exp(-k1 * t) - exp(-k2 * t))
>
> # calculate partial derivatives with respect to each parameter
> D(pk.mod, "k1")
-(exp(-k1 * t) * t)
>
> D(pk.mod, "k2")
exp(-k2 * t) * t
```

Next, plausible values for k_1 and k_2 need to be chosen based on earlier experiments, theory, or just an educated guess. We use $k_1 = 0.2$ and $k_2 = 3$, which were defined above to create the PK curve. Then, the partial derivatives are evaluated using these values of the parameters at each time point. The matrix `res` stores the results and we loop through the time points.

```
> # matrix to store results
> res <- matrix(NA, nrow=25, ncol=2)
>
> # evaluate partial derivs. at each time point
> for(i in 1:25){
+     res[i,1] <- -(exp(-k1 * t.vals[i]) * t.vals[i])
+     res[i,2] <- exp(-k2 * t.vals[i]) * t.vals[i]
+ }
>
> # put everything into one matrix
> res <- cbind(t.vals, res)
> colnames(res) <- c("t.vals","k1","k2")
> head(res)
     t.vals        k1          k2
[1,]      0  0.000000 0.00000e+00
[2,]      1 -0.818731 4.97871e-02
[3,]      2 -1.340640 4.95750e-03
[4,]      3 -1.646435 3.70229e-04
[5,]      4 -1.797316 2.45768e-05
[6,]      5 -1.839397 1.52951e-06
```

We can now use these values to find the optimal time points with the `optFederov()` function in the `AlgDesign` package. We specify the parameters (and include 0 to indicate that there is no intercept) and that there should be four time points (`nTrials=4`). We specify that `row=c(1,25)` and `augment=TRUE` to indicate that rows 1 and 25 of `res` need to be included as time points, that is, two of the four selected points should be the first and last (at $t = 0$ and $t = 24$ h).

```
> library(AlgDesign)
> set.seed(1)
> best.des <- optFederov(~ 0 + k1 + k2, data=data.frame(res),
+                        nTrials=4, criterion="I", nRepeats=100,
+                        row=c(1,25), augment=TRUE)
```

The output is a list and the information that we want is in the `design` slot. The results indicate that in addition to the baseline and 24 h time points, we should take observations at 1 and 5 h.

```
> best.des$design
   t.vals          k1          k2
1       0  0.000000 0.00000e+00
2       1 -0.818731 4.97871e-02
6       5 -1.839397 1.52951e-06
25     24 -0.197514 1.29124e-30
```

The code below creates the PK curve in Figure 5.16 with equally spaced time points and the optimal time points plotted with different symbols.

```
> # make equally spaced points and the optimal points
> eq.space <- seq(0,24, length.out=4)
> best <- best.des$design$t.vals
>
> par(las=1)
> plot(y ~ t, type="l",  ylab="Concentration", xlab="Time (h)",
+       lwd=1.5)
>
> points(exp(-k1 * eq.space) - exp(-k2 * eq.space) ~ eq.space,
+         pch=4, cex=2)
> points(exp(-k1 * best) - exp(-k2 * best) ~ best,
+         pch=1, cex=2)
>
> legend("topright", pch=c(1,4), cex=1.2,
+         legend=c("Optimal","Equal spacing"))
```

The optimal observation times are at 1 and 5 h, but these values depend on the values of k_1 and k_2 that we chose. But the purpose of the experiment is to estimate these values, which once again emphasises that the more you know about the experimental system the better the experiment you can design. Plausible initial values for k_1 and k_2 can be guessed, but much like selecting an estimate for the within group variability in a power calculation, there is uncertainty. Even if the values of k_1 and k_2 – and therefore the shape of the PK curve – are unknown, it is highly likely that the fast changes will occur early. Therefore, shifting the observations to earlier times will be better than an equally spaced design, even if the chosen time points are not optimal. Furthermore, experiments can be conducted sequentially, where initial time points are chosen, the experiment conducted, and estimates of k_1 and k_2 are obtained. Then, using the new values of k_1 and k_2 a better set of time points are selected for a second experiment (see Lawson for further details [213]).

An assumption of the above procedure was that a two compartment model with first order kinetics (represented by the model in Figure 5.14) was a good description of the biological system. The model itself may be a poor representation of the underlying biology. Nevertheless, the same principle applies: placing more observations where change is

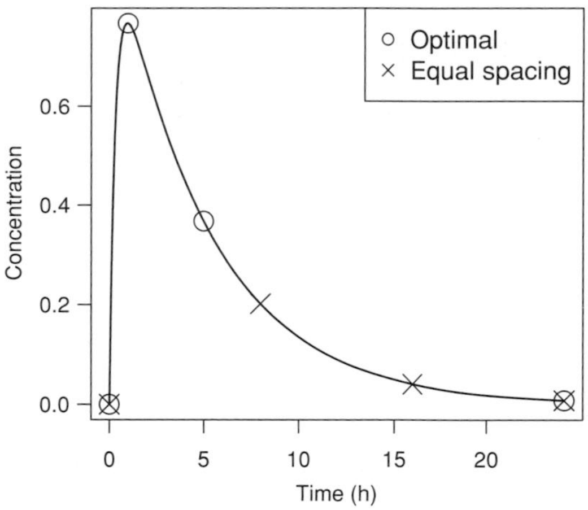

Fig. 5.16 The PK curve shows the concentration of the drug in the blood over 24 h. With an initial and final time point selected at 0 and 24 h, two more time points are required. The optimal values (circles) occur at 1 and 5 h. Spacing the observations out equally puts them at 8 and 16 h, but the early changes are missed.

predicted to be faster is more efficient than an equally spaced design. Although one can get fancy in trying to estimate an optimal set of time points, large improvements from an equally spaced design can be had with some rough estimates of where change will be fast and where it will be slow.

5.3.8 Make use of blocking and covariates

Section 2.4 described how to use blocking to remove variation in the outcome when the experimental units are heterogeneous or when technical variation is expected to influence the outcome. Here, the idea is illustrated and an alternative method of using covariate adjustment is also presented. Figure 5.17 shows the results of a hypothetical experiment where eight rats were randomly assigned to a control or new diet group. The outcome is the amount of food eaten (in arbitrary units), and we suspect that larger rats will eat more food, regardless of the treatment condition. Some of the variability in the outcome can be attributed to baseline body weight, and if rats differ widely in their body weights, we would expect proportionally larger variation in the outcome, making it harder to detect a treatment effect.

This example uses the fictitious `block.covars` data from the `labstats` package and the data are shown below. Each row is one rat and the rows are sorted by the baseline body weight (`weight` column). Suppose that we have measured the body weights before randomisation to the treatment groups and we need to decide on the design of the experiment. There are two options and the data set has values for both, but in a real experiment we could only choose one. First, the rats can be paired into blocks and then one member of each block can be randomly assigned to one of two diets. This is a randomised block design and the column `RBD` shows the assignments. Alternatively, the rats could be randomly

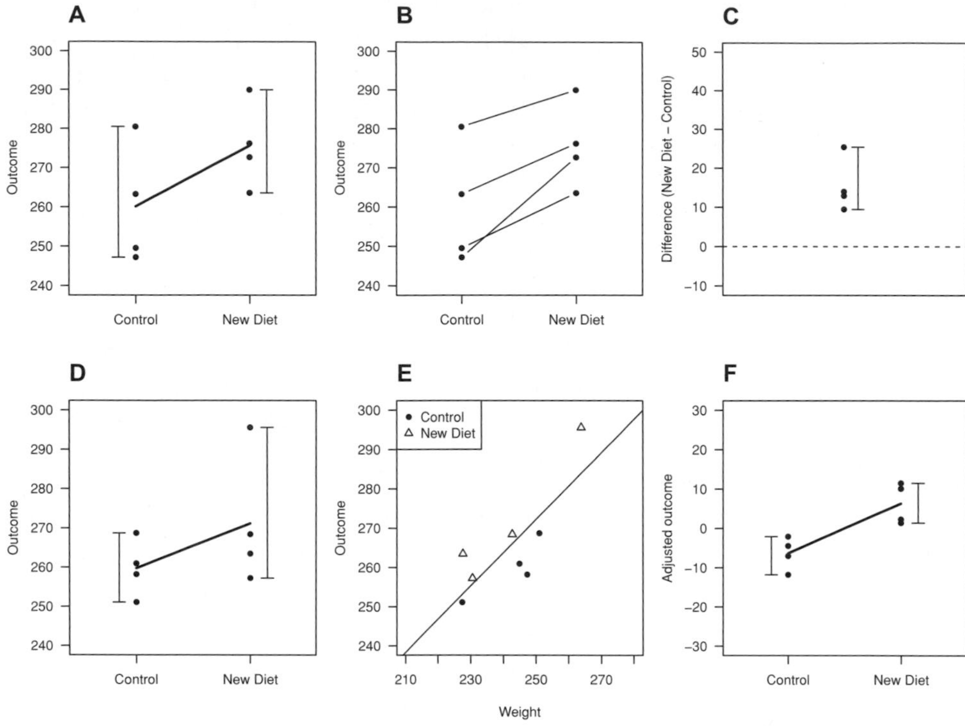

Fig. 5.17 Blocking versus ANCOVA. The top row of graphs are from a randomised block design where rats are paired according to baseline body weight and one member of each pair is randomised to each treatment group. The bottom row is a completely randomised design and the effect of baseline body weight on the outcome is removed statistically. The range of the *y*-axes is 60 units in all graphs, so the range bars can be directly compared.

assigned to the treatment groups without using information on baseline body weight. This is a completely randomised design and the column CRD shows the assignments. The baseline weight can then be used as a covariate in the analysis. The outcomes for each design are indicated in the y.RBD and y.CRD columns.

```
> block.covars
  weight block      RBD      CRD  y.RBD  y.CRD
1 227.47     1  Control  Control 249.54 251.10
2 227.69     1 New Diet New Diet 263.56 263.48
3 230.60     2  Control New Diet 247.19 257.24
4 242.75     2 New Diet New Diet 272.67 268.44
5 244.94     3 New Diet  Control 276.21 260.97
6 247.31     3  Control  Control 263.26 258.20
7 251.07     4 New Diet  Control 289.98 268.72
8 263.93     4  Control New Diet 280.50 295.58
```

One way to deal with variation in body weight is to only include rats that have similar body weight so that this variable is held fixed and will have minimal influence on the outcome. A drawback is that we cannot learn if the results (whatever they are) apply to rats having different body weights from those used in the experiment. In addition, it may not be possible to find enough rats with similar body weight.

If we have a heterogeneous group of rats, the first concern is to avoid having the heaviest rats predominately in one group and the lightest in the other – an example of confounding between weight and treatment condition. Confounding makes the results hard to interpret because the groups differ not only in their diet but also their weight. A lack of balance between weight and treatment group makes these predictors correlated and the analysis inefficient (Section 5.3.5). One way to achieve balance is to first sort the rats by weight and then group the rats into pairs as shown in Figure 2.2. The randomisation to treatment group occurs within each pair of animals, ensuring that the groups will be balanced with respect to body weight. The pairs are the blocks, allowing like with like comparisons because rats on the new diet are compared with rats of a similar weight on the control diet.

The experiment can be blocked in other ways. For example, instead of making four blocks of two rats we could have made two blocks of four rats, which would be appropriate if there are four heavy and four light rats. The randomisation is the same in that it occurs within each block, and then the blocking variable needs to be included in the analysis.

Figure 5.17A shows the blocked design but the pairing is ignored, both in the figure and the analysis. The rats in the new diet group ate more, but the difference between groups is tested against the large within-group variability, indicated by the range bars. The code below analyses the RBD data with the `aov()` function but the model does not include `block`. The p-value for this diet effect (`RBD` in the output) is not significant ($p = 0.15$) and the mean square residual is equal to 178.

```
> summary(aov(y.RBD ~ RBD, data=block.covars))
          Df Sum Sq Mean Sq F value Pr(>F)
RBD        1    479     479     2.7   0.15
Residuals  6   1065     178
```

Figure 5.17B plots the same data but connects the pairs of rats with a line. Rats connected by a line tend to eat a similar amount, and rats in the new diet group always eat more than their partner in the control group. Figure 5.17C plots the difference for each pair of rats and *the variation in these four data points is the relevant variability for testing the treatment effect*. Note how the range bar in Figure 5.17C is much smaller than those in A, because the variation in the outcome due to body weight has been removed. In A, we test the difference of the means, while in B, we test the mean of the differences. Since the randomisation was performed within blocks (pairs) the appropriate analysis should take this blocking structure into account. By using blocks the uncertainty in the estimate of the difference between groups is reduced by a factor of 0.37.

The code below is the same analysis as above, except that `block` is included as a variable in the model. Since block is a numeric variable, we have to convert it into a factor, otherwise

R will treat it as continuous. Including the blocking variable provides a more sensitive test for the treatment effect ($p = 0.021$), and the mean square residual equals 24, which is much smaller than the previous analysis. Blocking in this example was beneficial because we obtained a more precise estimate of the treatment effect.

```
> summary(aov(y.RBD ~ factor(block) + RBD, data=block.covars))
              Df Sum Sq Mean Sq F value Pr(>F)
factor(block)  3    993     331    13.7  0.029
RBD            1    479     479    19.9  0.021
Residuals      3     72      24
```

It was easy to form blocks in this example because there was only one variable that we wanted to balance across treatment groups. The `blockTools` and `MatchIt` packages can be used for more complex situations with multiple blocking variables.

A second option for dealing with large variations in body weight and its effect on the outcome is to use the weight values directly in an analysis, instead of indirectly by forming blocks and then using the blocking variable in an analysis (Figure 5.17D–F). The eight animals are randomly assigned to the two treatment groups and their weight played no part in the treatment assignment. Once again, we see a large within group variation as indicated by the range bars in Figure 5.17D. In Figure 5.17E, weight is plotted against the outcome variable and there is a clear association between the two. This is what we predicted when planning the experiment: rats that weigh more will eat more, regardless of the treatment group that they are in. The diagonal line is the regression line through all of the data points. Looking closer, we see that the four rats in the new diet group are above the line while the four control animals are below the line. The ANCOVA analysis removes the dependence on weight by taking the vertical distance from each data point to the regression line, and uses these distances as the adjusted outcome values, which are plotted in Figure 5.17F. Data points that lie above the regression line have positive adjusted values and those below the line have negative values because the vertical distances are calculated as 'data point minus value on the regression line'.[10] The adjusted values are centred around zero but the units are the same as the original values. When presenting adjusted values, one can add the overall mean of the outcome (which equals 265) to each adjusted point. This shifts all the values upward by a constant amount and puts them in a familiar range but has no influence on a statistical analysis. A large amount of variation in the outcome has been removed since the range bars in Figure 5.17F are much smaller than in D. By including weight as a covariate in the analysis, the uncertainty in the estimate for the difference between means is reduced substantially.

The code below analyses the experiment assuming that it was conducted as a completely randomised design, but baseline body weight is not included in the analysis. With a large p-value of 0.26, one would conclude that there is no effect of the new diet, which might be expected given the large variability in Figure 5.17D.

[10] These values are the residuals of a model that contains only the baseline body weights.

```
> summary(aov(y.CRD ~ CRD, data=block.covars))
           Df Sum Sq Mean Sq F value Pr(>F)
CRD         1    262     262    1.55   0.26
Residuals   6   1016     169
```

In the code below the baseline body weight is included in the model, and it is not surprising that it is a good predictor of final body weight ($p = 0.0026$). By including it in the analysis, much of the variation between rats is removed, making the estimate of the treatment effect more precise, and gives a much smaller p-value (0.0175).

```
> summary(aov(y.CRD ~ weight + CRD, data=block.covars))
          Df Sum Sq Mean Sq F value Pr(>F)
weight     1    823     823    31.1 0.0025
CRD        1    322     322    12.2 0.0174
Residuals  5    132      26
```

The adjusted outcome values (Figure 5.17F) are calculated in the code below by including only `weight` in the model and saving the residuals as a new variable.

```
> block.covars$adj.y <- resid(aov(y.CRD ~ weight, data=block.covars))
> block.covars
  weight block      RBD      CRD  y.RBD  y.CRD     adj.y
1 227.47     1  Control  Control 249.54 251.10  -2.08170
2 227.69     1 New Diet New Diet 263.56 263.48  10.11192
3 230.60     2  Control New Diet 247.19 257.24   1.40654
4 242.75     2 New Diet New Diet 272.67 268.44   2.31293
5 244.94     3 New Diet  Control 276.21 260.97  -7.01247
6 247.31     3  Control  Control 263.26 258.20 -11.79035
7 251.07     4 New Diet  Control 289.98 268.72  -4.45587
8 263.93     4  Control New Diet 280.50 295.58  11.50900
```

⚠ The ANCOVA method has several requirements and assumptions. First, *the treatment should not affect the covariate*. If the treatment affects the covariate, including the covariate in the analysis can remove a real treatment effect between groups. For example, if weight was measured at the end of the experiment instead of at baseline, and rats in the new diet group ate more and thus gained more weight during the experiment, then the ANCOVA would adjust for and remove this effect. Covariates should be measured before treatments are applied, which ensures that treatments cannot affect the covariate.

A second requirement is that the covariate needs to be associated with the outcome. If the regression line in Figure 5.17E was flat, then there would be no benefit of including groups within each block. The principle is identical to the example in Figure 5.17B, and the test for a treatment effect is performed within the blocks. The benefits of treating the groups as blocks is also the same: large differences between blocks are irrelevant for testing treatment effects. The same procedure applies if there are more biological units in a group than treatment groups.

In the right side of Figure 5.18 the grouping variable is nested within treatment, which results in two problems. The first is that the benefits of comparing like with like are lost, so the design is less efficient. The degree to which a nested design is less efficient than a crossed design is captured by this equation:

$$\rho = \frac{\sigma_b^2}{\sigma_b^2 + \sigma_w^2}, \tag{5.16}$$

where σ_w^2 is the variation within the groups (reflecting the degree to which pairs of biological units are similar within groups) and σ_b^2 is the variation between groups (reflecting how much the groups differ from each other). This equation is called the intraclass correlation coefficient (ICC), and denoted as ρ ('rho'). If there are no differences between groups $\sigma_b^2 = 0$ and therefore $\rho = 0$. The larger the group effect, the larger σ_b^2 becomes and ρ approaches a value of one. The key point is that as ρ gets larger, the nested design becomes less efficient.

The second problem with the nested design is that the definition of the experimental unit becomes ambiguous. All the biological units from the same group end up in the same treatment because they have been randomised together, and so the groups could be considered the experimental unit instead of the biological unit.

5.3.10 Add more samples instead of subsamples

The distinction between samples and subsamples or genuine replication and pseudoreplication is especially important when planning an experiment. All else being equal, it is better to increase the number of samples (experimental units) instead of subsamples [67]. Increasing the number of samples increases N, which we saw from Eq. (5.7) (p. 207) is one way of increasing power. Increasing the number of subsamples does not increase N and therefore has no direct effect on power. However, including more subsamples improves the precision of the estimate for each EU, and so can indirectly improve power, but only to a limited extent. There is usually little benefit to going beyond three subsamples for each sample (or three OUs for each EU). Increasing the number of subsamples is often less expensive than increasing the number of samples and subsamples are useful for quality control checks and to estimate measurement error. If a subsample is missing or needs to be excluded, the other subsamples provide information for that experimental unit and therefore the sample size is not reduced.

A related point is that for split-unit designs, where randomisation occurs at two or more levels in the hierarchy, it is better to put as many comparisons as possible – and certainly the most interesting comparisons – lower in the hierarchy where there are more EUs. Often this will not be possible, but it is an easy way of increasing power.

Box 5.3 Resource equation

- The left side of the equation is always the number of experimental units (N) minus one.
- For a categorical treatment variable with t levels $T = t - 1$.
- For a categorical biological variable with b levels $B = b - 1$.
- For a categorical technical variable with l levels $L = l - 1$.
- T, B, and L equal 1 if they are continuous and only a linear term is included.
- If interactions are included in the analysis they are calculated by multiplying the respective factors. For example, a treatment and biological factor interaction is $TB = (t - 1)(b - 1)$.

5.3.11 Have 10 to 20 samples to estimate the error variance

Planning exploratory studies is hard because there are multiple outcomes and many treatment, biological, and technical factors. In addition, little is known about the variability of the outcomes. A power analysis or sample size calculation in this situation may be of little value. How can a suitable sample size be determined? Mead *et al.* developed the *resource equation*, which has been adapted here to parallel the fundamental experiment design equation [274] . The fundamental experimental design equation (Section 2.2) is once again

$$\text{Outcome} = \text{Treatment effects} + \text{Biological effects} + \text{Technical effects} + \text{Error}. \quad (5.17)$$

The outcome can be influenced by the treatment effects that we are interested in testing, by inherent characteristics of the sample material, and by technical aspects of the experiment. Each of these effects that are included in the design and analysis will be estimated from the data. In addition, an estimate of the error variance will be obtained, which is the noise beyond which effects need to stand out; it is equal to σ^2 in Eq. (5.7). The number of samples available to estimate the error variance (E) is calculated from the following resource equation:

$$N - 1 = T + B + L + E, \quad (5.18)$$

where N is the sample size (number of EUs), and T, B, and L represent the number of parameters estimated for one or more treatment, biological, and technical factors, respectively. The number of parameters is equal to the number of factor levels (categories) minus one. E is the number of samples to estimate the error. This may sound familiar because E is also the error degrees of freedom. The rule of thumb is that E should be between 10 and 20, and the basis of this rule is that if E is less than 10 the error variance will be poorly estimated, and if it is greater than 20, resources have been wasted because additional questions could have been asked by including further treatment or biological variables. The rules for determining E are summarised in Box 5.3 and the examples below illustrate the calculations.

Suppose we have a simple experiment with 20 animals randomly assigned to two treatment groups ($N = 20$) and the BU = EU = OU. There are no biological or technical factors so $B = L = 0$. Since there are two treatment groups the number of treatment parameters is treatment status and sex). A one-way layout is neither the correct mental nor statistical structure.[11]

The resource equation applies mainly to exploratory studies because we want to discover as much as possible but are unsure of the sample size requirements because there are too many unknowns: the error variance, the size of the effects that might be seen, which factors are relevant, and which outcome will be the most sensitive. For confirmatory studies, there is a primary outcome and E may need to be much larger than 20 to have enough power.

5.4 When to stop collecting data?

Section 5.2 discussed methods for estimating the sample size required to meet the experimental objectives. Implicit in that discussion and in the calculations was the idea that the sample size is fixed in advance. Why is a fixed sample size necessary? Is it not possible to continue collecting data until the results are significant, or we run out of time, money, or patience, at which point we declare that no effect exists? For example, a large experiment may need to be divided into smaller batches, and if the results are significant after the first batch, why waste time and effort to run others when the answer is in hand? Such an approach increases the chance of false positive results because multiple statistical tests are conducted as the data become available. And what is to prevent a researcher from stopping the experiment when the results are in a favourable direction? This is called *optional stopping*, sampling to a foregone conclusion, or 'quitting while you are ahead'. If one is willing to collect data for long enough and perform multiple analyses, then eventually one of the results will be significant. If only the final sample size and statistical results are reported, then the readers will have been misled.

Another complication is that frequentist statistical methods require the sample size to be fixed in advance and to be independent of earlier results. Power analyses assume a fixed sample size because all of the standard statistical tests require it. Frequentist methods compare the observed results against a reference distribution, which is a distribution of other outcomes that could have occurred (Section 1.4). Since the sample size is used to create the reference distribution, it needs to be specified in advance. Bayesian methods are often simpler for experiments where the sample size is not fixed in advance [334, 339], although it is often still desirable for Bayesian methods to have good frequentist properties – meaning control of the false positive rate [340, 409]. Such Bayesian designs are becoming more common in the clinical trial literature [41].

An example is simulated below to illustrate how optional stopping affects the results. Assume that one clinical sample becomes available per week. Each sample is divided into a treated and control condition and a measurement is taken on each. After 5 weeks, the first analysis is conducted comparing the conditions with a sample size of five. If the result is significant the experiment stops and the results are reported. If not, another sample is

[11] The one-way layout does correctly partition the sources of variance and it may be useful when one or more factor level combinations are not included in the experiment are therefore missing.

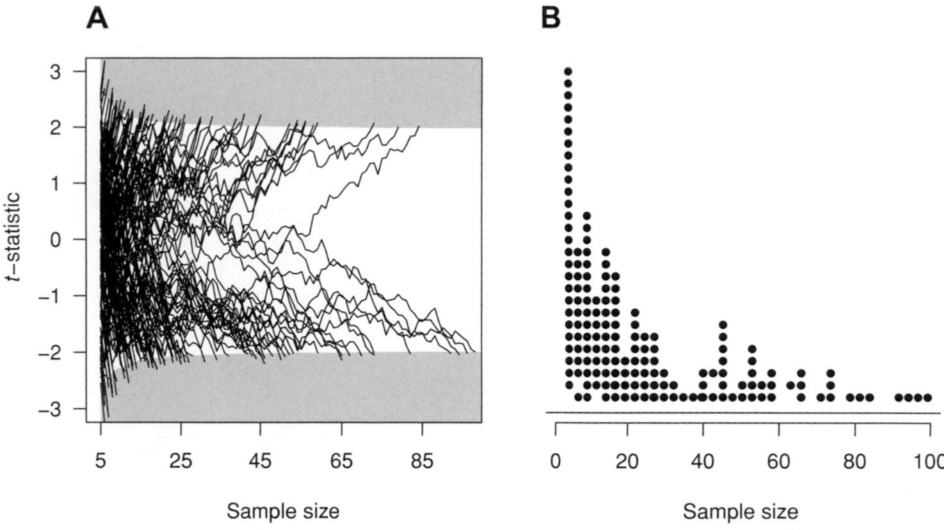

Fig. 5.20 Sampling until significance. Each line in (A) represents one simulated experiment that eventually obtained statistical significance. The grey area is the rejection region and once a line enters the grey area the result is significant and the experiment stops. The points in (B) correspond to the lines in (A) and show the size of the sample when the results became significant. Most of the false positives occur when the sample size is small.

collected each week and the experiment continues until the result is significant or until 100 weeks pass, at which point the experiment is ended. What is the probability of a false positive with this type of sampling procedure? What is the average number of weeks that we would have to wait until getting a false positive? To answer these questions, an experiment like the one just described was simulated 500 times, with a true difference of zero between conditions.

Figure 5.20 displays the results and the x-axis in Figure 5.20A is the sample size and the y-axis is the t-statistic. There is a one-to-one mapping between the absolute value of the t-statistic and the p-value, and the further the t-statistic is away from zero, the smaller the p-value. The grey regions indicate the t-statistics with associated p-values less than 0.05. Each line shows how one of the 500 experiments evolves over the weeks of data collection, and once the line enters the grey region the experiment stops.[12] Approximately 32% of the 500 simulations eventually obtained a significant result, which is a much higher error rate than the assumed value of 5%. If we only consider the first analysis that was done (after the first five samples), 5.6% of the simulated experiments were significant; it is the additional testing on subsequent weeks that increases the false positive rate. Figure 5.20B shows the distribution of the sample sizes (weeks) when the false positive result occurred. Most of the false positives occurred early in the experiment when the sample size is small (mean sample size = 24.8, median = 16). This is to be expected because when the sample size is small and the t-statistic is close to zero, it only takes a few extra samples favouring

[12] Lines for experiments that were not significant are not shown to avoid clutter, but they would be represented as lines that never enter the grey regions.

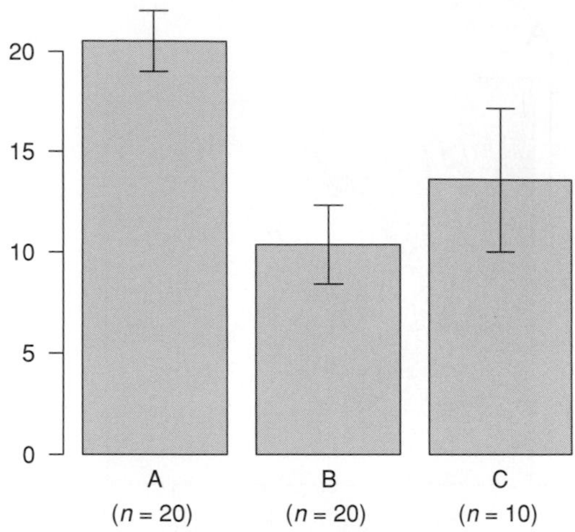

Fig. 5.21 Optional stopping bias. Group A differs from Group B ($p < 0.05$) but not from Group C ($p > 0.05$). Group C has half the sample size because further data were not collected after the desired non-significant result was obtained after the first analysis. Error bars are SEM.

one outcome to change the result. When the sample size is large and the t-statistic is close to zero, however, many samples are required to move the t-statistic into the grey region.

Optional stopping can be abused by continuing to collect data for groups where statistical significance is desired, and stopping early for those groups where a non-significant result is the desired outcome. Suppose a researcher wants to show that Group A differs from Group B, but is similar to Group C (Figure 5.21). After the first batch of data are collected with 10 samples per group, there are no significant differences between any of the groups. Further data are therefore collected but only for Groups A and B, since the desired non-significant outcome for the Group A versus Group C comparison has already been achieved. Increasing the sample size for Group C might make the difference from Group A significant. The researcher believes that the experimental objective has been met for the Group A and C comparison, and collecting more data for Group C would be a waste of effort. There are three problems with this reasoning. First, stopping collection when the 'right' outcome is achieved increases the chance of false positive results. Second, Group C has a smaller sample size and thus lower power for any comparison. Is there no significant difference between Groups A and C because there is no effect, or because the smaller sample size failed to detect it? The difference between Groups A and C could be the same magnitude as between Groups A and B, but the smaller sample size makes the second comparison significant and the first not. Third, bias can be introduced because the data are collected in two batches, and some experimental groups are not represented in every batch, making it hard to separate batch effects from treatment effects. One occasionally finds papers with unequal sample sizes between experimental groups, with groups that should be significant (to support the theory or hypothesis) having a large N while groups that should not be significant have a small N. This should raise warning bells, especially when the difference in sample sizes is large.

Despite the above drawbacks, collecting only as much data as necessary to answer a scientific question makes intuitive sense. Early work on this idea was done in the 1940s and is called sequential analysis or testing [388]. It was applied to situations where samples arrive one at a time, or in matched pairs like the above example. A variant of this idea is group sequential designs, where the data arrive in groups or batches [311]. More generally, the term *interim analysis* refers to analyses before all of the data have been collected. The false positive rate is controlled with 'alpha spending' functions, which involve using smaller *p*-values to conclude that an effect is present. Such designs are common in clinical trials because they allow for early stopping if a new drug is better than either the control or comparator drug, or if toxicities arise. Thus, fewer patients are assigned to dangerous or less efficacious treatments and the trials can be shorter and less expensive. The ethical considerations are fewer for animal studies but shorter and cheaper experiments are still desirable. These methods require that (1) the final sample size is fixed, (2) the number of interim analyses is defined in advance, and (3) a stopping rule to reject the null hypothesis at each interim stage. In other words, greater planning is required. These methods are not discussed here but the `gsDesign` R package has functions to calculate power and sample sizes for such designs.

5.5 Putting it all together

The previous three chapters examined the parts of an experiment and the principles of design, and here we bring all of the concepts together. This section is generic because the details depend on the planned experiment and the steps need not follow the order described below. A guiding principle is to keep the design as simple as possible, but ensure that the research question can be adequately addressed.

The first step is to decide if the experiment is (mainly) exploratory or confirmatory as this will influence subsequent decisions. Next, the outcome(s) need to be selected, and for a confirmatory study a primary and maybe a secondary outcome should be defined. Also consider what ancillary variables need to be measured or recorded to ensure the validity of the assay or to check assumptions. An example might be the body weight of rodents to assess their overall health or the total cell count in a cell culture experiment to ensure that cell death is similar across experimental conditions.

If the study is confirmatory, consider if a new experiment will add anything to what is already known. A systematic review and meta-analysis of the existing literature is often useful before conducting another study and an excellent example of this approach is by Kleikers *et al.* [191]. Several papers using animal models of stroke showed a beneficial effect of inhibiting NOX (NADPH oxidase) on infarct size and neurological and motor functioning. Based on their analysis of the literature, Kleikers *et al.* found that the quality of studies was low (few were randomised or blinded) and there was evidence of publication bias. Thus, another high quality confirmatory experiment was justified. The literature review also enabled them to obtain data for a sample size calculation for their

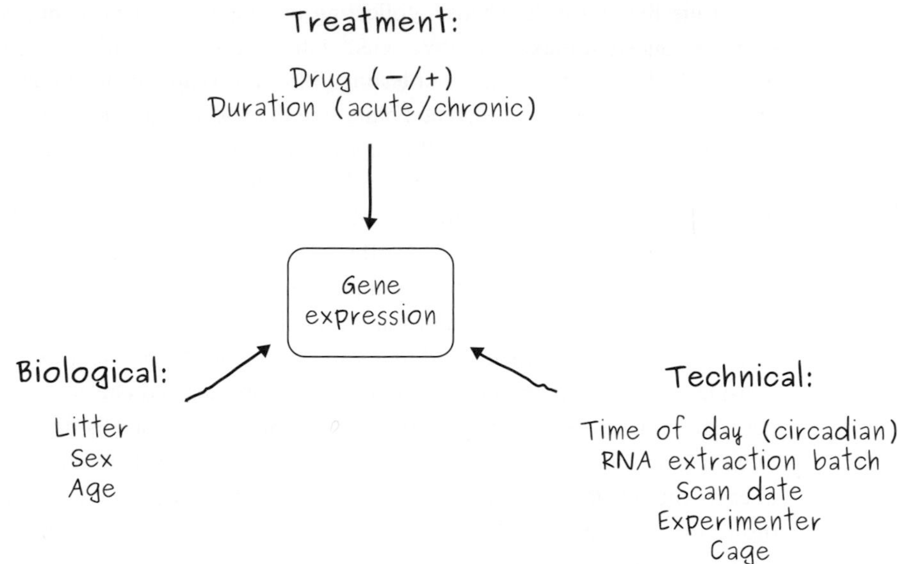

Fig. 5.22 Sketch of a mouse microarray experiment in the planning stage. The treatment effects are indicated, along with the biological and technical effects that might affect the outcome. These will need to be included as factors, covariates, or held constant.

experiment.[13] For an excellent introductory book on meta-analyses see Borenstein *et al.* [53].

The next step is to define the treatment effects that you are interested in testing, which directly relates to the goal or purpose of the experiment. Does a main effect or an interaction test the research hypothesis? That is, is the question 'does X affect Y' or 'does X affect Y only under condition Z'?

Next, identify the biological and technical effects that might influence the outcome. Are you interested in testing any of these as a hypothesis? Which effects will be allowed to vary and which will be held constant? Make a sketch like Figure 5.22 showing these variables. A microarray experiment is used as an example, with two treatment factors: the absence (−) or presence (+) of a drug and the duration of the treatment. Brainstorm and put anything that might be relevant. Think about the technical factors that might influence the outcome, such as the order of sample collection, the day on which the experiment is run, spatial effects on microtitre plates. Consider how samples will arrive: all at once, in batches (usually to make the experiment more manageable), or sequentially (e.g. clinical samples). If you are a junior scientist, discuss the sketch with the principal investigator, or with colleagues, to see if any important variables have been omitted.

[13] Kleikers *et al.* found that inhibiting NOX had little effect on infarct size and no effect on neurological or motor functioning. It is the same story once again; early studies without randomisation or blinding and plenty of researcher degrees of freedom show interesting and significant results. Properly conducted follow-up studies then fail to find an effect.

Exploratory studies will tend to have multiple factors varying (e.g. both sexes, multiple time points), whereas confirmatory studies will tend to hold more variables fixed. It will not be possible to control everything and the 80/20 rule for biological and technical effects applies.[14] Try to account for the major sources of variability in the outcome by using blocks or covariate adjustment and ensure that important biological and technical factors are not confounded with the treatment effects. If the experiment becomes too complex, consider confounding effects that are not of interest such as cage effects and day effects. Also consider which positive and negative control conditions will be included.

Make a layout of the design showing the factor level combinations like below. '−' and '+' are used to indicate the absence or presence of a factor (e.g. no drug/drug) or the lower and higher level of the factor without specifying any values. Suppose that in addition to the drug and duration treatment factors, we decide to include both sexes. Each of these factors has two levels, giving $2 \times 2 \times 2 = 2^3 = 8$ factor level combinations. This can be seen in the first eight rows in the layout below for the columns Sex, Duration, and Drug. Each row has a different combination of + and − signs and rows 1–8 show all possible combinations.

Suppose that we decide to keep age and most of the technical factors fixed at one level (e.g. one experimenter, all arrays scanned on the same day) but it is inevitable that multiple litters will be required and all animals cannot fit in one cage. In the table, we see that two litters will be used and that all animals from a litter will be housed together in the same cage (litter A in Cage 1; litter B in Cage 2). Litter and cage are thus completely confounded, which is an example of useful confounding because we are not interested in testing for litter or cage effects separately, only accounting for the variation they may introduce. The code below uses the `expand.grid()` function to generate all possible combinations of drug, duration, sex, and litters.

```
> # generate layout
> d <- expand.grid(Drug=c("-","+"), Duration=c("-","+"),Sex=c("-","+"),
+                  Litter=LETTERS[1:2])
>
> # add animal ID, cage, and reorder columns
> d <- data.frame("Animal ID"=1:nrow(d),
+                 Cage=rep(1:2, each=8), d[,4:1] )
>
> d
   Animal.ID Cage Litter Sex Duration Drug
1          1    1      A   -        -    -
2          2    1      A   -        -    +
3          3    1      A   -        +    -
4          4    1      A   -        +    +
```

[14] The 80/20 rule, also known as the Pareto principle, states that the majority (80%) of the technical and biological variation in the outcome will be the result of a small number (20%) of factors or causes.

5	5	1	A	+	−	−
6	6	1	A	+	−	+
7	7	1	A	+	+	−
8	8	1	A	+	+	+
9	9	2	B	−	−	−
10	10	2	B	−	−	+
11	11	2	B	−	+	−
12	12	2	B	−	+	+
13	13	2	B	+	−	−
14	14	2	B	+	−	+
15	15	2	B	+	+	−
16	16	2	B	+	+	+

Note how rows 1–8 for the Sex, Duration, and Litter columns are duplicated in rows 9–16. Litter and Sex are blocking variables and the eight animals within a litter will be randomly assigned to the treatment conditions, separately for each sex. Now that litter has been included as another variable with two levels, there are $2^4 = 16$ factor level combinations, meaning that a minimum of 16 animals are required to have one observation in each cell. Such tables are good for visualising how the factors relate to each other, whether the factors are uncorrelated, and to start thinking multidimensionally: this is not a one factor design with 16 levels but a $2 \times 2 \times 2 \times 2$ design. The multidimensional aspect is illustrated in Figure 5.24 for a different example.

At this point it can be useful to calculate the number of samples available to estimate the error using the resource equation. If all main and interaction effects are included in the analysis, there is no replication within the 16 factor level combinations and therefore there are no samples left to estimate the error.[15] Suppose we are only interested in the main effects and the drug-by-duration interaction. This gives:

$$\begin{aligned} N - 1 &= \text{Drug} + \text{Duration} + \text{Sex} + \text{Litter} + \text{Drug} : \text{Duration} + E \\ 16 - 1 &= 1 + 1 + 1 + 1 + 1 + E \\ 10 &= E \end{aligned} \tag{5.21}$$

samples remaining to estimate the error. This is probably too low because other interaction effects might be interesting to test and it is not uncommon for microarrays to fail quality control checks. It might be worthwhile to include another litter to increase the total sample size to 24. But now it will take longer to collect all the samples and genes that have a circadian rhythm will have a larger gradient of expression levels over time, which may be a problem for some experiments. One option to avoid circadian effects is to collect the samples from each litter on separate days so that all samples are collected around the same time of day, within a hour or two of each other. This introduces day as another variable, but since it is confounded with cage and litter, the experiment is not any more complex. The

[15] Think of it as fitting a straight line through two points; the fit is perfect and there is no variation remaining.

updated design layout is shown below with the additional litter and day included as a new variable. It is easy to see that day, cage, and litter are completely confounded, but it is hard to check the balance with these and the other variables.

```
> # make the layout
> d2 <- expand.grid(Drug=c("-","+"), Duration=c("-","+"),Sex=c("-","+"),
+                   Litter=LETTERS[1:3])
>
> # add animal ID, cage, and reorder columns
> d2 <- data.frame("Animal ID"=1:nrow(d2),
+                   Cage=rep(1:3, each=8), d2[,4:1] )
>
> d2
   Animal.ID Cage Litter Sex Duration Drug
1          1    1      A   -        -    -
2          2    1      A   -        -    +
3          3    1      A   -        +    -
4          4    1      A   -        +    +
5          5    1      A   +        -    -
6          6    1      A   +        -    +
7          7    1      A   +        +    -
8          8    1      A   +        +    +
9          9    2      B   -        -    -
10        10    2      B   -        -    +
11        11    2      B   -        +    -
12        12    2      B   -        +    +
13        13    2      B   +        -    -
14        14    2      B   +        -    +
15        15    2      B   +        +    -
16        16    2      B   +        +    +
17        17    3      C   -        -    -
18        18    3      C   -        -    +
19        19    3      C   -        +    -
20        20    3      C   -        +    +
21        21    3      C   +        -    -
22        22    3      C   +        -    +
23        23    3      C   +        +    -
24        24    3      C   +        +    +
```

It is good to confirm the balance by cross-tabulating the number of observations, for example:

```
> xtabs(~Litter+Drug, data=d)
      Drug
Litter - +
     A 4 4
     B 4 4
>
> xtabs(~Sex+Duration, data=d)
   Duration
Sex - +
  - 4 4
  + 4 4
>
> xtabs(~Litter + Duration, d)
      Duration
Litter - +
     A 4 4
     B 4 4
```

This experiment has duration of treatment as a variable, and a decision must be made about using a front- or end-aligned design (Section 2.11). A front-aligned design has the advantage of splitting the sample collection over 2 days with 12 animals on each day (Figure 5.23). The disadvantage is that the technical factor 'day of sample collection' is completely confounded with the treatment factor 'duration of treatment'. For a microarray study, this probably matters; for a behavioural study, it might be less important. Sketching a diagram is once again useful (Figure 5.23). Furthermore, if all animals are the same age when they start the experiment, the animals in the acute and chronic groups will be different ages with a front-aligned design. Thus, the age of the animal is confounded with the duration of treatment as well. This is a minor concern if the difference between acute and chronic treatments is only a few days. An end-aligned design lacks these problems and by confounding day with cage and litter, each block can be executed as a separate experiment. All comparisons of interest can be made within a block and are not confounded.

Next, define the design space for the treatment effects and the biological and technical factors that are not held fixed. Consider the rules of thumb for optimal designs. What ranges will the continuous variables take, how many levels will the factors take, what is the spacing between the factor levels (Section 5.3)? Will it be an equal N design or will some groups have a larger sample size? Ensure that factors are uncorrelated to maximise power. Define the factor arrangement, which factors are crossed and which are nested?

Define the biological, experimental, and observational units (Chapter 3). Ensure that the EUs are replicated. Will there be multiple OUs for each EU? Should there be replication at

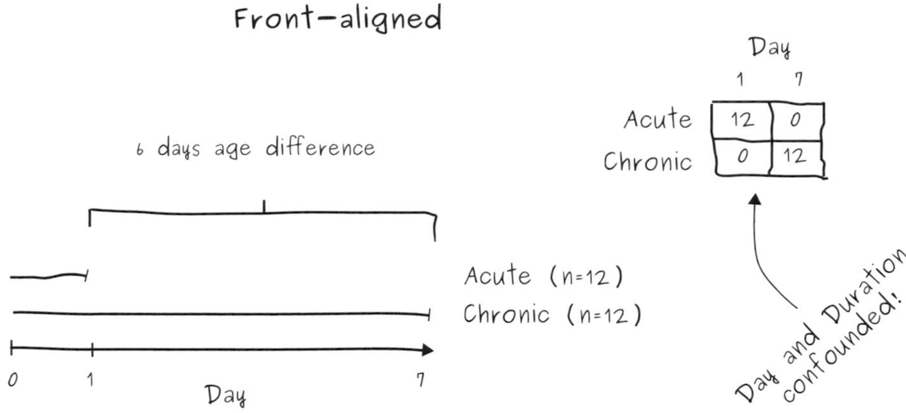

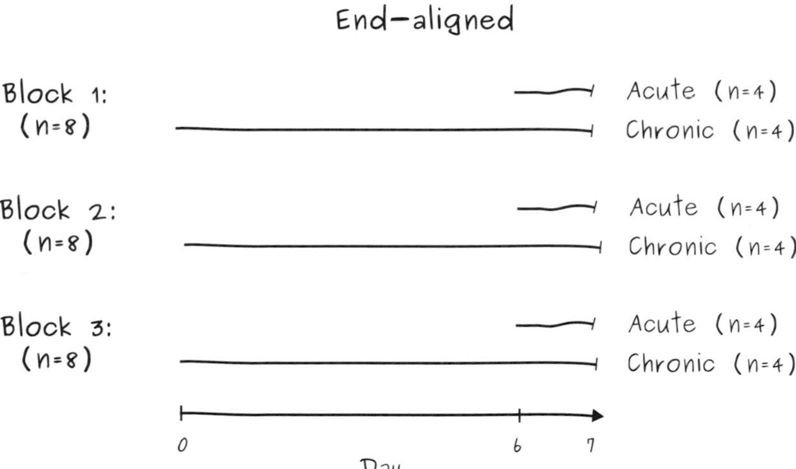

Fig. 5.23 Another sketch of the microarray experiment. The time line indicates the duration of drug treatment. A front-aligned design confounds the day of sample collection and the duration of treatment. There is also a slight age difference between animals (but 6 days is likely negligible). The end-aligned design can be executed as separate blocks over 3 days. Day, litter, and cage are all completely confounded and considered a block, but this is fine because these factors are not scientifically interesting. All relevant comparisons can be done within each block.

a higher level in the biological or technical hierarchy? Have a clear plan of randomisation and blinding.

A power analysis or sample size calculation may be useful, especially for a confirmatory study. Consider the probability of missing data due to drop-out or low quality samples and plan for this in the calculations. When will you stop collecting data? Will the sample size be fixed in advance, will there be interim analyses?

postdocs, students, technicians, collaborators from other groups or institutions, and contract research organisations. Reducing misunderstandings and improving communication is becoming increasingly important as science becomes more collaborative and as group members become more diverse. A SAP is especially useful when wet-lab groups collaborate with computational or bioinformatics groups, as there may be little shared knowledge, experience, or terminology.

Second, describing all the details in one document allows people to point out constraints on what is feasible, weaknesses, and suggestions for improvement. For example, a collaborator might suggest the inclusion of a positive control from their recent experience with a manuscript submission. A technician might mention that it will not be possible to conduct the experiment over five consecutive mornings because other groups have booked the equipment or facilities for the next 4 months. It might then be decided to conduct the experiment over two full days instead, to check if other groups are flexible with their bookings, or to wait until the next available slot. If large day effects are expected, then moving from 5 days to 2 days will be a major design change; in particular, how the treatment effects and any biological effects are balanced across days. This cannot be decided after the experiment is underway.

Third, once the information is written, it is easy to include it in the methods section of a manuscript or thesis. Since much of this information has to be written anyway, why not take advantage of the benefits of writing it before conducting the experiment?

Fourth, a SAP encourages experimenters to be honest. If the expression of a particular gene was stipulated as the primary outcome variable, then it is harder to fool yourself (and others) that another gene was predicted all along. After seeing the data, it is easy to say 'I would have picked this as my primary outcome anyway, therefore it is fine if I present it as such' (see hindsight bias; Section 1.2). When primary outcomes are specified in advance, it is remarkable how often another outcome turns out to be more interesting, or that the effect for the primary outcome is much smaller than predicted. Once written, the SAP can be pre-registered. Pre-registering protocols for preclinical studies is becoming more common because of concerns over reproducibility and questionable research practices. For example, the BioMed Central series of journals have an option to publish a protocol[17] and several journals have recently introduced a new type of research article called a Registered Report. For a Registered Report, methods and analyses are pre-registered and peer reviewed. If the protocol passes peer-review, the full study will be published so long as it adheres to the specifications of the protocol, regardless of the outcome. Further information can be found on the Open Science Framework website.[18] There is some debate about the usefulness of pre-registering exploratory studies, but publishing a protocol for a confirmatory study gives results much more weight.

Fifth, a SAP makes the experimenter aware that they may not know how to analyse the data that the experiment will generate, or if two variables are nested or crossed for example. This will prompt them to do a simpler experiment that they can analyse and understand,

[17] `http://www.biomedcentral.com/authors/protocols`

[18] `https://osf.io/8mpji/wiki/home/`. AsPredicted is another place to pre-register experiments (`https://aspredicted.org/`)

or to seek advice. Figuring out how to analyse the data – or finding someone who can – should not be done once the experiment is completed.

Finally, a SAP allows the relevant information to be quickly and easily shared. This might be important if the Animal Welfare Officer needs information for an inspection. Giving others the impression that you are an organised scientist is never a bad idea.

5.7.2 What to include in the SAP

Below is a suggested list of items to include in a SAP, in the approximate order that they should appear. Some items may be irrelevant for some experiments and there may be items not included here that should be added. When deciding what to include in the SAP, as well as the amount of detail, the main criteria is whether the information is useful to you and others involved with the experiment.

Aim or hypothesis: This could be a specific hypothesis or a general research question such as 'What is the effect of a high fructose diet on gene expression in the brains of mice?'

Type of experiment: Classification of the experiment as either exploratory or confirmatory (or the parts that are exploratory and confirmatory).

Outcome variable(s): Definition of the primary outcome variable (if any), as well as secondary and tertiary outcome variables. Also include ancillary variables such as body weight. If the experiment is exploratory, you could mention that the outcome is gene expression or behavioural measures of anxiety and depression. The point is to list variables that will be measured.

Treatments and experimental conditions: This section lists the treatment effects, including the names of the treatments or experimental interventions and the factor levels. Positive and negative controls can also be listed. See Section 2.2 and Eq. (2.1) for information on writing this and the next three points.

Subject/Sample information: This section lists the biological effects, both those that are varied and those that are held constant, including species and strain of animals, litter, age, sex, and cell line.

Technical effects: This section lists all of the important technical effects that vary and that are held constant. For example, if the experiment will be conducted on one day or over several; the number of experimenters; if there will be any batching, and so on. In addition, you might include other details such as not using the outer wells on 96-well plates to avoid edge effects. Section 2.12 on heterogeneity and confounding is useful to consider when writing this section.

Design: The design indicates how the treatment, biological, and technical effects from the previous three points are related. One could write a simple equation such as: y = Dose + Litter + Day. Then, indicate which factors are random and which are fixed, and if the factors are crossed or nested. It would also be good to include the justification for the design; for example, why a variable was used for blocking. The name of the design can be provided (e.g. randomised block design), and if any effects are aliased (Section 2.12.9). One can also include justifications for the choices made; for example, based on optimality criteria (Section 5.3).

Randomisation and blinding: Indicate where randomisation occurs and how it will be done. This includes randomisation of experimental units to treatment groups and also the order of sample collection or processing or spatial locations on a microtitre plate (Sections 2.12.7 and 2.12.8).

Sample size and units: Define the biological, experimental, and observational units. Report the number of experimental units and observational units (subsamples). The results of a power analysis or sample size calculation can be included in this section. In addition, the stopping rule should be reported (Section 5.4).

Preprocessing: Describe any modifications of the data such as normalisations, transformations, or the calculation of new variables from measured variables (e.g. change scores; Section 6.2). Also, indicate how missing data will be addressed.

Exclusion criteria: Indicate any rules used to exclude data. For example, animals with a body weight below a given value will be excluded. Also indicate how outliers will be detected and dealt with.

Analysis: Describe the models (the conventional name of the test can also be used, such as a '*t*-test'). Examples are given in Chapter 4. It is hard to know what the best model will be before seeing the data, and so multiple models can be described, along with the method of choosing the final model. For example, one can state that sex will be included as a predictor in an initial model, and if it is not significant ($p < 0.05$), then the final model will exclude sex. Thus, if sex is an important predictor, then inferences about treatment effects will be made with sex included in the model, otherwise inferences will be made by ignoring sex. This allows some flexibility in data analysis while still restricting the scope of all of the analyses that could be conducted. A pre-specified model is critical for a confirmatory experiment, but still useful for exploratory studies. Including the R code for the analysis is useful if you are uncertain how to model the data, as others may be able to comment on it.

Names and dates: It is useful to include the names of the people involved with the project, who is responsible for each aspect of the experiment, who has reviewed the SAP, and the date of each version (it will likely be revised several times). This gives everyone involved ownership of the project and can also be used as a reference should any dispute over authorship arise.

The larger and more complex the experiment the more useful a SAP becomes. After the SAP is completed, share it with others involved in the project to get feedback and comments, and revise if necessary. Once the design and statistical aspects of the SAP are defined, any deviations from the protocol should be noted. Even with the best planning experiments sometimes need to be modified after they are underway and large technical effects might arise that need to be included in the model. Once the first SAP is written, subsequent SAPs for similar experiments can be created quickly by making minor modifications. SAPs require a small investment in time and effort, but pay for themselves many times over in the longer term.

Further reading

If you design and conduct experiments for a living, learning as much as possible about experimental design is a wise investment. The formal training that biologists receive in DoE is less than 5% of the potentially relevant material. What if pilots learnt only 5% of the controls in a cockpit, or surgeons only how to use 5% of instruments in an operating room? In addition to the books suggested on page 93 the following are useful resources.

DoE with R: Lawson is an applied book with R code integrated throughout the text [213]. It would be a logical choice as a next book after completing this one, but few examples are from biology.

Optimal designs: The introductory text on optimal designs by Berger and Wong provides many of the details that were omitted in Section 5.3 because they were presented as rules of thumb to make them as widely accessible as possible [36].

DoE in other fields: The book *Improving Almost Anything: Ideas and Essays* is an annotated collection of papers from George Box and colleagues [54]. It is not directly related to biological experiments, but with chapters such as 'Statistics as a catalyst to learning', 'How to get lucky', 'Scientific method: the generation of knowledge', and 'Sequential experimentation and sequential assembly of designs', it provides worthwhile information for any scientist.

6 Exploratory Data Analysis

It is the unusual observation made by the prepared mind that often paves the way to fundamental new advances.

Sir Walter Bodmer, FRS

You can observe a lot by just watching.

Yogi Berra

In Section 2.1, we made the distinction between learning/exploratory experiments and confirming experiments. A related distinction is between exploratory and confirmatory data analysis. Exploratory data analysis (EDA) is also called initial data analysis, preliminary data analysis, or cross-examination of data and it has two purposes. First, to understand the data before a formal statistical analysis, including quality control checks for impossible or implausible values and assessing whether the planned statistical model is appropriate. It is always useful to plot the data before an analysis and Anscombe's famous data set illustrates why [11]. Suppose we have two continuous variables and the Pearson correlation between them is $r = 0.81$ ($p = 0.002$). Is this enough to conclude that a relationship exists? Is there anything else you would like to know if you viewed this result in a journal? Anscombe created four variables that have the same correlation, slope, intercept, and p-value with a fifth variable, but the relationships are different.

The data are in the `anscombe` data set that comes with the base R installation and the code below calculates the correlation between the first pair of variables (`x1` and `y1`). The correlation is sensible if the data look like the values in Figure 6.1A. The other pairs of variables are plotted in panels B–D, and despite having the same statistical summaries, a linear correlation does not tell the whole story.

```
> cor.test(~y1+x1, data=anscombe)

Pearson's product-moment correlation

data:  y1 and x1
t = 4.241, df = 9, p-value = 0.00217
alternative hypothesis: true correlation is not equal to 0
95 percent confidence interval:
 0.424391 0.950693
sample estimates:
     cor
0.816421
```

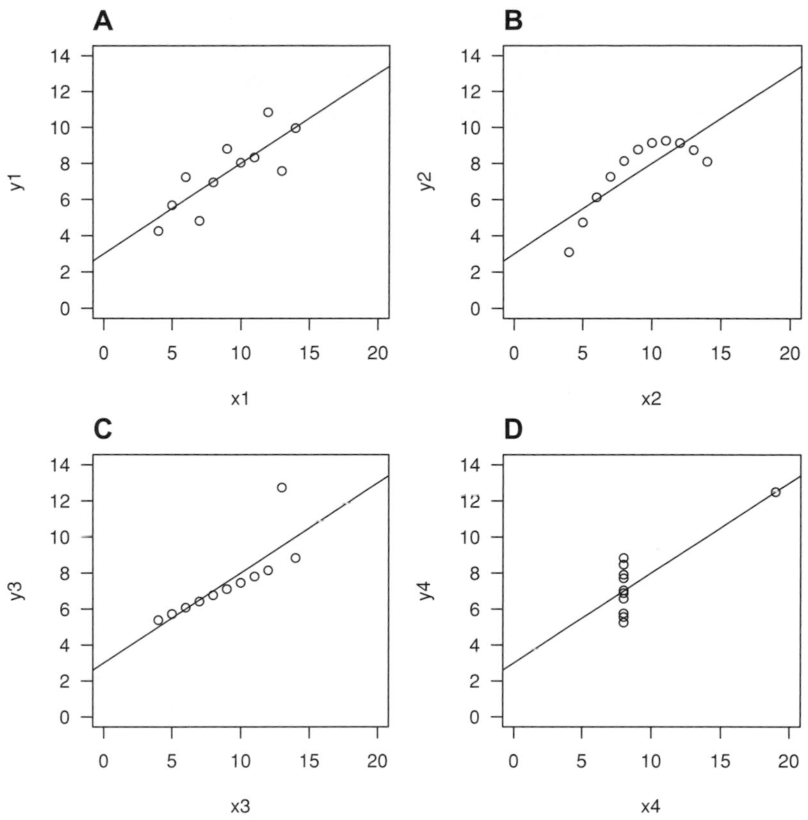

Fig. 6.1 Anscombe data. The data in all four panels have the same correlation, *p*-value, slope, and intercept, but a correlation or linear regression is only appropriate for the top left graph.

The curvilinear relationship in Figure 6.1B is not captured with a Pearson correlation. Figure 6.1C contains an outlier, and it might be of interest to see how the results change if it is excluded. Finally, a single data point is responsible for the significant result in Figure 6.1D, and so support for a linear relationship is weak. This classic example shows how a simple graphical display provides more information to interpret the results.

The second purpose of EDA is to discover new and unanticipated relationships, but controlling the false positive rate is hard when the data are used both to find and then test relationships. For example, maybe a linear relationship was predicted, but the results show a strong curvilinear relationship (Figure 6.1B), which we now want to test. This is an unexpected feature of the data that alters the analysis plan.

6.1 Quality control checks

Before jumping into an analysis it is always useful to perform quality control (QC) checks. Data quality control receives little attention in statistics books or courses and applied statisticians and data analysts learn it informally on the job. The larger the data set, the greater the need to perform QC checks because it is harder to spot unusual features by eye, and with more data there is a greater chance of errors. QC checks are even more important if the data were generated by someone else and given to you to analyse. When you have collected the data yourself, you are aware of all the important features of the experiment that might affect the results: you know the design of the experiment, what all of the variables mean, the units of measurement, and what values are impossible or implausible. When someone else has conducted the experiment and collected the data, assumptions are inevitably made and they should be verified if possible. For example, were all of the data collected on the same day? By the same person? Were the data averaged or normalised? What is the experimental unit, how are missing values indicated? And what on earth does the variable 'XF.tt1' represent!?

In the following examples, assume the data sets are large enough so that QC checks cannot be performed by glancing at the data. Also assume that the data were generated by someone else and given to us to analyse, so we know little about the experimental details. Statisticians often find themselves in this situation, but assume that you are a principal investigator and one of your students has conducted an experiment in the lab of a collaborator, using an assay or instrument that is new to you. You ask for the data so that you can analyse it yourself. Since this is a new assay we have to spend time to understand the data, which would be known or obvious if you conducted the experiment yourself or if it was a method routinely used in your lab. Many QC checks are described below but they won't all be necessary for every data set.

6.1.1 Data layout

Tabular data are usually organised so that rows contain the cases, subjects, or experimental units and columns contain the variables, features, attributes, or measurements. This is a standard format for most statistical software and is assumed for all examples here. When multiple outcomes are measured on subjects – including the special case of one outcome measured at multiple time points – the data can be organised in either a *long* or a *wide* layout. In a long layout, the multiple measurements are stacked in a single column and additional columns are required to indicate what the values represent, such as the time the measurement was taken. This is shown below using the `hypertension` data set in the `labstats` package, where the outcome (`Y`) is measured on three occasions for each subject and `Time` indicates the time point. Information for each subject appears on multiple rows and in this data set there are 10 subjects and 3 time points, giving 30 rows.

```
> library(labstats)
>
> # check dimensions
> dim(hypertension)
[1] 30  4
>
```

```
> head(hypertension)
  Subject   Diet Time   Y
1       1 HighCa    1 133
2       1 HighCa    2 141
3       1 HighCa    3 100
4       2 HighCa    1 130
5       2 HighCa    2 122
6       2 HighCa    3 102
```

Most of R's modelling and plotting functions require the long layout. The wide layout, however, is easier to view in a spreadsheet, and is therefore preferred by biologists. The code below shows how to convert the `hypertension` data into the wide layout. This process is called *reshaping* and there are several functions and whole packages available. The `reshape()` function can convert data into either layout, and the `direction` argument specifies the layout to be converted to. The `timevar` argument specifies the variable indicating the multiple measurements on each subject. The `idvar` argument specifies the variables that are constant for each subject. These are usually properties of the subject such as their age, sex, litter, cage, and their experimental condition (assuming that each subject is only in one condition).

```
> # convert to wide layout
> wide.hyper <- reshape(hypertension,
+                       timevar="Time",
+                       idvar=c("Subject","Diet"),
+                       direction="wide")
>
> # check dimensions
> dim(wide.hyper)
[1] 10  5
>
> wide.hyper
   Subject   Diet Y.1 Y.2 Y.3
1        1 HighCa 133 141 100
4        2 HighCa 130 122 102
7        3 HighCa 151 152 144
10       4 HighCa 144 135 129
13       5 HighCa 171 142 128
16       6  LowCa 104 139 153
19       7  LowCa 139 174 190
22       8  LowCa 114 116 151
25       9  LowCa 131 153 175
28      10  LowCa 147 167 157
```

Y is now in three columns instead of one, and the number in the column name indicates the time point (e.g. Y.1 is the first time point). To go from a wide to a long format direction must be set to "long". In the code below the varying argument specifies the variables that should be combined into one variable in the long layout. The v.names argument specifies the name of this new variable and BP (for blood pressure) is used instead of the original name (Y). The new BP variable needs another variable to indicate which time point the measurement was taken. This is created automatically and the timevar argument allows us to specify a name for this variable.

```
> long.hyper <- reshape(wide.hyper,
+                       varying=c("Y.1","Y.2","Y.3"),
+                       v.names="BP",
+                       timevar="Time",
+                       direction="long")
>
> # check dimensions
> dim(long.hyper)
[1] 30  5
>
> # reorder by subject, then time
> long.hyper <- long.hyper[order(long.hyper$Subject, long.hyper$Time), ]
>
> head(long.hyper)
    Subject   Diet Time  BP id
1.1       1 HighCa    1 133  1
1.2       1 HighCa    2 141  1
1.3       1 HighCa    3 100  1
2.1       2 HighCa    1 130  2
2.2       2 HighCa    2 122  2
2.3       2 HighCa    3 102  2
```

The rows of the new data frame may not be ordered in the best way so the order() function reorders them by subject and then by time. The reshape() function has other arguments that are not discussed but might be useful. The stack() and unstack() functions perform similar transformations and the melt() and cast() functions from the reshape2 package are popular alternatives.

6.1.2 Possible and plausible values

Once the data layout is known, one of the first things to check is that the data contain no impossible values such as negative ages, or implausible values such as ages greater than 100. Unusual values will need to be resolved before analysis can proceed.

Minimum and maximum values

The summary() function is useful for checking the range of the data as it provides the minimum and maximum values for each variable. In the cats data set below we see that the minimum body weight (Bwt) and heart weight (Hwt) values are greater than zero, which is sensible because weight cannot be negative.

```
> data(cats, package="MASS")
> summary(cats)
 Sex        Bwt             Hwt
 F:47   Min.   :2.00   Min.   : 6.30
 M:97   1st Qu.:2.30   1st Qu.: 8.95
        Median :2.70   Median :10.10
        Mean   :2.72   Mean   :10.63
        3rd Qu.:3.02   3rd Qu.:12.12
        Max.   :3.90   Max.   :20.50
```

Unless we are familiar with feline anatomy, we may not know what sensible lower or upper values are for these variables, but the heart weights are greater than the body weights. This is suspicious because a part of cat – the heart – cannot weigh more than the whole cat. The units of measurement should therefore be checked for correctness and consistency. The documentation for the data set indicates that heart weight is measured in grams and body weight in kilograms, which clarifies this unusual feature. Expressing the weight variables in the same units may be beneficial for some analyses, but we keep them as they are.

Data type

Many R functions require variables to be a certain type, such as a number or a factor. We might also have expectations about variable types; for example, we expect that a variable called 'cell count' should have whole numbers because it is impossible to have half a cell. If cell counts are decimal numbers we need to ask the experimenter if the values have been adjusted or transformed.

The summary() function provides information about variable types because factor levels are listed for factors and summary statistics are given for numeric variables. Another option is to check the class of each variable in a data frame using the sapply() function, shown below. The cellcount data set from the labstats package has a variable called cell.count, which we can see is an integer.

```
> head(cellcount)
    plate row column cell.count
1 Plate_1   1      1        165
2 Plate_1   1      2        235
3 Plate_1   1      3        105
4 Plate_1   1      4        142
```

```
> # convert the date from a string into a "Date" format
> date.data$obs.date <- as.Date(date.data$obs.date, format="%d-%m-%Y")
>
> # check order
> date.data
  subject visit.number   obs.date
1       1            1 2015-03-01
2       1            2 2015-03-08
3       1            3 2015-03-15
4       2            1 2015-03-01
5       2            2 2015-08-03
6       2            3 2015-03-15
```

Checking for incorrect dates by looking at a list of numbers is painful and so the `tapply()` function calculates the difference (using the `diff()` function) between consecutive dates for each subject. For this to work the rows of the data must be ordered by subject and then by visit number. The output below shows that for subject 1 (`$'1'`) the difference between the second and first visit is 7 days, and the difference between the third and second visit is also 7 days. For subject 2, however, the difference between the second and first visit is 155 days, and the difference between the third and second visit is −141 days, which is impossible because the third visit cannot be before the second visit.

```
> # check difference between observation dates
> with(date.data, tapply(obs.date, subject, diff))
$`1`
Time differences in days
[1] 7 7

$`2`
Time differences in days
[1]  155 -141
```

A closer look at the date values shows that visit number 2 has a day/month swap. It is 2015-08-03 (August 3rd) but should be 2015-03-08 (March 8th). There are two things to look for with this output. The first is negative numbers, and the second is unusually long or short times between consecutive dates. Not all day/month swaps or incorrect date entries will have negative differences, but unusual values should still be checked. If subjects are assessed at fixed intervals (e.g. weekly, monthly, annually) the difference between dates should be similar. Thus, the difference of 155 days between the second and first visit for subject 2 also indicates a problem. Similarly, if subjects are assessed every 3 months, two assessments a few days apart is suspicious.

If subjects are assessed at multiple times, it is likely that researchers are interested in changes over time. Usually the date is recalculated as 'time since entry into the study' and is one of the main predictor variables in a longitudinal design. Errors in the predictor can have a large influence on the analysis.

6.1.3 Uniqueness

Understanding the uniqueness of values is not as critical as finding impossible or implausible values, but it can also flag data entry errors and it provides a better understanding of the data.

Subject IDs and other unique values

Each subject or sample should be assigned a unique identification number. We saw earlier how non-unique IDs can give incorrect results (the `glycogen` data set analysed in Section 4.3.4, p. 157). The three functions described below can be used for these checks. But first, a vector of female names is created that are the subject identifiers, which we expect to be unique and therefore to appear only once in the vector. The `length()` function counts the number of entries, which is five. The `unique()` function returns only the unique elements of a vector and thus removes duplicate entries. If there are no duplicate entries `length(person)` and `length(unique(person))` should return the same value. Below we see that there are only three unique entries and therefore some duplication is present, but we do not know where in the vector the duplication occurred.

```
> person <- c("Anna","Brynn","Carey","Brynn","Brynn")
>
> # number of entries
> length(person)
[1] 5
>
> # unique entries
> unique(person)
[1] "Anna"  "Brynn" "Carey"
>
> # number of unique entries
> length(unique(person))
[1] 3
```

The `duplicated()` function returns a vector of `TRUE` (is duplicated) and `FALSE` (not duplicated) values with the same length as the input vector. The first occurrence of `Brynn` (second entry) is `FALSE`, because even though `Brynn` is duplicated, this is the first occurrence. By putting the *not* operator (`!`) in front of the `duplicated()` function the values of `TRUE` and `FALSE` are reversed (because not TRUE = FALSE, and *vice versa*). This enables the vector of TRUE and FALSE values to be used as a filter, shown in the last line of code below.

```
> # is a value duplicated?
> duplicated(person)
[1] FALSE FALSE FALSE  TRUE  TRUE
>
> # how many duplications?
> sum(duplicated(person))
[1] 2
>
> # not duplicated?
> !duplicated(person)
[1]  TRUE  TRUE  TRUE FALSE FALSE
>
> # filter duplications
> person[!duplicated(person)]
[1] "Anna"  "Brynn" "Carey"
```

If the data are in the long format then there will be multiple entries for unique subject identifiers, and so this check is less useful. There may, however, be other things to check such as sample IDs, for example if a blood sample was taken at each time point and given a unique assay number.

Another uniqueness check is for whole rows of duplicated data, which can arise if data are pasted into a spreadsheet twice by accident. The strategy is to combine all the variables together into one large new variable, and then test for uniqueness. The `hypertension` data are used for this example and only the first three lines are shown below. The `apply()` function pastes together the values across a row and `collapse="_"` indicates that an underscore should be inserted between the entries pasted together. The results are stored in `combos` – a character vector as long as the number of rows in `hypertension`. The first few entries of `combos` is shown and the first is `"1_HighCa_1_133"`, which we can verify is the first line of the `hypertension` data (output from the `head()` function) separated by underscores. The final line of code checks for duplications, and there are none.

```
> head(hypertension, 3)
  Subject   Diet Time   Y
1       1 HighCa    1 133
2       1 HighCa    2 141
3       1 HighCa    3 100
>
> # combine rows into one long string
> combos <- apply(hypertension, 1, paste, collapse="_")
>
> head(combos)
[1] " 1_HighCa_1_133" " 1_HighCa_2_141" " 1_HighCa_3_100" " 2_HighCa_1_130"
```

```
[5] " 2_HighCa_2_122" " 2_HighCa_3_102"
>
> # check for duplicated row entries
> sum(duplicated(combos))
[1] 0
```

Consistent factor levels

Another check is for inconsistent naming of factor levels. This is often detected when the `summary()` function is used on a data frame but inconsistencies can be missed if there are many factor levels because by default `summary()` only shows the first seven (but the number can be increased with the `maxsum` argument).

The code below generates a vector of group labels – three treated samples and three control – but each treated sample has a different spelling. The first has a capital T, the second a lower case t, and the final one has a white space after the final t. Since R is case-sensitive, these are three distinct factor levels. There are several ways to correct the labels and here the `tolower()` function converts all the characters to lower case. This also converts `cond` from a factor to a character vector. Next, `gsub()` finds a single white space (indicated by the first set of quotes with a space between them), and replaces it with nothing (second set of quotes with no space). This removes *all spaces* and is not a problem here, but there might be other spaces that we would like to keep. The `gsub()` function has options for more complex pattern matching (see `help(gsub)` for details). The final line of code converts the character vector back into a factor.

```
> cond <- factor(c("Treat","treat","Treat ","Cntrl","Cntrl","Cntrl"))
> summary(cond)
 Cntrl  treat  Treat Treat
     3      1      1      1
>
> # convert to lowercase (factor also converted to character)
> cond <- tolower(cond)
>
> # "find and replace" white space with nothing
> cond <- factor(gsub(" ", "", cond))
> cond
[1] treat treat treat cntrl cntrl cntrl
Levels: cntrl treat
```

Data granularity

Another thing to check is the *granularity* of the data – a general term encompassing the discreteness, resolution, or precision of the measurements. The `cats` data set in the `MASS` package is used for illustration. Referring back to the graph of the body weights in

Figure 4.12 (top right graph on page 167), we see that the measurements appear at discrete values. The `table()` function below counts the number of observations with the same values. The minimum body weight is 2 kg and 5 cats have this weight. The next heaviest cats weigh 2.1 kg and there are 10 of them. Looking through the values we see that the weights are measured to the nearest 10th of a kilogram or 100th of a gram.

```
> table(cats$Bwt)

  2 2.1 2.2 2.3 2.4 2.5 2.6 2.7 2.8 2.9   3 3.1 3.2 3.3 3.4 3.5 3.6
  5  10  14  13   9  10   9  12   7   8  11   6   6   5   5   5   4
3.7 3.8 3.9
  1   2   2
```

Why does this matter? It is inappropriate to report values, such as the difference between sexes, to more significant figures than the precision of the measurements. The results in this example should be reported to one decimal place or two significant figures, that is, a mean difference of 0.5 kg and not 0.5404 kg.

If the data are coarser than expected, as in this example, it might indicate that the values have been rounded. Suppose we know that the scale used to weigh the cats reports values to one more decimal place. It would be preferable to obtain the original more precise data if available. If this is impossible because the data were rounded as they were written in a lab notebook, we could still ask the experimenter to record all of the digits in future experiments.

Suppose that approximately half the values in the data are recorded to three decimal places and the other half to one decimal place. The example below has six values saved in the variable `prec`. When `prec` is printed, zeros are appended to the first, third, and sixth measurements so it appears that all are measured with the same precision. This is a quirk of R that you need to be aware of.

```
> # the 1st, 3rd, and 6th entry have only one value after the decimal
> prec <- c(2.1, 2.254, 2.3, 2.376, 2.450, 2.2)
>
> # the output is padded with zeros
> prec
[1] 2.100 2.254 2.300 2.376 2.450 2.200
```

The first measurement might have been exactly 2.100, but it would be suspicious if there are many values with the last two digits equal to zero (or with only one digit after the decimal if looking at the data before reading it into R). Suppose that in the `cats` data set about half the values have the pattern X.XXX, where X can represent any digit, and the other half have the pattern X.X00. Think about how data could be generated such that the first two digits can be any number but the last two are zero. One hypothesis is that about half of the measurements just happened to be nice round numbers. Another hypothesis is that the data have been collected differently. Perhaps two people collected the data and one rounded the values while the other did not. Maybe one person collected the data over 2 days and they were inconsistent with the number of digits they recorded. Or maybe two weigh scales with different precision were used. The 'nice round numbers' hypothesis is unlikely compared with the other possibilities. It would be even more peculiar if the precision differed between the first half and second half of the data, as it might indicate that two files were merged. If information about experimenters, dates, and instruments are unavailable it is impossible to check if these factors account for the different precisions. We would have to ask the experimenters for this information, and this is where horror stories originate and post-mortems are conducted (recall the quotations opening Chapter 1).

Suppose the experimenters tell us that the male and female cats are housed separately and that one technician measured the females and another the males using the scales available in the respective rooms. We are interested in sex differences but the cats differ not only on sex but on (1) their housing, (2) the person taking the measurements, (3) the measuring device. Here we have not one but three variables completely confounded with sex – the variable of scientific interest. We know that male cats weigh more than female cats and may believe that housing animals in separate rooms has little influence on body weight. We might be less certain about how two technicians take measurements or how well calibrated the two scales are, but we suspect that the contribution to differences in body weight are minimal, relative to the biological effect of sex. Although the experiment is a disaster from a design perspective, the correct qualitative conclusion was still reached (males weigh more), confirming a well-known and large effect. But if the treatment effects or biological effects are less certain, then the person, measuring device, and other technical factors are alternative explanations that cannot be so easily dismissed.

The code below shows how to follow up on our suspicions, even if no other data are available. First, the numeric outcome values (`prec`) are converted into character values. The standard way is to use the `as.character()` function, but the trailing zeros are lost, which are of primary interest. The `sprintf()` function is used instead to format the output to retain three decimals by specifying `"%.3f"`.

```
> # converting to a character removes trailing zeros
> as.character(prec)
[1] "2.1"   "2.254" "2.3"   "2.376" "2.45"  "2.2"
>
> # format character output to keep zeros
> char.prec <- sprintf("%.3f", prec)
> char.prec
[1] "2.100" "2.254" "2.300" "2.376" "2.450" "2.200"
```

Next, `grep()` finds the location (the position in the `char.prec` vector) of values that end in two zeros. `grep()` is a pattern matching function that takes the pattern as the first argument and the vector to search as the second argument. The dollar sign in the "00$" pattern indicates that the two zeros must match at the end of the string. Otherwise, the number 2.001 will be a match. The result is saved in index and positions 1, 3, and 6 have the necessary pattern, which is easy to confirm visually.

```
> # find location of pattern matches
> index <- grep("00$", char.prec)
> index
[1] 1 3 6
```

The final step is to create a categorical variable (group.prec) indicating if the pattern matched or not. The ifelse() function tests if the numbers 1 to 6 (the length of the vector prec) are in index. If so, a value of X00 is returned, otherwise a value of XXX. These are the levels of the new categorical variable and are arbitrary but they indicate the two patterns, where X represents any number and 0 represents zero. The original data are combined with the new categorical factor and we can visually confirm the matching.

```
> # make a factor for pattern type
> group.prec <- ifelse(1:length(prec) %in% index, "X00", "XXX")
> group.prec <- factor(group.prec)
>
> prec.dat <- data.frame(prec, group.prec)
> prec.dat
   prec group.prec
1 2.100        X00
2 2.254        XXX
3 2.300        X00
4 2.376        XXX
5 2.450        XXX
6 2.200        X00
```

Let's recap what we are doing. We noticed the variable prec contained some values rounded to one decimal place and others rounded to three, and this made us suspicious that the data were collected differently, but we don't know how. We created a new categorical variable called group.prec that indicates if a value was rounded to one (X00) or to three (XXX) decimal places. Now we can check if the outcome values differ between these groups. The rational is that if the data were collected differently the measured values might be different. The code below generates the graph in Figure 6.2 and the values in XXX group tend to be higher. As this is a fictitious example, we do not interpret the results but the differences between groups indicate that a biological or technical variable might be affecting the outcome. If there are no differences between groups then we can be more confident in the data quality and therefore the results.

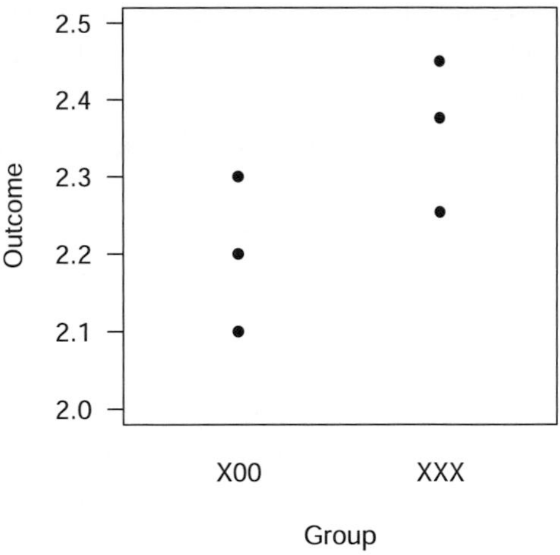

Fig. 6.2 A categorical variable is made based on the precision of the measurements for the outcome. Then, the values of the outcome are plotted by group to see if there are systematic differences.

```
> library(beeswarm)
> par(las=1)
> beeswarm(prec ~ group.prec, data=prec.dat, pch=16,
+           ylim=c(2, 2.5), xlab="Group", ylab="Outcome")
```

We could also check if `group.prec` is associated with other variables in the data set, as this might indicate how the groups were formed and might provide an explanation of why the groups differ. For example, if there is a variable called 'Day' and the `X00` values are associated with Day 1 and the `XXX` values with Day 2, then we have some idea about how the differences were generated. All of this started because we noticed an unusual feature of the data and decided to investigate further.

Near-zero variance variables

Nowadays, more outcomes can be measured than we know what to do with, or even understand what they mean. Examples include output from high content image analyses, large-scale behavioural phenotyping experiments, and molecular descriptors of compounds. Just because you can measure it, does not mean that it's useful or relevant. One of the first steps with such data is to filter out measured variables that are unlikely to be useful, and one criterion is whether the outcome has zero or near-zero variance. If an outcome has the same value across all samples, time points, or experimental conditions, it provides no information; for example, if the experiment uses only male rats the variable *sex* is not a useful predictor. There are other cases where the variance is close to zero; for example, there is only one female in the experiment. The variance of each variable could be calculated and those with near-zero variances could be considered for removal. But a problem with this approach is that the variables are often on different scales and have different units, so variances cannot be compared directly. Another approach is to use the `nearZeroVar()` function in the `caret` package, which we apply to the `cats` data.

```
> caret::nearZeroVar(cats, saveMetrics = TRUE)
    freqRatio percentUnique zeroVar   nzv
Sex   2.06383       1.38889   FALSE FALSE
Bwt   1.07692      13.88889   FALSE FALSE
Hwt   1.33333      50.69444   FALSE FALSE
```

The `zeroVar` column will equal `TRUE` if a variable is constant across all samples (rows) and `FALSE` otherwise. Similarly, the `nzv` column will equal `TRUE` if the variable has either zero variance or near-zero variance. The `percentUnique` column shows the percentage of unique values for a variable and will have a value of 100 if there are no duplicated values and 0 if the values are all the same. The percentage uniqueness can be calculated 'by hand' using the following code, which is the number of unique values divided by the total number of values, times 100.

```
> # percent unique
> length(unique(cats$Bwt))/nrow(cats) * 100
[1] 13.8889
```

Sex has a low percentage unique value because there are only two sexes and so most of the values are duplicates. Since body weight measurements are measured to the nearest 100th of a kilogram, they have a lower percentage unique value than the heart weight measurements. A low percentage unique value for a continuous measurement is not a cause for concern, but it is useful to know to better understand the data and how they were generated.

The `freqRatio` column calculates the ratio of the number of the most frequent value to the number of the next most frequent value. If the body weight data are tabulated and sorted, 2.2 is the most frequent value, occurring 14 times and 2.3 is the next most frequent value, occurring 13 times. The ratio of these two numbers equals 1.076923, which is calculated below and the same as the output from the `nearZeroVar()` function above.

```
> # frequency ratio
> sort(table(cats$Bwt), decreasing=TRUE)

2.2 2.3 2.7   3 2.1 2.5 2.4 2.6 2.9 2.8 3.1 3.2   2 3.3 3.4 3.5 3.6
 14  13  12  11  10  10   9   9   8   7   6   6   5   5   5   5   4
3.8 3.9 3.7
  2   2   1
>
> 14/13
[1] 1.07692
```

A high freqRatio indicates that one value occurs much more often than the others. Variables with both a high frequency ratio and low percentage unique value might be candidates for removal when creating predictive models.[2] Here we use nearZeroVar() to highlight samples for further examination and to better understand the data. For example, if the most common value is the lowest or highest, it might indicate that measurements are censored, that is, the measurement has a lower or upper value that cannot be exceeded. This might indicate, for example, that measurements below the lower limit of detection have been assigned a minimum value.

6.1.4 Missing values

The first thing to determine about missing values is how they are defined in a data set. In R, a missing value is indicated with NA; this is not a string or factor but a special indicator for a missing value. If you are analysing data with R then using NA as a missing value indicator during data collection and in lab notebooks (either paper or electronic) minimises the chance of errors and reduces later work to convert the missing value indicator to NA. Other people and other software might indicate missing values differently, such as using a value of 0, −1 (if the non-missing data are positive), or 999 (if this value is out of the normal range of the data). If others have generated the data, it might be necessary to confirm how missing values are indicated.

Using numbers to indicate missing values is asking for trouble; how is the software supposed to know what is a measurement and what is an indicator of 'no data available'? Zero is especially ambiguous because zero indicates the absence of something, but the absence of the thing being measured is not the same as the absence of data because a measurement was not taken. The code below calculates the mean of the same three numbers using four different missing value indicators for the first value. The means differ and only the first calculation is correct.

```
> mean(c(NA , 10, 20), na.rm=TRUE)   # NA indicates missing value
[1] 15
> mean(c(0  , 10, 20))               # 0 indicates missing value
[1] 10
> mean(c(-1 , 10, 20))               # -1 indicates missing value
[1] 9.66667
> mean(c(999, 10, 20))               # 999 indicates missing value
[1] 343
```

The second thing to determine is what a value of NA means for this experiment, does it mean the same thing for all variables, and does it always mean the same thing for a

[2] Predictive models are not covered in this book but Kuhn and Johnson discuss how the nearZeroVar() function is used in this context [205]. Their website also provides more information: http://topepo.github.io/caret/

Box 6.1 Missing data mechanism

There are three ways that data can go missing and the distinction is important because it determines which corrective measures are appropriate [336]. If the probability of missingness is the same for all data and does not depend on other variables, then the missing values are *missing completely at random* (MCAR). For example, suppose some samples are accidentally dropped and destroyed. Since the dropped samples are unrelated to the value of the outcome that we would have observed, the mechanism that generated the missing values (clumsiness) is said to be *ignorable*. Ignorable missingness is useful because inference can proceed in the usual manner and the missing data will not bias the estimates. Whether the missing data mechanism is ignorable is an assumption that cannot be verified with the data.

Data are *missing at random* (MAR) when the probability of missingness depends on a known or measured variable. For example, suppose two technicians are processing the samples and one is much clumsier than the other. Although missingness is not completely random because it depends on the technician, each technician randomly drops the samples with a different probability. When the data are MAR, the missing data mechanism is also ignorable.

Data are *missing not at random* (MNAR) when the probability that a value is missing depends on the value; the fact that a value is missing tells us something about what that value might have been. MNAR occurs when values are below the limit of detection, when outliers are routinely excluded (e.g. any value beyond $3 \times$ SD from the mean), when the treatment kills the most severely affected animals, when cells are selected for quantification that have certain electrophysiological properties, or when heavier people are less likely to report their body weight. With MNAR, missingness is not ignorable and a naive analysis can lead to biased estimates. Analysis of missing data is a large topic and van Buuren provides a nice introduction with examples in R [372].

given variable? For example, suppose the expression of a single gene is measured and there are several NA values. A NA value could mean 'sample was lost and no measurement taken', or 'RNA quality was low, the measurement unreliable, and so the measurement was removed', or 'the expression level was below the limit of detection (LOD)'. The last case includes the situation where the measuring device provides no numeric value and where a value was provided but was manually removed. Knowing what NA means matters because it determines how the missing values are treated. If the sample was lost then the expression of the gene could be anything, and removing the sample from the analysis might be the only option.[3] Box 6.1 discusses three missing data mechanisms.

If the measurement is below the LOD then we know that the value is small and somewhere between the LOD and zero. Removing the sample from the analysis will bias results upwards and a solution is to substitute a value for each NA. Common options for values to substitute are the LOD, LOD/2, LOD/$\sqrt{2}$, or zero. Another option is to impute a value such

[3] Methods exist to impute values for missing data based on other variables. They are not considered here but are discussed by van Buuren [372].

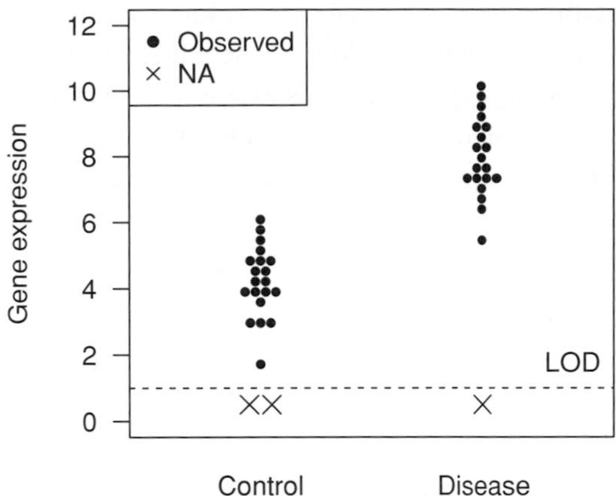

Fig. 6.3 Missing values and the limit of detection (LOD). Values below the LOD were substituted with a value of LOD/2 = 0.5. The substitutions appear reasonable for the control group but not the disease group. Could there be another reason that values are missing?

as drawing a number from a uniform distribution between zero and the LOD, the rational is that we know the value must be between these limits and assume that all values are equally likely. Lubin *et al.* compared several methods for substituting values and their recommendation is that substituting all NAs with the same value (e.g. LOD/2) is inadvisable unless the proportion of NAs is low ($<$ 5–10%) and randomly imputing a value is inadvisable unless the proportion of NAs is $<$ 30% [248]. Their preferred approach is multiple imputation (see van Buuren for more on multiple imputation [372]) but randomly generating values from a uniform distribution below the LOD and a lower value will usually be good enough.

Suppose we are told that genes below the LOD are assigned a value of NA. It does not follow that *all* NA values represent genes below the limit of detection. Some samples may have been lost or had low RNA quality. It is therefore useful to verify that substituting or imputing a low value for all NAs makes sense, for example by plotting the results against other variables in the data. The graph in Figure 6.3 shows gene expression data for two groups. The LOD for this assay is one (horizontal line) and the $\times$s indicate three NA values that were substituted with a value of LOD/2 $=$ 0.5. Do these substituted values make sense? The two values for the control group do not appear dissimilar from the other observed control values. However, the single substituted value for the disease group looks disconnected from the others. Maybe the gene in this sample is indeed below the LOD, but an alternative explanation is that NA means something different for this sample and it would be useful to confirm with the experimenter. Otherwise, our substitution may have generated an outlier (if gene expression is an outcome) or a value with high leverage (if gene expression is a predictor).[4]

[4] A value with high leverage can be an influential observation, meaning that the results can differ markedly if this observation is included or excluded from the analysis.

Once the missing data indicator is known (converted to NA if necessary) and what NA means, the next step is to look at the pattern of missing values. The `sleep` data set from the `VIM` package is used for this example. The study examined correlations between sleep characteristics and ecological variables in 62 species [8]. `summary()` returns the number of NAs for each variable (column). It is also sensible to check the number of missing values for each row, that is, for each species. In the code below the `apply()` function uses the `is.na()` function to test if a value is missing, and `sum()` adds the number of missing values.

```
> library(VIM)
> summary(sleep)
    BodyWgt            BrainWgt              NonD            Dream      
 Min.   :   0.00   Min.   :   0.14   Min.   : 2.10   Min.   :0.00  
 1st Qu.:   0.60   1st Qu.:   4.25   1st Qu.: 6.25   1st Qu.:0.90  
 Median :   3.34   Median :  17.25   Median : 8.35   Median :1.80  
 Mean   : 198.79   Mean   : 283.13   Mean   : 8.67   Mean   :1.97  
 3rd Qu.:  48.20   3rd Qu.: 166.00   3rd Qu.:11.00   3rd Qu.:2.55  
 Max.   :6654.00   Max.   :5712.00   Max.   :17.90   Max.   :6.60  
                                     NA's   :14      NA's   :12    
     Sleep            Span              Gest             Pred      
 Min.   : 2.60   Min.   :  2.00   Min.   : 12.0   Min.   :1.00  
 1st Qu.: 8.05   1st Qu.:  6.62   1st Qu.: 35.8   1st Qu.:2.00  
 Median :10.45   Median : 15.10   Median : 79.0   Median :3.00  
 Mean   :10.53   Mean   : 19.88   Mean   :142.4   Mean   :2.87  
 3rd Qu.:13.20   3rd Qu.: 27.75   3rd Qu.:207.5   3rd Qu.:4.00  
 Max.   :19.90   Max.   :100.00   Max.   :645.0   Max.   :5.00  
 NA's   :4       NA's   :4        NA's   :4                     
      Exp            Danger     
 Min.   :1.00   Min.   :1.00  
 1st Qu.:1.00   1st Qu.:1.00  
 Median :2.00   Median :2.00  
 Mean   :2.42   Mean   :2.61  
 3rd Qu.:4.00   3rd Qu.:4.00  
 Max.   :5.00   Max.   :5.00  

>
> # number of missing values by row (species)
> apply(sleep, 1, function(x) sum(is.na(x)))
 [1] 2 0 2 3 0 0 0 0 0 0 0 0 2 2 0 0 0 0 1 1 2 0 0 2 0 2 0 0 0 2 3 0 0 0 1
[36] 1 0 0 0 0 2 0 0 0 0 0 2 0 0 0 0 0 2 0 2 1 0 0 0 0 0 3
```

The above summaries examined each variable on its own, but it is often useful to examine patterns of missingness across two or more variables. A simple check is to cross-tabulate

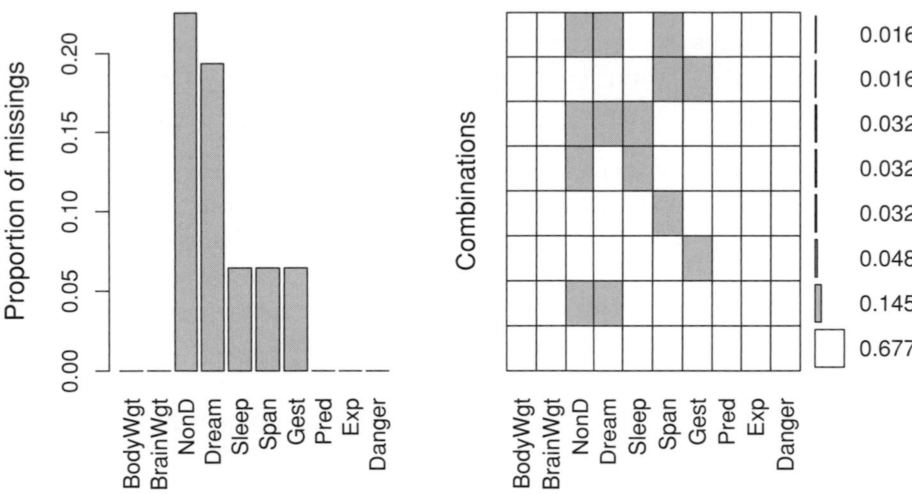

Fig. 6.4 Missing data. The proportion of missing values for each variable (left) and the pattern of missing values (right). Grey squares indicate missing values and white squares indicate observed values.

two variables, based on whether they are missing instead of their values. The code below uses the `is.na()` function to test if values are missing for the variables `NonD` and `Dream`. `is.na()` returns `TRUE` if a value is missing, `FALSE` otherwise. `xtabs()` then cross-tabulates the `TRUE/FALSE` values and the results are displayed below. Forty-eight species (rows) of the `sleep` data contain no missing values for these two variables, and 12 rows have missing values for both variables.

```
> # cross-tabulation of missing values
> xtabs(~is.na(NonD) + is.na(Dream), data=sleep)
             is.na(Dream)
is.na(NonD) FALSE TRUE
      FALSE    48    0
      TRUE      2   12
```

The above code is fine for checking two variables, but the `aggr()` function from the `VIM` package is better when there are many. The graph on the left in Figure 6.4 shows the proportion of missing values for each variable. The graph on the right is more interesting and shows the pattern of missing variables. Starting from the bottom of the graph we see a row of white squares and the number 0.677 on the right. A white square indicates observed data and this tells us that 67.7% of the sleep data have no missing values. Grey squares indicate missing values and the row above has grey squares for the NonD and Dream variables, with a value of 0.145 on the right. This tells us that 14.5% of the sleep data have missing values for both the NonD and Dream variables. The same interpretation applies to the other rows. The rows are sorted (bottom to top) by the frequency of the pattern, and therefore the predominant patterns are at the bottom.

```
> miss <- aggr(sleep, plot=FALSE)
> plot(miss, col=c("white", "darkgrey"), numbers = TRUE)
```

The right graph in Figure 6.4 enables a better understand the data. For example, why are the variables `NonD` and `Dream` missing together in almost 20% of the cases ($0.145 + 0.032 + 0.016 = 0.193$), either on their own or in combination with other missing values? It is because they are both sleep variables and tend to be measured together (or not). The `VIM` package contains other plots for understanding missing data and the `tableplot()` function in the `tabplot` package is also useful.

6.1.5 Factor arrangement

In Section 2.7 (p. 66), a distinction was made between crossed and nested factors. Recall that when two factors are crossed every level of one factor occurs with every level of the other factor. When two factors are nested some factor level combinations do not occur. The factor arrangement determines the statistical analyses and an appropriate model cannot be fit to the data unless the factor arrangement is known. An example was shown in Section 4.3.4 (p. 157) of how incorrect results can be obtained if the factor arrangement was incorrectly specified. The `xtabs()` function can help assess the factor arrangement but it may not provide a definitive answer. Recall that in the `glycogen` data the rats did not have unique identification numbers and it appeared that the rats were exposed to all treatments.

Summary of quality control checks

A data set with many errors and inconsistencies might indicate sloppy experimentation and data management. Even if the inconsistencies are resolved there may be others that have been missed (e.g. wrong values but within a normal range) or others that could not be checked. It is not uncommon to spend 80% of the time on QC checks and preprocessing (discussed in the next section). If the true value of an incorrect entry cannot be verified, it should be entered as a missing value, or the subject should be removed if you suspect that other values for that subject are incorrect.

⚠ If discrepancies are found, try to determine their cause, and *consider if they could lead to or indicate larger problems.* For example, one person has a BMI of 22 but is classified as obese (a BMI of 22 is in the normal range). This might be a transcription error or a one-off careless mistake. If several people have labels that do not match their BMI then either the people responsible for the data collection and entry are exceptionally careless, or there might be another explanation. For example, often data are combined into a master file from several smaller files. If the master file already contained the BMI data and the labels were copied and pasted from another file, the order of subjects in the two files might be different. Or the pasted values might be shifted up or down by one row so the data are misaligned.

Box 6.2 **List of quality control checks**

- Are maximum and minimum values for each variable reasonable/allowable?
- Are units correct and consistent (e.g. mmol/L vs mg/L).
- Are factor names consistent (case sensitivity)?
- Are annotations and factor levels correct?
- Are derived variables correct (e.g. does BMI = weight/height^2)?
- Is the difference between consecutive dates constant or similar, are all values positive?
- Are subject IDs unique and the number of observations per subject similar?
- Are there unusual duplications in values or whole rows?
- Is there differential rounding of data?
- Is there censoring or truncation of data; have values been imputed?
- How are missing values indicated?
- Is there a pattern to the missing values?
- How are the values distributed for each variable?
- Are there any perfectly or highly correlated variables?
- Are there any constant or near-zero variance variables?
- Are there linear combinations of variables?
- Are there outliers or unusual clusters?
- Are there spatial, temporal, or other technical artefacts?
- What is the factor arrangement: crossed or nested?
- Are variables time-varying or time-fixed?

Row shifts can occur if the data are in the same order in the two files but the number of rows differs. This could occur if there are no data for a subject in one file (maybe the recording device was broken and instead of including the subject with a row of missing values, the subject was excluded entirely). Row shifts are more severe if they occur early in the file because all subsequent data are incorrect. This may be easier to detect because much of the data may fail QC checks. If the error occurs near the end of the file then only some of the data will be incorrect but the error may be harder to detect. One way to minimise the above errors is to avoid copying and pasting data; it is error prone and leaves no record of how the data were combined. It is better to merge data from several files or sources based on a unique identifier, usually a subject or animal ID.[5] If a row shift occurred, all of the data between the merged files are misaligned – a major problem – even though we could only detect problems with the BMI data. Thus it is important to consider how QC failures indicate wider problems with the data.

A simple experiment with one outcome and two groups of three samples will not require extensive QC checks. The probability of a data set having errors is proportional to the:

[5] The `merge()` function in R can be used.

- number of variables
- number of rows
- number of people involved in data collection
- number of derived variables
- number of files integrated into a master file
- amount of copying and pasting
- use of spreadsheets.

Box 6.2 summarises the above points.

6.2 Preprocessing

Direct measurements may be unsuitable for analysis. Data preprocessing is any calculation, transformation, or manipulation of the recorded data that occurs before formal statistical inferences are made. Preprocessing includes removing or adjusting for technical artefacts, removing bad samples or values, imputing missing values, calculating derived variables, or rearranging the data in a format suitable for the statistics software.

Preprocessing requirements and methods depend on the experiment and instruments; sometimes the methods are simple and standardised and other times they are complex with many options. Five preprocessing options are discussed and regardless of the methods used, consider the following points. First, documenting the preprocessing steps enables the workflow to be reproduced. Given the raw data, anyone should be able to generate the preprocessed data. A written description is better than nothing, but all preprocessing should be done algorithmically, not manually. For example, if data are copied and pasted, rearranged, and manually deleted, there is no record of how the preprocessed data were generated. Scripts provide an unambiguous description of the preprocessing and the ability to recreate the preprocessed data. Second, the same preprocessing steps should be applied to all samples and to all conditions. Bias can be introduced if controls are preprocessed differently from treated samples. Third, only use preprocessing when necessary. Expressing the outcome variable as a percentage of the control condition is pointless if the only reason is to have the mean of the control group equal 100%.

Software from instrument manufacturers often preprocess data in ways that are unsuitable, not optimal, or make untenable assumptions. Interesting features can be removed or artefacts introduced, and they will never be discovered if only the preprocessed data are  available. *Always ask for the raw data*. Many of the quality control checks described above can and should be applied to both the raw and the preprocessed data.

6.2.1 Aggregating and summarising

Aggregation is the process of simplifying and reducing the amount of data by summarising the raw values – while still retaining the key features. Summarising can be done by row, column, or both. We used aggregation in Section 4.3.4 (p. 157) to average multiple glycogen measurements (subsamples) on each rat (experimental unit) and also to calculate the slope of blood pressure measurements over time in a repeated measures design, to reduce the number of data points per subject (Section 4.6, p. 181). Aggregation also includes calculating a total clinical score or disease severity from several subscales or clinical outcomes, or calculating areas or volumes from measurements of lengths. Once the derived variables are calculated the original variables may be of little interest and can be removed.

6.2.2 Normalising and standardising

Normalisation – also called standardisation – is the process of making the data 'the same' by some criterion and often involves equating distributions or properties of distributions across samples or across variables. The mean and variance are properties of distributions that are often equated. Normalising can be done by row or by column. Examples include making the distribution of genes from all microarrays the same (quantile normalisation), converting several outcomes to z-scores so they are on the same scale,[6] or scaling data to lie between zero and one.

6.2.3 Correcting and adjusting

Data correction or adjustment is the process of removing known sources of bias or variation in the data. Often the values or distributions become more alike, but this is a side effect and is distinguished from normalisation. A common example is correcting people's body weight for their height to give a body mass index (Eq. (6.1), p. 279). Other examples of correction include adjusting for background fluorescence intensity in microarrays, removal of spatial artefacts from microtitre plates (see Section 6.3.3), removal of batch effects, subtracting a baseline measurement from a final measurement.

6.2.4 Transforming

Any modification of the data in some sense transforms it, and so both normalisation and correction are transformations in the everyday meaning of the term. *Transformation* is used here in a more restricted sense to mean the application of a mathematical function to only one variable, and the same function is applied to all elements in that variable. A common example is taking the logarithm of positively skewed data. Normalising and correcting are not transformations because they involve other variables, such as background measurements, or a different function is applied to different parts of the data, such as subtracting a different mean from each plate.

Transformations are used to put data on a more relevant scale, to meet the requirements of a statistical model such as normality or equal variances, or to deal with outliers. Other examples of transformation include changing units such as grams to kilograms or °F to °C,

[6] Raw values can be converted to z-scores by first calculating the mean and standard deviation of the raw values, and then for each value subtracting the mean and dividing by the standard deviation. The distribution of z-scores will have a mean of zero and a standard deviation of one.

Table 6.1 Suitable and poor transformations for different types of data. ln = natural logarithm.

Data type	Transformation	Avoid	References
Count	Square root: $\sqrt{x}$	Log	[298]
Proportion	Logistic: $\ln\left(\frac{x}{1-x}\right)$	Arcsin	[389]
Latency	Reciprocal: $1/x$		
Continuous, positive skew	Log: $\log_2(x)$		[259]

square root and reciprocal transformations, and converting values into ranks. Other less common examples include smoothing, binning (not recommended, see Section 5.3.4, p. 231), and converting from the time domain into the frequency domain for digital signal processing.

Some transformations work well with certain types of data and others should be avoided, even though they are frequently used. Table 6.1 lists several types of data that often have non-normal distributions, along with good and bad transformations. Count data often have a positive skew and can have values of zero. A square root transformation is often suitable because the square root of zero is still zero, whereas the log of zero is undefined. However, instead of transforming data to meet the assumptions of a standard statistical model, it is often better to use a statistical model that is more appropriate for the data; that is, change the model to fit the data instead of changing the data to fit the model [220]. Generalised linear models (GLMs) were developed in the 1970s to deal with count and proportion data and are available in most statistics software [291]. The `glm()` function in R can be used for such data and their use is discussed in most statistics with R books [85, 86, 109]. For count data. Hilbe wrote an excellent introductory book suitable for biologists [152], and a more comprehensive but technical book [151].

6.2.5 Filtering

Filtering is the process of removing data, including removing whole subjects (rows), variables (columns), or data from individual cells. There are two main reasons for filtering. The first is that the data do not pass QC checks. For example, gene expression studies require intact RNA, but RNA is rapidly digested by enzymes. The amount of RNA degradation can be measured and expressed as an RNA integrity number (RIN), and samples with a RIN below a threshold can be removed [345]. A sample may be just above the threshold for acceptable RNA quality and thus retained, but the expression values may be unlike the high quality RNA samples, and removing the microarray from the analysis could be the best option. Another quality related reason for removing a value is when it is so distant from the rest of the data or outside the expected range that it is known to be an artefact. Also, sometimes a variable or a sample has too many missing values and the simplest solution is to remove it from the data. When whole rows or columns are filtered the dimension of the data set is reduced and when individual cells are filtered they are usually set to NA.

The second reason for removing data is when the variables are redundant or uninformative, which can occur because variables have zero or near-zero variance, are highly correlated, or are linear combinations of each other. On page 287, we discussed checking for zero or near-zero variance variables as a QC check, and depending on the research question and the analysis that is to be conducted, they may be candidates for removal. A variable might be uninformative if it is highly correlated with other variables. High correlation is not a problem *per se* and it depends on why the variables are highly correlated. Recall the example from Chapter 1 measuring subjects' strength on the bench press, deadlift, and squat (Figure 1.7, p. 13). We want to keep these measures of strength even though they are highly correlated because they are providing different information about the subjects' strength. But suppose we have a high-content imaging experiment and one output is the mean fluorescent intensity of cells in a well, and a second output is the median fluorescent intensity. These are different summary statistics of the same set of pixels and often have a correlation > 0.99. Only one of these variables needs to be retained in the data or used in an analysis.

Variables that are linear combinations of other variables are also candidates for removal. A linear combination is made by summing and multiplying other variables. For example, if we measure the lengths (L) and widths (W) of several objects, their perimeters (P) can be calculated as $P = 2L + 2W$. P is a linear combination of L and W and this matters because ⚠ *it is not possible to fit a model with predictors that are linear combinations of each other.* This is a technical problem because division by zero occurs in the calculations. In the R code below an outcome (Y) and two predictor variables (L, W) are generated from a normal distribution. P is another predictor generated from a linear combination of L and W, and all three predictors are entered in the model.

```
> Y <- rnorm(10)
> L <- rnorm(10)
> W <- rnorm(10)
> P <- 2*L + 2*W
>
> combo.mod <- aov(Y ~ L + W + P)
> summary(combo.mod)
            Df Sum Sq Mean Sq F value Pr(>F)
L            1   3.42    3.42    2.24   0.18
W            1   0.12    0.12    0.08   0.79
Residuals    7  10.68    1.53
```

The output from the summary() function is missing the variable P – it disappeared from ⚠ the model! R addresses the problem by quietly removing the last variable and provides no error message or warning. Other software packages have alternative solutions.

Linear combinations can occur in the process of creating derived variables such as summing clinical subscales to get a total clinical score. The findLinearCombos() function in the caret package can find linear combinations, and the code below uses the cbind()

function to collect all four variables into a matrix.[7] The output shows that a linear combination was found involving columns 4, 2, and 3, corresponding to variables P, L, and W, and that by removing column 4, the remaining variables will be linearly independent.

```
> caret::findLinearCombos(cbind(Y,L,W,P))
$linearCombos
$linearCombos[[1]]
[1] 4 2 3


$remove
[1] 4
```

Removing column 4 (P) is only a suggestion. P might be preferred and L and W could be removed instead. Linear combinations do not necessarily need to be removed, as long as you are aware that such dependencies exist and where they can create problems.

6.2.6 Combining

The last preprocessing method we consider is combining data. Data can be combined with other experimental data; for example, combining behavioural data for an *in vivo* experiment with histological data. For a gene expression experiment, information about pathways and gene ontology classifications can be added from databases. Metadata – data about the data – can also be added. Examples include information about who conducted the experiment, when it was conducted, which instrument was used, and the order of sample processing. Some of this information might be part of the design and already available, but sometimes experiments do not go as planned and the actual order of sample processing differs from the planned order. This information would then need to be added. Such metadata is relevant if there are multiple experimenters, if the experiment was conducted over several days, and if multiple instruments were used. Metadata can be used to check assumptions, such as no differences between days, but are rarely included with the data. This information usually has to be requested from the experimenters.

6.2.7 Pitfalls of preprocessing

Preprocessing is often necessary, but rarely easy. The data are altered, and therefore so are the statistical results. There are often more ways to preprocess data than to statistically analyse it, and there is little guidance on how preprocessing should be done [49]. Below we discuss several ways that preprocessing can change the data for the worse.

[7] The caret package has many functions for preprocessing, including findLinearCombos(), findCorrelation(), and nearZeroVar().

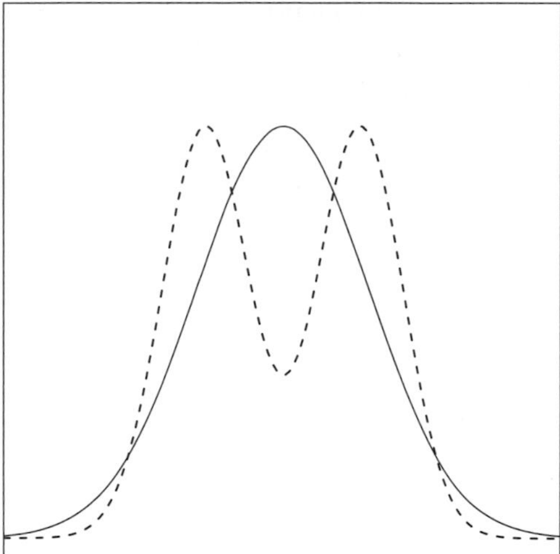

Fig. 6.5 Averaging can remove information. Both distributions have the same mean and variance but one is bimodal.

Information is lost

The first pitfall is that preprocessing may remove important information, and a common example is expressing outcome variables as a percentage of the control condition. When the measured values are meaningful, converting them into percentages loses the units of measurement and the actual values. How can we know if the controls have unusually high or low values, or that there was a 12 g difference in body weight between the two experimental groups? The data have no context and cannot be compared across studies. If the measured values are in arbitrary units however, such as a fluorescence or grey-level pixel intensity, then little information is lost.

Another example of information loss is when researchers routinely remove data from the tails of a distribution; for example, beyond two or three standard deviations from the mean. Some researchers use such a rule to remove outliers, but by definition, 5% of the data is outside of a 2 SD threshold (assuming the distribution is Gaussian), and this filtering step often throws away good data.

A third example of information loss is when data are aggregated by calculating a mean or median. These summaries capture all of the information in the data if the raw values are Gaussian, but the mean and median may be poor summaries when the raw values are non-Gaussian. Figure 6.5 shows two distributions that have the same mean and variance, but one is bimodal. Information about the two distinct populations is lost when the distributions are averaged.

Signal to noise ratio is worse

A second pitfall is that preprocessing can remove signal or add noise – the opposite of what is intended. Take the example of measuring gene expression in histological sections with *in situ* hybridisation and autoradiography [215]. Oligonucleotide or RNA probes with

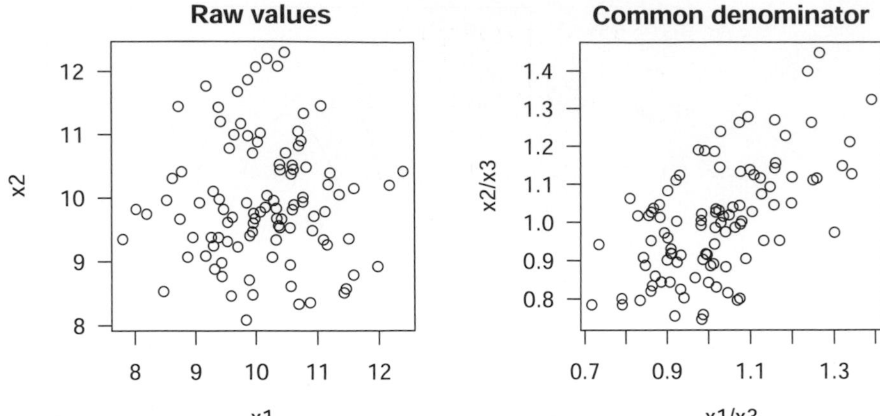

Fig. 6.6 Spurious correlation. Two uncorrelated variables can become correlated when 'corrected' for a common third variable.

a sequence complementary to the gene of interest are labelled with radioactive atoms. The location of the bound probe in the tissue is determined by exposing the tissue and probes to photographic film. The darkness of the film is proportional to the amount of gene expression and is captured as a digital image for quantification. The anatomical structure of interest is then located in the image and the darkness of the structure is measured. Without justification, many researchers multiply or divide the darkness values by the size of the structure and then nonlinearly transform the data to an optical density using one of several equations. These steps only add noise to the darkness values; multiplying or dividing the darkness values by the size of the structure – which is measured with error – adds noise. The nonlinear transformations tend to increase the variance of the darkness values and can create outliers. The best results from these experiments are obtained with the least amount of preprocessing [215].

Bias is introduced

A third pitfall is adding signal where none exists, in other words, introducing bias that is then mistaken for a real effect. Continuing with the *in situ* hybridisation example, suppose the size of the anatomical structure differs between experimental groups, but gene expression remains constant. Multiplying or dividing the darkness values by the size of the structure generates ratio values that differ between groups, but not because of differences in gene expression. A related example is when cell counts in histological sections are expressed as counts per unit area or volume. It is impossible to tell if differences between groups are caused by differences in cell counts, in the size of the structure, or both.

Spurious associations can be introduced between two unrelated variables when they are divided by a third [6, 102, 119, 200]. In the code below three variables (`x1`-`x3`) are generated from a normal distribution with a mean of ten, a standard deviation of one, and a sample size of 100. The three variables are uncorrelated by construction and we verify the correlation between `x1` and `x2` by calculating the Pearson correlation ($r = -0.001$, $p = 0.992$). The data are also graphed in Figure 6.6 (left).

```
> # generate 3 unrelated variables
> set.seed(1)
> x1 <- rnorm(100, 10)
> x2 <- rnorm(100, 10)
> x3 <- rnorm(100, 10)
>
> # x1 and x2 are uncorrelated
> cor.test(x1, x2)

Pearson's product-moment correlation

data:  x1 and x2
t = -0.009843, df = 98, p-value = 0.992
alternative hypothesis: true correlation is not equal to 0
95 percent confidence interval:
 -0.197374  0.195462
sample estimates:
        cor
-0.00099432
```

In the code below we divide both x1 and x2 by x3 and calculate the correlation between the ratios (x1/x3 and x2/x3). Now there is a strong correlation and small p-value ($r = 0.6$, $p < 0.001$; right graph in Figure 6.6), but this is driven by our attempt at correcting x1 and x2.

```
> # when divided by x3, x1 and x2 are correlated
> cor.test(x1/x3, x2/x3)

Pearson's product-moment correlation

data:  x1/x3 and x2/x3
t = 7.363, df = 98, p-value = 5.65e-11
alternative hypothesis: true correlation is not equal to 0
95 percent confidence interval:
 0.453543 0.709988
sample estimates:
     cor
0.596796
>
> par(las=1,
+     mfrow=c(1,2))
> plot(x2 ~ x1, main="Raw values")
> plot(I(x2/x3) ~ I(x1/x3), ylab="x2/x3", xlab="x1/x3",
+      main="Common denominator")
```

The following references discuss real examples of such spurious correlations [6, 102, 119, 200], and the most relevant is Kronmal [200]. He discusses medical examples where both outcome and predictors are ratios like our example, only the outcome is a ratio, and only the predictor is a ratio. Some parts of Kronmal's paper are technical (it is in a statistics journal) but the examples are clearly described and can be understood from the text. The conclusion from these papers is that correction is often best done by including the variable that we want to adjust for (e.g. x3) as covariate in a statistical model, and that ratios should be avoided. An example of this approach was discussed in Section 4.3.5 (p. 166) when analysing the heart weight of cats, and see Vickers for a comparison of these and other correction methods [379].

Another example is from Lew, who discusses a fictitious but realistic case with two dose–response curves whose magnitudes change their order after correcting for baseline values [233]. With the raw data, the control group is greater than the test group and, with the corrected data, the test group is greater than the control group. The wrong conclusion would be reached if only the corrected data were plotted and analysed. The main lesson from this paper is that *both the raw and corrected data should be plotted and examined.*

Sometimes normalisation methods can create differences in some parts of the data while overall making distributions more alike. For example, functional genomics experiments assume that the total amount of RNA is constant across all samples and that most genes are not differentially expressed between groups. These assumptions are not always true and standard preprocessing methods can introduce differences where none exist [247].

Assumptions are no longer met

A fourth pitfall is that preprocessing can add unusual features to the data, such that statistical assumptions are no longer met. We saw an example of this in Figure 4.18 (p. 182) where the measurements were corrected for baseline differences so that at $t = 0$ the values were 100% for all rats. Thus the variance of the data at $t = 0$ is zero (variances are plotted in Figure 4.19, p. 184). In this experiment there is nothing gained by equating baseline measurements, and by doing so we have lost the units of measurement (the force of muscle contraction), the variation in baseline values (information on biological variability), and have made the variances between time points unequal.

Another related example is shown in Figure 6.7. The left graph shows the raw data for a fictitious cell culture experiment that was conducted independently on 3 days (blocks), which are distinguished by symbol and line type. There are three experimental groups, each point is a well in a microtitre plate that we will treat as a genuine replicate, and the lines show the group means. On all 3 days, Group 1 has lower values than the control group, and Group 2 has higher values. These differences are small compared with the day-to-day variation. The other graphs show two ways of removing the day effects. In the middle graph, the mean of the control group from each day is calculated and subtracted from all values for that day. Hence, the values for the control group are centred around zero and all three lines meet at exactly zero. Further calculations can re-express the values so the controls are centred at another value (e.g. 100), but this does not affect the point being

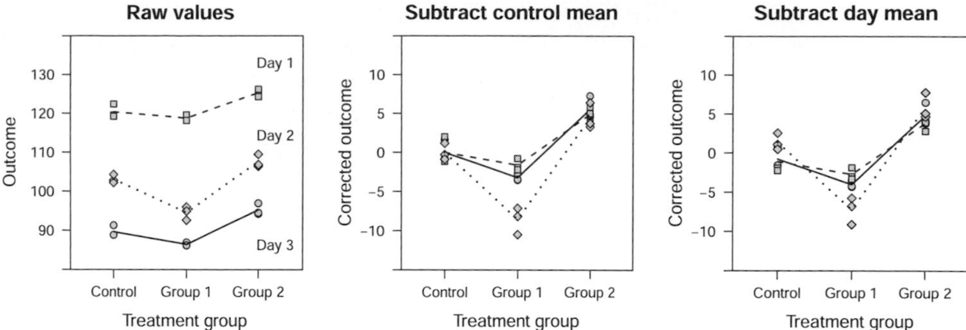

Fig. 6.7 Correcting for block effects. The variances of the treatment groups become unequal when using only the control samples to remove differences between days ($p = 0.007$, middle graph). When all samples are used, the variances are similar ($p = 0.531$, right graph).

made and the damage has already been done: the variances of the three groups are now unequal (Bartlett's test: $p = 0.007$). The graph on the right is similar, but instead of using only the control groups, the mean of all groups for each day is calculated and subtracted from each point for that day. The variances are now more alike ($p = 0.531$), and this is the preferred method if you want to remove block effects to highlight the treatment effects in graphs. *This correction is unnecessary for an analysis because it is equivalent to including day as a blocking factor in the model.* The right graph in Figure 6.7 therefore corresponds to the statistical model and is preferred to the middle graph. Lew makes a similar argument and provides a nice example with data expressed as a percentage of the control group [234].

When graphing data, removing effects that are of little scientific interest emphasises the effects of the remaining variables – compare the treatment effects in the left and right graphs of Figure 6.7. For an analysis, however, removing effects from the data is questionable because parameters have been estimated and effects have been quietly removed without decreasing the degrees of freedom. Recall from Section 4.1.2 (p. 132) that the total df is $N - 1$ and that a df is removed for every parameter that is estimated. This gives the residual df, which is used to calculate p-values. Removing effects without decreasing the residual df is therefore equivalent to inflating the sample size by the number of dfs that should have been removed. More complex experiments could have multiple effects removed, thereby overestimating the sample size even more. There is a blurry line between preprocessing and formal inference and this point has not received much attention. Removing unwanted effects is probably fine for graphing data but plotting error bars is inappropriate because they are calculated from the sample size. Since the sample size is inflated, the error bars will be too narrow, giving a misleading impression of the precision. Manually removing effects is unnecessary for an analysis, just include the variables in the statistical model. This does not remove the unwanted effects from the data, only from the conclusions or inferences that we make about the treatment effects.

A related point is that raw data should be provided in the supplemental material for a publication or in a public repository. The preprocessed data could be included as well,

Box 6.3 Key points about the pitfalls of preprocessing

- Do not preprocess data for the sake of it, ensure that each step is necessary.
- Know the assumptions of preprocessing methods and ensure they hold.
- If you receive data that has been preprocessed, know what was done and why.
- Both raw and preprocessed data should be examined and require quality control checks.

but is optional. This suggestion is not unreasonable and many journals require that raw Western blot or histological images are submitted, along with any enhanced images that will appear in the figures. Preprocessing data irreversibly removes information and limits the data's usefulness as part of the scientific record. You do not know what others might want to do with the data; your technical effect might be someone else's main effect of interest, so it is better to retain all effects. This is a problem with some microarray studies when only highly preprocessed data are submitted to public repositories. These data cannot be processed in a way more suitable for the new application and it is impossible to use the latest gene annotation information to improve inferences [127, 243, 406, 410]. Jaynes puts it succinctly: 'The First Commandment of scientific data analysis publication ought to be: "Thou shalt reveal thy full original data, unmutilated by any processing whatsoever"' [175].

A final example where preprocessing can distort the data so that statistical assumptions are no longer met is when adjusting for baseline values using ratios, such as when calculating percentage change from baseline. Even if both the numerator (final values) and denominator (baseline values) are normally distributed, their ratio often will be skewed.

Preprocessing is ineffective

A final pitfall is that corrections do not work as advertised [351]. If a preprocessing method has been developed, published in a top journal, and is routinely used, it does not follow that it is good. For example, electrical conduction in the heart can be measured with an electrocardiogram, from which several values are calculated. An important value for drug development is the QT interval, which represents the time between depolarisation and repolarisation of the ventricles. A prolonged QT interval is a marker of dangerous ventricular arrhythmias and compounds are checked during drug development for their ability to increase the QT interval. The QT interval, however, cannot be used directly because it is dependent on the heart rate (the slower the heart rate the longer the interval), which is measured as the RR interval from the electrocardiogram. The QT interval therefore needs to be corrected for the RR interval and around 20 formulae have been developed. Although they are better than using the raw QT interval values, most do not remove the dependency on heart rate and are therefore inadequate [257]. Senn and Julious refer to these as *crude corrections* and one example is dividing the QT interval by the square root of the RR interval [351]. This is another example of a ratio adjustment and once again a regression or ANCOVA approach using the RR interval as a predictor is a better alternative [257].

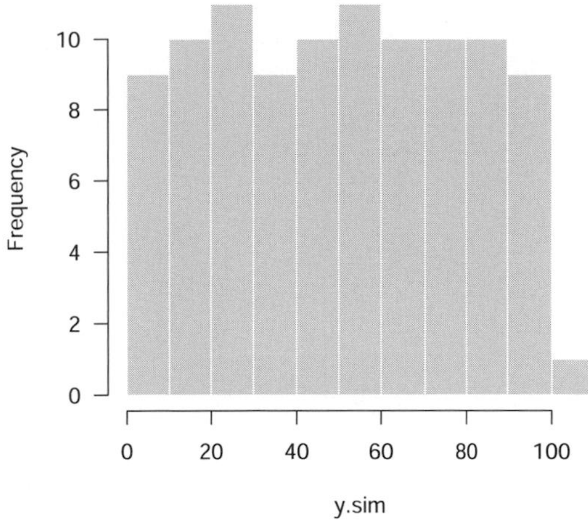

Fig. 6.8 Non-normal data generated from a normal distribution.

Correcting or adjusting outcomes for other variables by division has been criticised several times in this chapter because this approach often performs poorly. The preferred method is usually the ANCOVA approach because it is more efficient (makes better use of information), is more flexible, and does a better job of correcting.

6.3 Understanding the structure of the data

This section describes graphical methods that can be used to understand the structure of the data. This is useful for quality control and to understand the relationship between the biological and technical factors with the outcome, as well as the relationship between the outcomes.

6.3.1 Shapes of distributions

Examining the shape of a distribution is often done to assess if the data are normally distributed – a requirement of many statistical tests. *A common misunderstanding is that the data should be normally distributed, but the statistical models only require the data to be generated from a normal distribution.* Non-normal data can be generated from a normal distribution, and need not be a cause for concern. In the code below, 100 samples are generated from a normal distribution (using `rnorm()`) with a standard deviation of 0.25. The mean of each data point depends on another variable `x`, which ranges from 1–100. Thus, each data point is drawn from its *own* normal distribution with a common standard deviation of 0.25, but the mean depends on the value of `x`. A histogram of the data is plotted in Figure 6.8 and the distribution is uniformly distributed between 0 and 100.

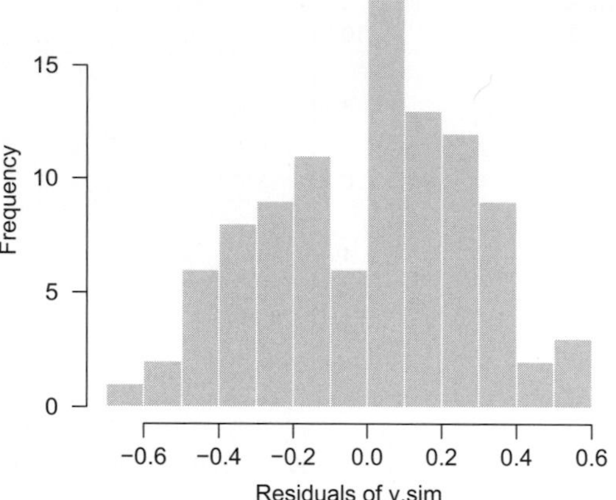

Fig. 6.9 Residuals are normally distributed even though the data are not.

```
> # mean for each person
> x <- 1:100
>
> # within group standard deviation
> sigma <- 0.25
>
> # data generated from a normal distribution
> y.sim <- rnorm(n=100, mean=x, sd=sigma)
>
> # mean of simulated data
> mean(y.sim)
[1] 50.5359
>
> par(las=1)
> hist(y.sim, col="grey", border="white", breaks=10,
+     main="", xlab="y.sim")
```

The distribution is non-normal because each data point was generated from a normal distribution with a different mean. If we could somehow remove the dependency of `y.sim` on `x`, then the data points will be normally distributed. We can do this by fitting a model using `aov()` with `y.sim` as the outcome and `x` as the only predictor. The residuals are extracted with the `resid()` function and plotted in Figure 6.9, and they appear normal. The key point is *that the distribution of the raw data is irrelevant, it is the distribution of the residuals that needs to be checked for normality.*

There are two reasons why the residuals may not be normal. The first is if the data (`y.sim`) were generated from some other distribution, say a log-normal distribution (e.g. using the `rlnorm()` function). Second, important predictor variables or an interaction term are not in the model. If the model below excluded x (`resid(aov(y.sim ~ 1))`) then the residuals would look like the raw values in Figure 6.8, except they would be centred at zero.

```
> # fit a model and save the residuals
> resid <- resid(aov(y.sim ~ x))
>
> # residuals are normally distributed
> par(las=1)
> hist(resid, col="grey", border="white", breaks=10,
+      main="", xlab="Residuals of y.sim")
```

In the above example, the shape of the distribution was determined by looking at a histogram. Histograms are useful when the sample size is large, but the impression about the shape of the distribution partly depends on the number of bins (bars in the plot). Other graphs are better for assessing the shape of a distribution. The code below generates data from a normal (`n.dist`), uniform (`u.dist`), *t* (`t.dist`), and log-normal distribution (`l.dist`) using the built-in R functions.

```
> set.seed(123)
> n.dist <- rnorm(100, 100, 10)
> u.dist <- runif(100)
> t.dist <- 10 * rt(100, df=3) + 100
> l.dist <- rlnorm(100, 4.5, 0.65)
```

Figure 6.10 shows the normal data (`n.dist`) plotted with five different graphs. The first is a histogram without binning, where each unique value has its own bar. Because the data are continuous and there are no duplicate values, this graph would be a uniform distribution with all bars having a height of one, were it not for the following trick. In the code below the `round()` function rounds the values to the nearest whole number, allowing duplicates to occur, and the `table()` function aggregates similar values together for plotting. Such a graph provides a high-resolution view of a distribution when the data do not have too many unique values and the amount of data is not excessive. This graph is suitable for count data because the values are whole numbers and duplicates are likely (see Figure 6.20 on page 327 for an example with cell count data).

```
> library(BHH2)
> par(mfrow=c(2,3),
+     mar=c(5,4,3,1),
+     las=1)
>
> plot(table(round(n.dist,0)), ylab="Frequency",
```

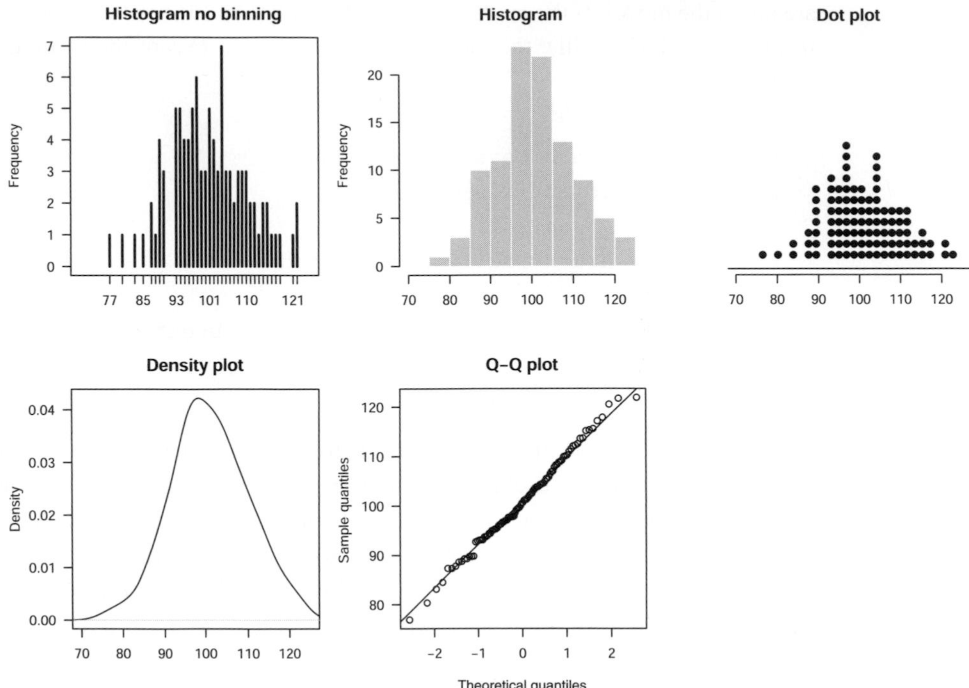

Fig. 6.10 Graphs to assess the shape of a single variable.

```
+        main="Histogram no binning", xlim=c(70, 125))
>
> hist(n.dist, col="grey", border="white", breaks=10,
+        main="Histogram", xlab="", xlim=c(70, 125))
>
> dotPlot(n.dist, pch=19, main="Dot plot", xlab="",
+           xlim=c(70, 125), cex=1.1)
>
> plot(density(n.dist), main="Density plot", xlab="", xlim=c(70, 125))
>
> qqnorm(n.dist, main="Q-Q plot"); qqline(n.dist)
```

The second graph in Figure 6.10 is a standard histogram for comparison. The third graph is a dotplot from the `BHH2` package. Each value is plotted as a point and similar values are stacked on top of each other. An advantage of this graph is that the sample size is easy to see. Binning of the values occurs and depends on the size of the plotting symbol.

The fourth graph is a density plot, which is a smoothed histogram. The `density()` function performs the calculations and passes them to the `plot()` function. The `density()` function has several options and the `adjust` option controls the smoothness. It has a default value of one, and the higher the value, the smoother the plot. An advantage of a density plot is that several distributions can be compared by plotting them on top of each other. A disadvantage is that the sample size cannot be estimated from the graph. Also, the *y*-axis, 'Density', is irrelevant for interpreting the shape and tends to confuse those unfamiliar with density plots. It is often better to suppress the *y*-axis by setting `yaxt="n"` and `ylab=""` in the `plot()` function.

The final graph is a quantile–quantile plot (Q–Q plot) and is a good way to assess the shape of a distribution. The `qqnorm()` function compares the actual data (*y*-axis) with data from a theoretical normal distribution that has the same mean and standard deviation as the actual data (*x*-axis). If the data are perfectly normal, all of the points will fall on the diagonal line. Since `n.dist` was generated from a normal distribution the points are all close to the line.

It takes practice to interpret the information in a Q–Q plot and the code below and the next set of graphs (Figure 6.11) compare dotplots and Q–Q plots for the three non-normal distributions we generated above. When the data are uniformly distributed (top graphs) the Q–Q plot has an 'S' shape because there are too many points below the diagonal line on the right and too many points above the line on the left. This shape indicates that there are not enough extreme values for a distribution with this standard deviation. A uniform distribution has a lower and upper limit (0 and 1) but a normal distribution has no constraints, and the 'S' shape of the Q–Q plot highlights that the data are bounded.

```
> par(mfrow=c(3,2),
+     mar=c(5,4,3,1),
+     las=1)
> dotPlot(u.dist, pch=19, main=~Uniform, xlab="")
> qqnorm(u.dist, main=~Uniform); qqline(u.dist)
>
> dotPlot(t.dist, pch=19, main=~t[(3)], xlab="")
> qqnorm(t.dist, main=~t[(3)]); qqline(t.dist)
>
> dotPlot(l.dist, pch=19,main=~log~normal, xlab="")
> qqnorm(l.dist, main=~log~normal); qqline(l.dist)
```

The second pair of graphs in Figure 6.11 shows a *t*-distribution with three degrees of freedom, indicated as $t_{(3)}$. A *t*-distribution resembles a normal distribution but has heavier tails and thus more extreme points.[8] The Q–Q plot shows that there are points well below the diagonal line on the left and points far above the line on the right. This is what outliers look like in a Q–Q plot.

The final pair of graphs in Figure 6.11 shows a log-normal distribution, which can have only positive values and is skewed to the right. For the Q–Q plot the points are above the

[8] The degrees of freedom is unrelated to the sample size, it is a parameter that affects the shape of the distribution. A better term might be 'shape parameter' to avoid confusion with the degrees of freedom of a statistical model, which does depend on the sample size. A *t*-distribution becomes more like a normal distribution as the degrees of freedom increases, and a rule of thumb is that the approximation is good enough when df = 30.

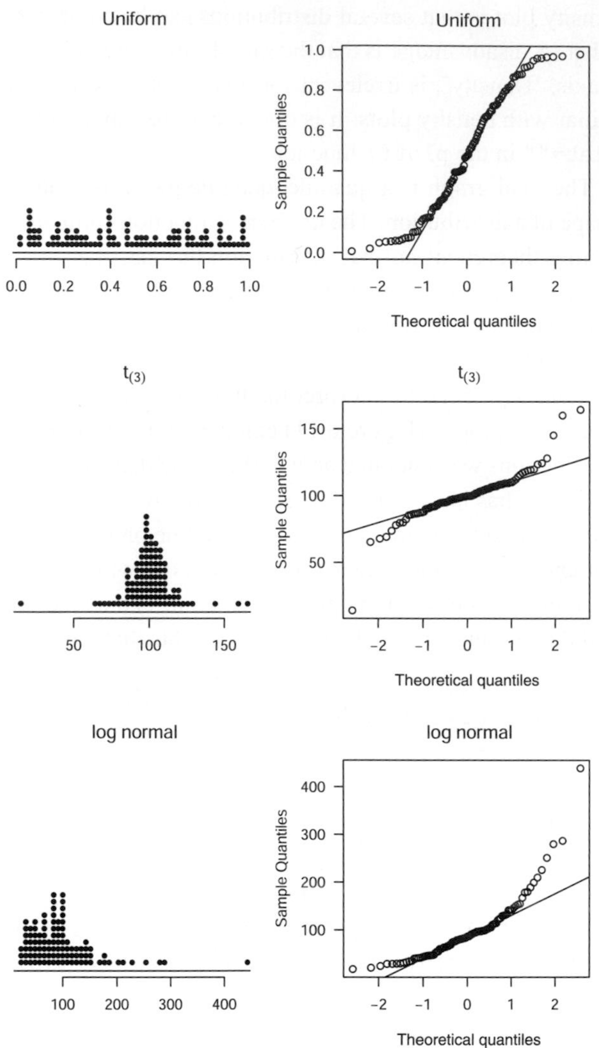

Fig. 6.11 Dotplots and Q–Q plots for three non-normal distributions.

diagonal line on the left, much like the uniform distribution, reflecting the bounded nature of the distribution. The points are above the line on the right, much like the *t*-distribution, indicating that the observed values are larger than expected for a normal distribution and that there are outliers. Interpreting Q–Q plots and understanding how a distribution deviates from a Gaussian becomes easier with practice.

In addition to graphical assessments, the shape of a distribution can be formally tested with the `ks.test()` function (Kolmogorov–Smirnov test). `ks.test()` requires three items to be specified and the code is below. The first item is the data to be tested (`n.dist`). The second is the distribution the data are hypothesised to have (`pnorm` for a normal distribution). The last item is the values of the parameters for that distribution. Since we are hypothesising a normal distribution, we need to specify a mean and standard deviation, and these are calculated from the data (`n.dist`). The null hypothesis is that the distribution is normal (or which ever distribution we are testing) and therefore a small p-value means that we reject the null. In other words, a small p-value implies that the distribution is not normal. The p-value for `n.dist` is large ($p = 0.888$) and we conclude that the distribution is close enough to normal. This procedure is the opposite of a standard hypothesis test because we usually want a small p-value to reject a hypothesis, but here we want to demonstrate normality and so desire a large p-value.

```
> ks.test(n.dist, "pnorm", mean=mean(n.dist), sd=sd(n.dist))

One-sample Kolmogorov-Smirnov test

data:  n.dist
D = 0.0581, p-value = 0.888
alternative hypothesis: two-sided
```

Assessing normality using only a KS-test is often unhelpful because large departures from normality will go undetected with a small sample size and negligible departures from normality will have a small p-value with a large sample size.

6.3.2 Effects of interest

The most interesting plots are those that enable us to visually test our hypotheses; for example, if the outcomes differ by group or if there are relationships between variables.

Two variables

A popular graph in biology is the mean and error bar plot. Bars or points indicate the group means and the error bars represent the standard error of the mean (SEM).[9] This graph is terrible for understanding the data. The problem with plotting the mean is that it hides important features of the data, such as skewness, outliers, clusters, and the number of samples in the groups.

Error bars representing the SEM are also unhelpful. First, they are a function of both the variability and the sample size, and unless the groups have the same number of samples, it is hard to compare variances across groups. Second, error bars are symmetric about the mean and can include impossible values if the data are skewed or bounded. Third, they are not designed to help us infer if a difference between two groups is statistically significant. A rule of thumb is that if the SEM is doubled, it is approximately a 95% CI, and if CI

[9] The SEM is the standard deviation divided by $\sqrt{n}$, where n is the number of samples in the group.

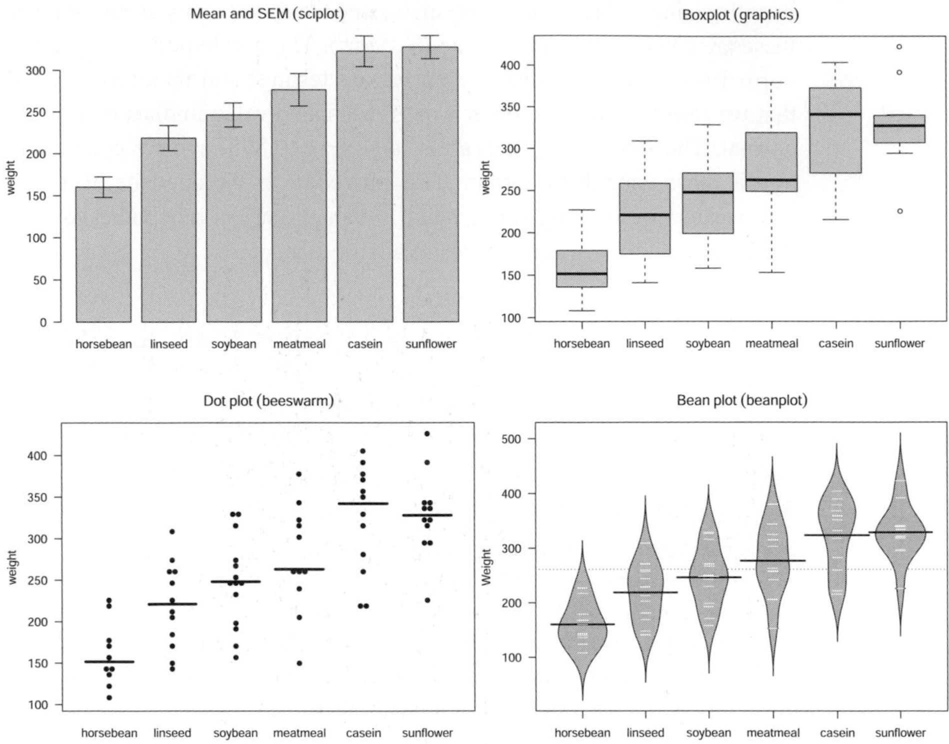

Fig. 6.12 Graphs of one continuous versus one categorical variable from the `sciplot`, `base`, `beeswarm`, and `beanplot` packages.

bars from two groups do not overlap, then the difference between groups is significant.[10] However, the difference may be significant even if the 95% CI overlap. Furthermore, this informal approach to inference ignores problems with multiple testing. Finally, the width of the error bars is not the same width that is used for inference. Recall in Section 4.1.3 (p. 135) on multiple comparisons that the `pairwise.t.test()` function had a `pooled.sd` argument that determined if the within group variability was estimated from all groups in the experiment or from the two groups being compared. A standard analysis always pools across groups and so a graph that reflects the analysis would have error bars of the same size for all groups, but by default graphs estimate the SEM using only data from each group.

Figure 6.12 shows three alternative graphs to a mean and SEM plot. This experiment compares the effect of feed supplements on the growth of chickens and the outcome is body weight. The data are in the `chickwts` data frame in the `datasets` package. The feed supplements are ordered alphabetically by default, making it easy to find an entry in a long list but is not ideal for understanding the data. The `reorder()` function uses the group means to reorder the supplements from low to high.

[10] The SEM is approximately a 68% confidence interval with a large sample size [75], but nobody is interested in a 68% CI.

```
> data(chickwts)
>
> # reorder groups by mean weight
> chickwts$feed <- reorder(chickwts$feed, chickwts$weight, mean)
```

The top left graph in Figure 6.12 is a standard mean and SEM plot drawn with the `bargraph.CI()` function in the `sciplot` package. The top right plot is a boxplot (also called a box-and-whisker plot) and is made with the `boxplot()` function in the `graphics` package (part of the base installation). A boxplot displays a five number summary for each group. The thick horizontal line is the group median, the lower and upper edges of the box are the 25th and 75th percentile, meaning that 50% of the data points lie within the box. This is called the interquartile range (IQR). The 'whiskers' are the lines extending above and below the box and can represent several summaries, depending on the software. In R, the whiskers extend to the most extreme data point that is no more than 1.5× the IQR. For the horse bean feed supplement, the ends of the whiskers coincide with the minimum and maximum values, since these are within 1.5× the IQR. If some values are outside of the 1.5× limit, they are plotted as separate points, and the whiskers extend to the next point that is within the 1.5× limit, as seen in the sunflower group. Boxplots provide more information than a mean and SEM plot and asymmetrical distributions can be detected. A drawback of boxplots is that they cannot detect clusters or bimodal distributions, and since they are a five number summary of the data, there should be at least five observations in each group for the graph to make sense, but ideally many more. With few observations, the summaries (medians, IQRs, and whiskers) are unstable, meaning that if the experiment was conducted again, these values would be different. As a rule of thumb, if there are fewer than 30 observations per group it is better to plot the individual data points, as in the bottom left graph of Figure 6.12. A final problem with boxplots is that it is hard to visually compare two groups to get a feel for whether they differ (unless the differences are large).

```
> library(sciplot); library(beanplot)
> par(mfrow=c(2,2),
+     mar=c(4,3.8,3,0.5),
+     las=1)
>
> bargraph.CI(feed, weight, data=chickwts, main=~Mean~and~SEM~(sciplot),
+             ylab="weight")
>
> plot(weight ~ feed, data=chickwts, col="grey", main=~Boxplot~(graphics),
+      xlab="")
>
> beeswarm(weight ~ feed, data=chickwts, method="center",
+          pch=16, main=~Dot~plot~(beeswarm), xlab="")
> bxplot(weight ~ feed, data=chickwts, probs=0.5, add=TRUE)
```

```
>
> beanplot(weight ~ feed, data=chickwts, main="Bean~plot~(beanplot),
+          what=c(1,1,1,1), col=c("darkgrey","white","black","black"),
+          ylab="Weight", border="black")
```

The bottom left graph of Figure 6.12 plots all the data using the beeswarm() function in the beeswarm package. The horizontal lines represent the group medians. Since there are 10–14 observations per group, this is the preferred plot for quality control checks because clusters and outliers are easy to see. This graph is also suitable for publication because all of the data are shown, although the overall message might be harder to communicate because there is more information in the graph.

The bottom right graph in Figure 6.12 shows a beanplot. The small horizontal white lines are the raw data, and they contain the same information as the beeswarm plot. The longer horizontal black lines are the group means. The grey blobs are density plots (turned sideways compared with Figure 6.10 and reflected vertically) and thus provide information on the shape of the distributions and enable bimodal distributions to be detected. A related plot is the violin plot found in the vioplot package.

The data in Figure 6.12 have no unusual features and so the shortcomings of mean and SEM plots are not highlighted. Section 6.3.4 (p. 335) shows an example where error bars obscure important trends in the data and Cleveland [75, Figure 3.76] provides an example with four groups that have identical means and standard deviations but the underlying data differ: one looks approximately normal, another has equally spaced points (uniformly distributed), the third has two clusters of points, and the final group has two outliers.

The greatest virtue of mean and SEM plots is what they hide: outliers, skewed distributions, clusters of points, and missing values (the data points cannot be counted and compared with the sample size stated in the methods). For this reason, they will not go out of fashion. A distinction should, however, be made between graphing data to understand its structure and to present the results of an analysis. Presenting results involves communicating a message, and there is value in condensing the results to summary statistics such as the mean, which can help the message stand out. The key point is that mean and error bar plots should not be the only ones used to explore data, and more informative displays can often be made for publications.

The above graphs had one continuous outcome and one categorical predictor. For two continuous variables, scatterplots are excellent graphs and have been used earlier in this book – for example Figure 5.3 (p. 200) – and so are not described again. Recall that when the two variables are observations on the same samples at two time points (e.g. pre and post), under two conditions, or comparing two methods of measurement (e.g. new method with a gold standard), then the Tukey mean-difference plot is a better alternative (Figure 5.4, p. 202).

Three or more variables

Most experiments have multiple continuous and categorical variables and this section describes graphs for understanding complex relationships between them.

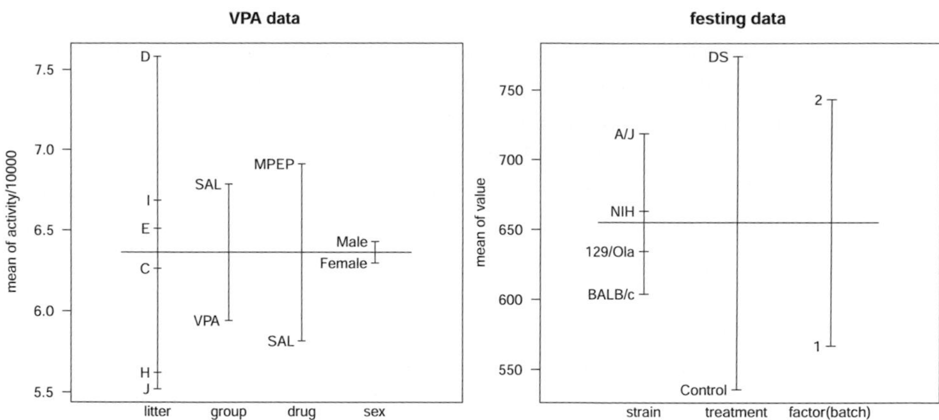

Fig. 6.13 A design plot is useful for ANOVA models.

Design plot: one outcome, many factors

The graphs in Figure 6.13 are suitable for designed experiments and show a single continuous outcome variable plotted against many categorical predictors. The `plot.design()` function in the code below uses the formula syntax to specify the variables for plotting. The left graph shows the `VPA` data from the `labstats` package (analysed in Section 4.5, p. 175). The outcome is the amount of locomotor activity and the *y*-axis shows the mean for each level of each factor; the horizontal line is the overall mean. This graph provides a quick impression of the size of the main effects and we can see that (1) the difference between sexes is small, (2) the difference due to MPEP and VPA are of similar magnitude, and (3) the greatest variation is between litters.

```
> par(mfrow=c(1,2),
+     mar=c(1,4,3,0.5),
+     las=1)
>
> plot.design(activity/10000 ~ litter + group + drug + sex,
+             data=VPA, main="VPA data")
>
> plot.design(value ~ strain + treatment + factor(batch), data=festing,
+             main="festing data")
```

There are a few caveats when interpreting these graphs. First, when calculating the mean for each factor, the other factors are ignored, making the graph hard to interpret when the data are unbalanced. Suppose that animals from litter D are more likely to be in the MPEP condition than the SAL condition. Are animals in litter D highly active because of some special characteristic of litter D, or because most animals tend to be in an experimental condition that induces locomotor activity? Second, no information about interactions is provided. Even though sex appears unimportant in Figure 6.13, it might interact with another variable. Third, groups with smaller sample sizes will tend to have a greater variation around the mean because of sampling variability (Section 1.2.4, p. 8). There are four animals in each litter but 12 in each of the other groups (e.g. 12 males and 12 females), and we therefore expect the litters to vary more around the horizontal mean line. We cannot estimate from the graph if the variation between the litters is greater than expected given their smaller sample size. Fourth, the graph provides no information on the factor arrangement (nested versus crossed). Recall that the VPA experiment is a split-unit design where litters H, I, and J were assigned to the VPA condition and litters C, D, and E to the saline condition. The litters are nested within 'group' but this information is hard to take into account when interpreting the graph.

Despite these caveats, design plots provide a quick overview of the data. The right graph in Figure 6.13 shows the results for the `festing` experiment (analysed in Section 4.4.2, p. 173). Since batch is a numeric variable it is converted into a factor for plotting.

Scatterplot matrix: many continuous outcomes

The correlation between many continuous variables can be calculated with `cor()` function, but the pattern of relationships is hard to see. A scatterplot matrix is one method of examining the correlation between several continuous variables. The `Soils` data from the `car` package is used for this example, which measures physical and chemical characteristics of 48 soil samples. Suppose we are interested in three properties of the soil: `pH`, sodium levels (`Na`), and conductance (`Conduc`). The code below loads the data and calculates the correlation between the variables containing the relevant data (columns 6, 13, and 14). The three variables are highly correlated and the last line of code reorders the rows to make the output in the same order as Figure 6.14.

```
> data(Soils, package="car")
>
> # all pairwise correlations
> all.cors <- cor(Soils[,c(6,13,14)])
>
> # reorder rows to make the same as the graph
> all.cors[3:1,]
              pH        Na    Conduc
Conduc -0.764810  0.972409  1.000000
Na     -0.693261  1.000000  0.972409
pH      1.000000 -0.693261 -0.764810
```

The code below uses the `splom()` function from the `lattice` package for the scatterplot matrix.[11] The `Soils` data frame is passed to `splom()` and the three variables are selected.

[11] The `pairs()` function in the base `graphics` package makes a similar graph.

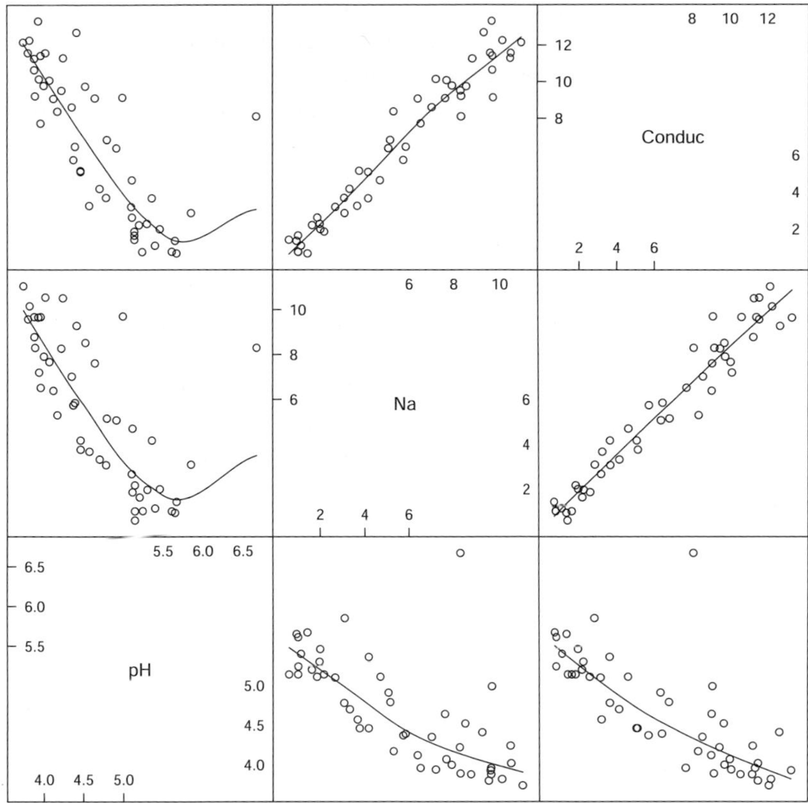

Fig. 6.14 Scatterplot matrix.

The type argument allows us to specify multiple options for plotting; "p" indicates that the points should be plotted and "smooth" indicates that a smoothed regression line should be added.

```
> library(lattice)
> splom(~Soils[,c(6,13,14)], cex=0.8, col="black",
+        type=c("p","smooth"))
```

Figure 6.14 shows all possible correlations between the variables. The data are laid out in a 3 × 3 grid, which mimics the 3 × 3 output of `all.cors`. The top left panel shows the correlation between pH (*x*-axis) and conductance (*y*-axis). To determine the variable on the *x*-axis in any panel, move vertically until a box with a label appears, which is `pH`. To determine the variable on the *y*-axis, move horizontally until a box with a label appears, which is `Conduc`. The values in the top left panel are the same as the bottom right panel, but the axes are swapped – now pH is on the *y*-axis and conductance is on the *x*-axis, which can be determined using the same procedure of moving vertically and horizontally to find the box with the labels. All pairs are therefore plotted twice.

Conductance, sodium, and pH have a strong linear correlation, but there is an outlier: the point with the highest pH value should have a low value for sodium and conductance but instead has an average value. Each point corresponds to one sample – that is, one row in the data frame. Unusual points raise two questions: 'which sample is it?' and 'which point corresponds to this sample across all variables (in all panels)?' To answer these questions the graph must become interactive.

The code below sets the interactive session with `trellis.focus()`, and the outer box in Figure 6.14 turns red. After the `panel.brush.splom()` function is run, left clicking on the unusual point in any panel will highlight that sample in all other panels. Repeat to highlight multiple points. When all the desired points have been selected, right clicking anywhere on the graph ends the interactive session.[12] The R command line then reports the row numbers in the data frame for the selected samples in the order that they were selected (output not shown). Using this method we find that the unusual sample is in row 24, which can now be examined further.

```
> trellis.focus()
> panel.brush.splom()
```

A scatterplot matrix can also indicate categorical variables with different symbols or colours. The soil samples were taken at four depths, and specifying `groups=Depth` in the code below indicates that the symbols should encode the depth. Although it is customary to use different symbols we use the numbers 1–4 because they have an easy to understand natural ordering. The plotting symbols are set with `trellis.par.set()`, and the values to `pch` need to have quotation marks. Shallow samples (depth = 1) have a high pH, low sodium, and low conductance (Figure 6.15), while deeper samples (depth = 4) have a low pH, high sodium, and high conductance.

```
> trellis.par.set(superpose.symbol=list(col="black", pch=c("1","2","3","4")))
>
> splom(~Soils[,c(6,13,14)], data=Soils, groups=Depth,
+        auto.key=list(columns=4, title="Depth"), cex=1.2)
```

3D scatterplot: three continuous outcomes

A 3D scatterplot is another plot to examine three continuous variables. The `cloud()` function from the `lattice` package is used and shown in Figure 6.16. Information on the depth

[12] R cannot run other commands during an interactive session and right clicking on the graph restores R's normal functioning.

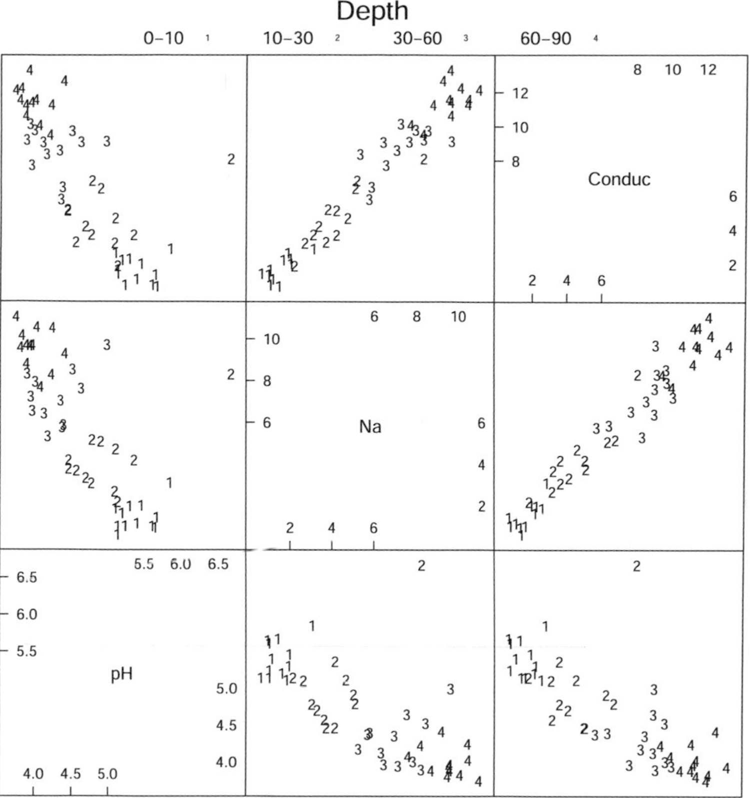

Fig. 6.15 Scatterplot matrix with information on sample depth encoded by symbol type (1 = shallow; 4 = deep).

of the sample is indicated once again by symbol type. By default, `cloud()` uses arrows on the axes to indicate the direction of increasing values (base of the arrow is low, arrowhead is high). Specifying `scales=list(arrows=FALSE)` in the `cloud()` function displays the numeric values.

```
> trellis.par.set(superpose.symbol=list(col="black", pch=c("1","2","3","4")))
>
> cloud(Conduc ~ Na + pH, data = Soils, col="black", group=Depth, cex=1.2,
+       R.mat = matrix(c(-0.448, 0.308, -0.841,
+           0, -0.894, -0.173, 0.413, 0, -0.017, 0.939,
+           0.353, 0, 0, 0, 0, 1), nc = 4), screen = list())
```

3D scatterplots usually need to be rotated to find a good viewing angle. The viewing angle is controlled with the `Rmat` argument – a matrix of numbers impossible to interpret. A good way to find a suitable viewing angle is to make the graph interactive with the

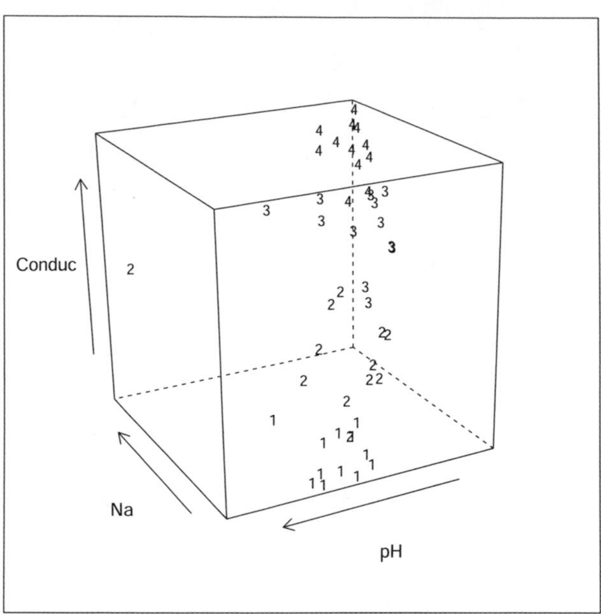

Fig. 6.16 3D scatterplot with information on sample depth encoded by symbol type (1 = shallow; 4 = deep).

playwith() function in the playwith package.[13] The code below shows how to wrap the cloud() function within playwith(). The dots represent the normal arguments to cloud, which are excluded to save space. When the interactive window opens, click on the 'Pan' button. Then, left click and drag the graph to rotate. Once a suitable angle is found, click on 'Tools' → 'Edit call', which opens a new window with the R code to generate the plot with the current viewing angle. Then, copy and paste the code into your R script file. This is how the above values for R.mat were obtained.

```
> library(playwith)
> playwith(
+     cloud(...)
+     )
```

Scatterplots with conditioning: one outcome, multiple predictors

When experiments have several continuous and categorical variables researchers want to visualise them together. The two main functions when the outcome is continuous are xyplot() in the lattice package and coplot() in the base graphics package. Using the Soils data from the previous section, suppose we are interested in the association between conductance (the outcome variable) and sodium. From the previous graphs we saw

[13] rgl is a another popular package for interactive 3D graphics.

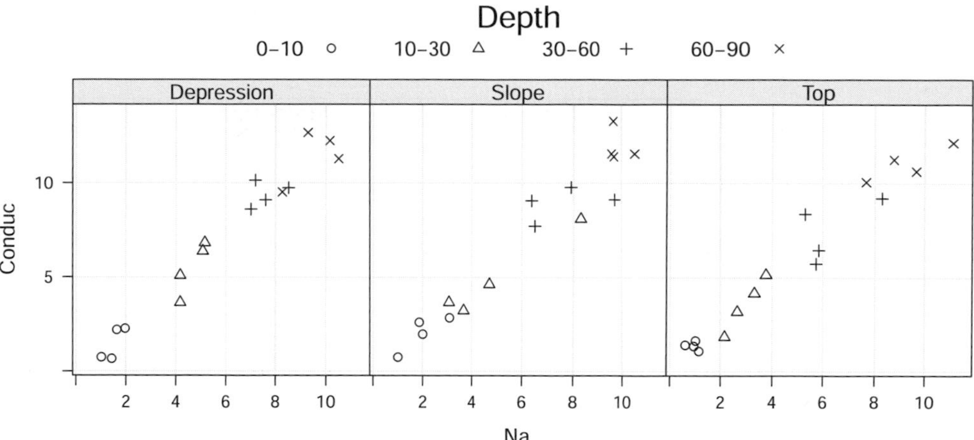

Fig. 6.17 Scatterplot with three predictor variables. Sodium and conductance are conditioned on contour.

that both values depend on the depth, which will need to be included in the graph. Another variable in the data set is `Contour` – a factor with three levels that describes the topography of the soil sample location. The code below generates the plot in Figure 6.17 and the vertical bar `|` is the conditioning operator. It indicates that the variables to the left of it – conductance and sodium – should be plotted separately for each level of the variable to the right of it – contour. The `layout` argument specifies the layout of the three panels using the format `c(number_of_columns, number_of_rows)`. In Figure 6.17, we see that the relationship between conductance and sodium is similar for the three contours.

```
> trellis.par.set(superpose.symbol=list(col="black", pch=1:4))
>
> xyplot(Conduc~Na|Contour, data=Soils, group=Depth, type=c("g","p"),
+        auto.key=list(columns=4, title="Depth"),
+        scales=list(alternating=FALSE), layout=c(3,1))
```

When experiments have blocking factors, it is a good idea to check the magnitude of the block effects. Figure 6.18 includes `Block` as a fifth variable, and the symbol type distinguishes the blocks by specifying `groups=Block` in the code below. `Contour` and `Depth` are to the right of the vertical bar, separated by a plus sign, indicating that the relationship between conductance and sodium is conditioned on two variables. The `reorder()` function reorders the levels of `Contour` by the mean value of conductance instead of the default alphabetical ordering. It is easier to detect patterns when the levels of the conditioning variables are ordered by their mean or median. `depth` is not reordered because it already has a natural ordering. The `useOuterStrips()` function from the `latticExtra` package creates the 4×3 grid of factor levels for depth and contour. Otherwise, the factor levels for depth are drawn nested under contour (not shown).

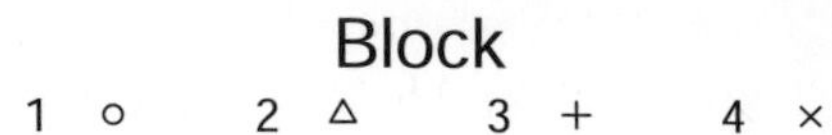

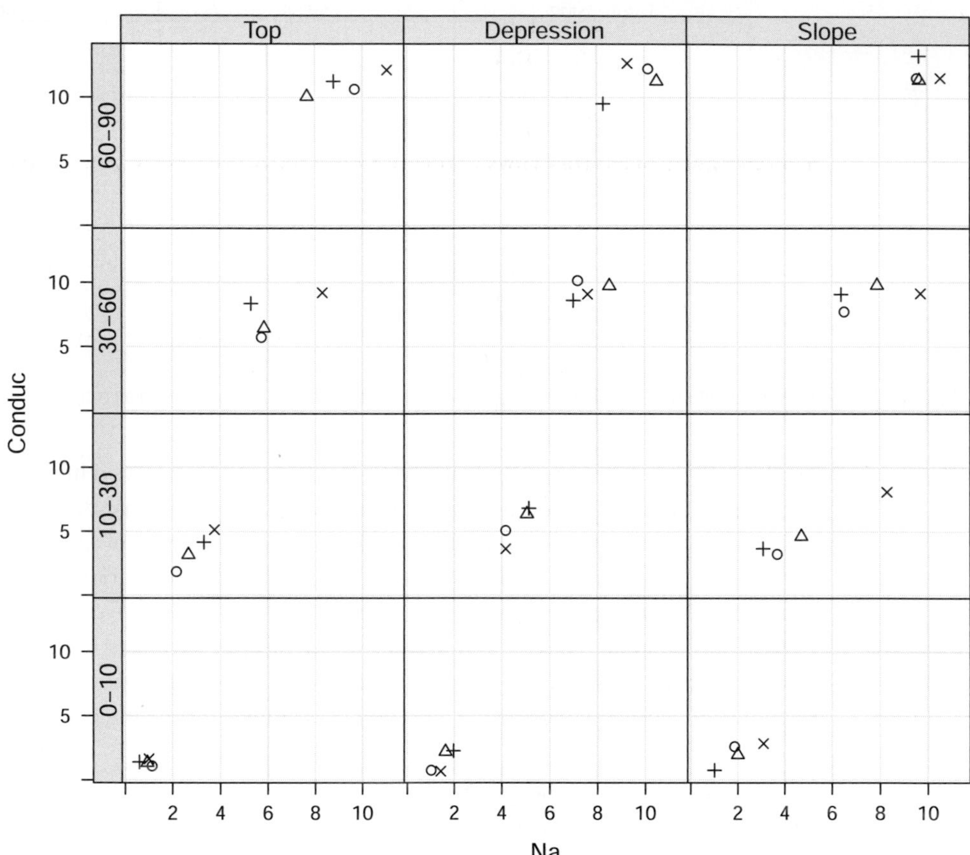

Fig. 6.18 Scatterplot with four predictor variables.

```
> library(latticeExtra)
>
> trellis.par.set(superpose.symbol=list(col="black", pch=1:4))
>
> useOuterStrips(
+ xyplot(Conduc~Na|reorder(Contour,Conduc,mean)+Depth, data=Soils,
+        groups=Block, type=c("g","p"), scales=list(alternating=FALSE),
+        auto.key=list(columns=4, title="Block"))
+     )
```

Figure 6.18 may be overwhelming until you know what to look for. The key relationships are listed below, in no particular order.

Look down columns (across rows): Looking down the column 'Top', the points shift from high to low (on the y-axis). This means that conductance depends on the depth, and the same is true for the other columns. The points also shift to the left as we go from top to bottom, indicating that sodium levels also depend on depth.

Look across columns (within rows): Looking across the row '60–90', the points have similar values on the y-axis. This means that conductance is independent of contour. The same is true for the other rows (depths).

Look at patterns across rows and columns simultaneously: Compare the values across the row '60–90' with those in the row below ('30–60'). The values shift down by an equal amount in both rows. The 'Depression' values do not, for example, shift down more than those in 'Top' or 'Slope'. The same is true when looking at the next row ('10–30'). Not only are values constant within rows (across columns) but the downward shift in values from row to row is constant. This tells us that there is no depth by contour interaction.

Look at relationships within panels: There appears to be a positive association between sodium and conductance within most panels, although it is stronger in some and non-existent when sodium varies little (e.g. bottom left panel).

Look at the order of symbols: There is no strong or consistent block effect, which would be seen if one plotting symbol is the highest in all panels.

It is often necessary to create multiple graphs of the same data to understand all of the relationships – some graphs highlight certain relationships better than others. The options consist of which variables are (1) on the x-axis, (2) conditioned on (appear after the `|`), and (3) used for grouping (supplied to the `groups` argument). The code below plots the same data but excludes the sodium variable, plots block on the x-axis, groups by depth, and still conditions on contour. The result is shown in Figure 6.19, where it is easier to see the block effects compared with Figure 6.17.

```
> trellis.par.set(superpose.symbol=list(col="black", pch=1:4),
+                 superpose.line=list(col="black"))
>
> xyplot(Conduc~Block|reorder(Contour,Conduc,mean), data=Soils,
+        type=c("g","b"), scales=list(alternating=FALSE), layout=c(3,1),
+        groups=Depth, auto.key=list(columns=4, title="Depth"))
```

The above graphs should be examined before a formal analysis because they will help determine which variables and interactions to include in the model. Such graphs also guide expectations about the statistical results. If, for example, the analysis indicates a strong effect of contour, then it might be worthwhile double checking the results because this was not the impression obtained from the graphs. Was the model correctly specified? Was an error made somewhere?

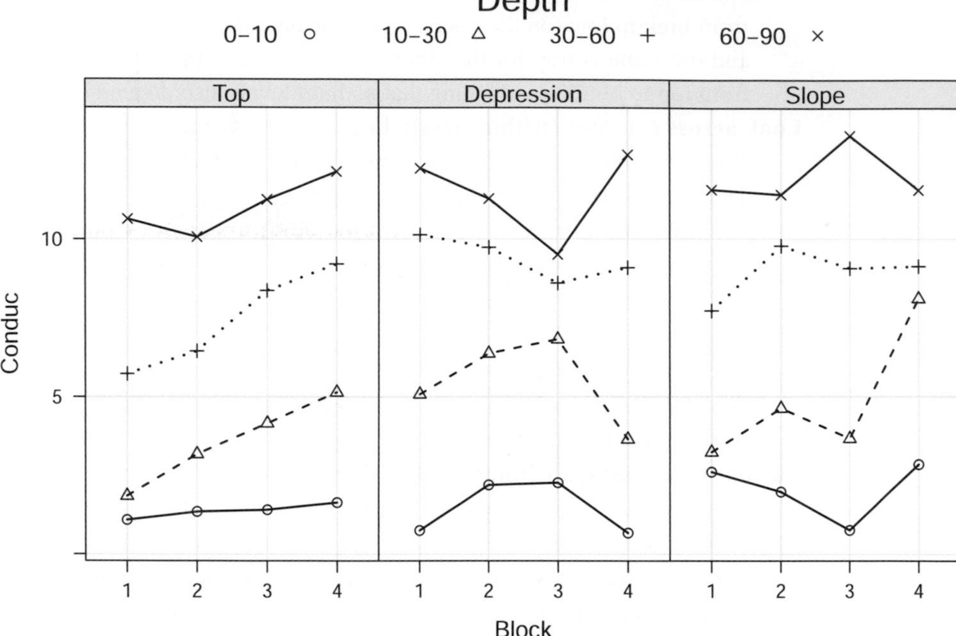

Fig. 6.19 Another scatterplot with three predictor variables but varying the grouping and conditioning variables. This graph allows block effects to be easily seen.

6.3.3 Spatial artefacts

Many *in vitro* experiments use multi-well microtitre plates and the position of samples on these plates can be a source of technical artefacts (Section 2.12.8, p. 89). Potential artefacts include edge-effects, gradients, stripes, and checker-board patterns. There are several plots that can be used to examine these effects.

The `cell.count` data set from the `labstats` is used for this example. The data are from a high-content screen and the only outcome variable is the number of cells in each well. Cell counts were not the primary outcome for the experiment but are useful for quality control checks. The experiment used six 1536-well plates and a summary of the data is below. There are no missing values but the minimum cell count is zero, indicating that some wells had no cells. There are 32 rows and 48 columns in 1536-well plates, and the minimum and maximum values for the row and column variables indicates that none have been excluded, such as the control wells. The variable `plate` is a factor and the summary shows that there are six plates with a complete set of 1536 observations.

```
> summary(cellcount)
    plate            row              column         cell.count
 Plate_1:1536   Min.   : 1.00   Min.   : 1.0   Min.   :  0
 Plate_2:1536   1st Qu.: 8.75   1st Qu.:12.8   1st Qu.:344
```

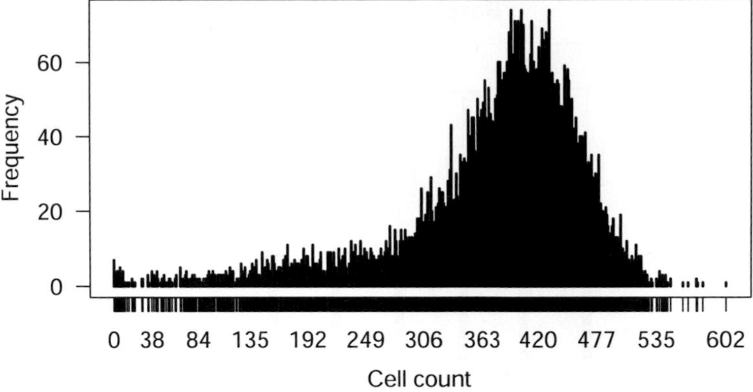

Fig. 6.20 Cell count across all plates.

```
Plate_3:1536   Median :16.50   Median :24.5   Median :395
Plate_4:1536   Mean   :16.50   Mean   :24.5   Mean   :376
Plate_5:1536   3rd Qu.:24.25   3rd Qu.:36.2   3rd Qu.:434
Plate_6:1536   Max.   :32.00   Max.   :48.0   Max.   :602
```

Since cell counts are integers the `table()` function in the code below counts the frequency of wells with 0, 1, 2, 3, etc. cells and the results are stored in `cell.num`. Looking at the first few entries of `cell.num` shows that seven wells have zero cells, three wells have one cell, and so forth. The data are plotted as a histogram with no binning (Figure 6.20) and the distribution appears normal except for the long tail to the left.

```
> cell.num <- table(cellcount$cell.count) # seven wells with zero cells
> head(cell.num)

0 1 2 3 4 5
7 3 2 4 4 1
>
> par(las=1)
> plot(cell.num, xlab="Cell count", ylab="Frequency")
```

Another useful graph is to look at the distribution of cell counts on each plate, and Figure 6.21 shows a boxplot and a density plot of cell counts. The plates have similar distributions in that the median, boxes, and whiskers are similar across plates, and the shape of the density curves are similar.

```
> par.set <- list(box.umbrella=list(col="black", lty=1),
+                 box.dot=list(col="black"),
+                 box.rectangle = list(col="black"),
```

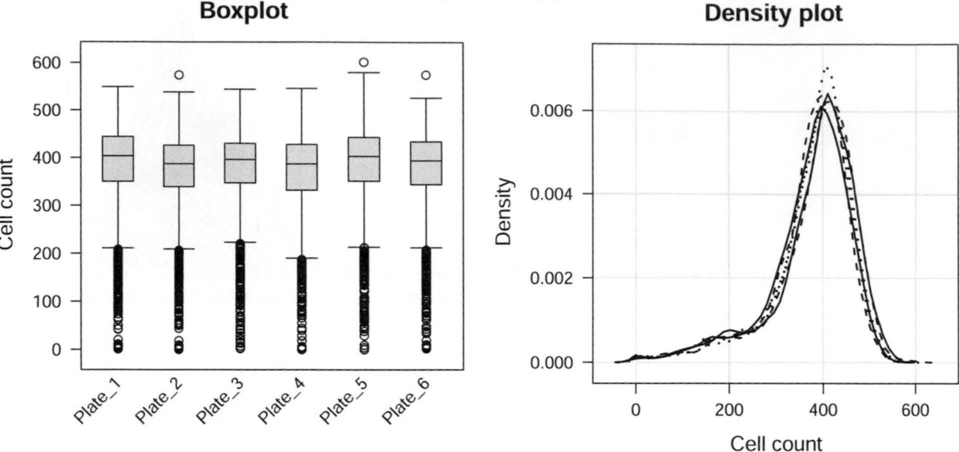

Fig. 6.21 Plate effects. Distributions are similar across all plates indicating the absence of large plate effects.

```
+                     plot.symbol=list(col="black"))
>
> p1 <- bwplot(cell.count ~ plate, data=cellcount,
+                 ylab="Cell count", scales=list(x=list(rot=45)),
+                 col="black", pch="|", fill="lightgrey",
+                 main="Boxplot", par.settings=par.set)
>
> p2 <- densityplot(~cell.count, data=cellcount, groups=plate,
+                plot.points=FALSE, col="black", type=c("g","l"),
+                     xlab="Cell count", main="Density plot")
>
> print(p1, split=c(1,1,2,1), more=TRUE)
> print(p2, split=c(2,1,2,1))
```

The above graphs were preliminary looks at the data and now spatial effects are examined. The code below calculates the mean of each row and the mean of each column separately for each plate. `row.means` is a matrix with 6 rows (one for each plate) and 32 columns (because the 1536-well plates have 32 rows). The first few columns of `row.means` are shown below. Similarly, `col.means` has 6 rows and 48 columns (because the 1536-well plates have 48 columns).

```
> # calculate row and column means
> row.means <- with(cellcount, tapply(cell.count, list(plate,row), mean))
> col.means <- with(cellcount, tapply(cell.count, list(plate,column), mean))
>
> dim(row.means)
```

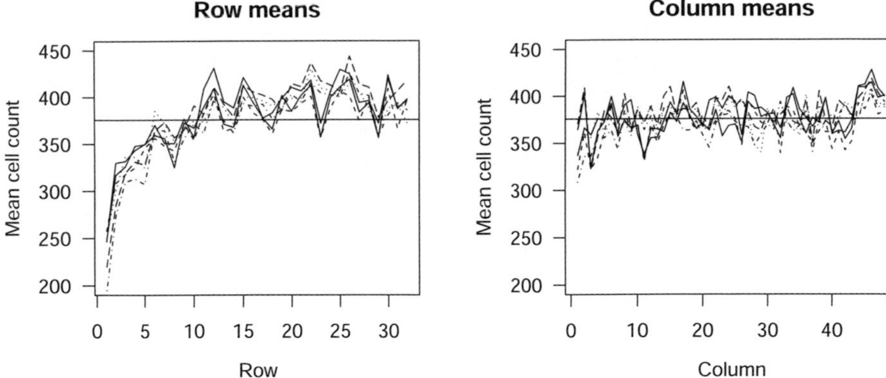

Fig. 6.22 Spatial effects. Each line is one plate and row numbers 1–10 have lower cell counts. There also appears to be some zig-zagging across rows. The horizontal line is the overall mean cell count (across all plates).

```
[1]  6 32
>
> row.means[,1:5]
              1       2       3       4       5
Plate_1 246.812 317.000 325.979 347.938 349.583
Plate_2 257.729 308.417 317.896 324.729 346.000
Plate_3 249.979 299.833 337.146 336.125 324.500
Plate_4 194.958 273.583 309.750 313.104 307.167
Plate_5 219.833 284.792 319.333 331.021 327.854
Plate_6 246.417 329.750 331.750 343.417 349.938
>
> dim(col.means)
[1]  6 48
```

In the code below the mean values are plotted with the `matplot()` function. The data matrices have to be transposed with the `t()` function so that each plate corresponds to one line in the graph (Figure 6.22). Otherwise the x-axis would be the plate number and the lines would represent the rows or columns. The spatial gradient across the first 10 rows is easy to detect (left graph), and it is consistent across all six plates. The final few columns tend to have higher values for all plates (right graph), but the effect is not as large as the row effects. The horizontal line is the mean cell count across all plates and is used as a reference line.

```
> par(mfrow=c(1,2), las=1)
> matplot(t(row.means), type="l", col="black", ylim=c(200, 450),
+          xlab="Row", ylab="Mean cell count", main="Row means")
> abline(h=mean(cellcount$cell.count))
>
```

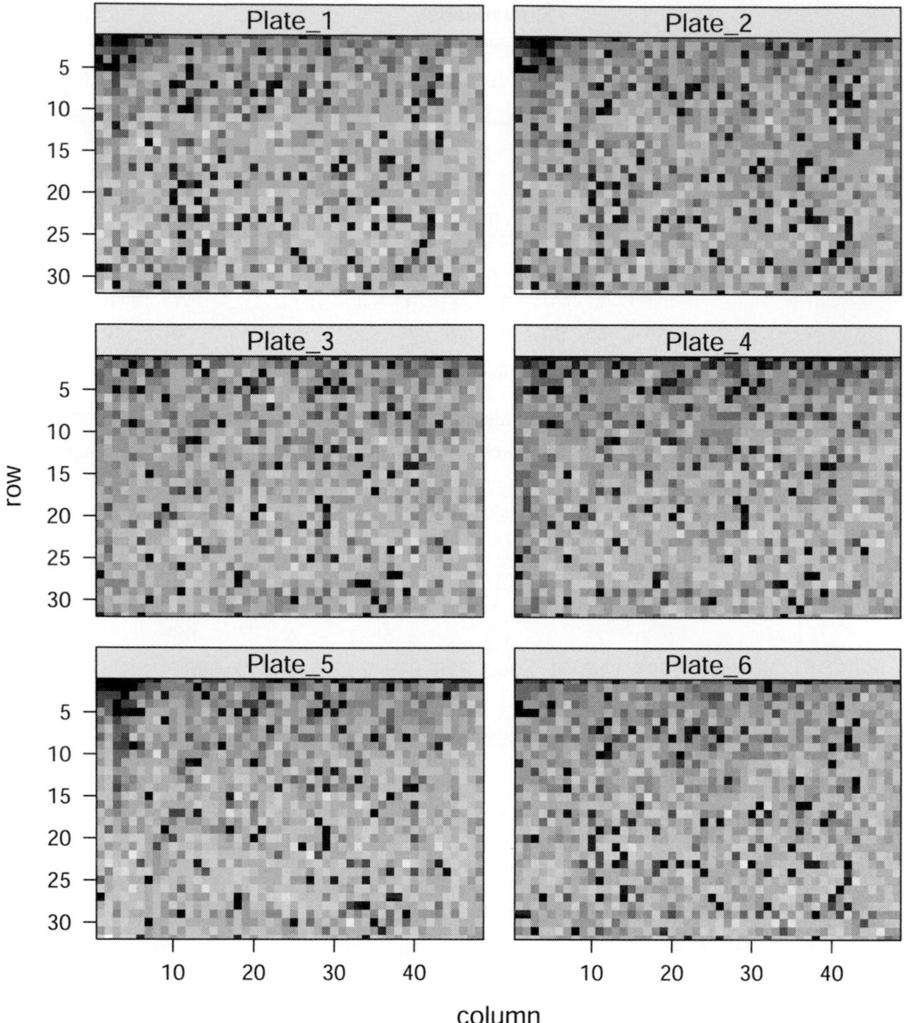

Fig. 6.23 Spatial effects. A level plot shows that the top left part of some plates tend to have lower cell counts (darker shades).

```
> matplot(t(col.means), type="l", col="black", ylim=c(200, 450),
+         xlab="Column", ylab="Mean cell count", main="Column means")
> abline(h=mean(cellcount$cell.count))
```

The `matplot()` function looks at slices of the data but the `levelplot()` function from the `lattice` package displays a physical representation of the layout of a 1536-well plate, where the rows and columns of the image represent the rows and columns of the plate. Figure 6.23 shows the results for all six plates and each small square within a plate represents a well. The darkness of a small square is proportional to the cell count. In the code below the `colorRampPalette()` function provides a range of colours that are mapped to cell count values. The values range from black (minimum cell count) to white (maximum cell count), with grey values indicating intermediate values. Spatial effects are easier to see with colours, and a blue–white–red colour scheme is provided in the code below but is commented out. Darker shades in the top left corner of plates one, two, and five are noticeable, indicating lower cell counts.

```
> # nice colour scheme (not used for book)
> # levelcols <- colorRampPalette(c("darkblue", "blue", "lightgreen",
> #                                   "white", "orange", "red", "darkred"))
>
> greycols <- colorRampPalette(c("black","white"))
>
> levelplot(cell.count ~ column*row|plate, data=cellcount, aspect=0.67,
+           ylim=c(32,1), between=list(x=1,y=1), layout=c(2,3),
+           as.table=TRUE, scales=list(alternating=FALSE),
+           col.regions=greycols(100), colorkey=FALSE)
```

The `levelplot()` function has many arguments to improve the display, most of which are not discussed. Two key arguments are `ylim=c(32,1)`, which reverses the y-axis so that the top of each image is row one, thus reflecting the physical layout. The second option is the `aspect`, which controls the height to width ratio of a plate. Since a 1536-well plate has 32 rows and 48 columns, the ratio is $32/48 = 0.67$. Setting the aspect to 0.67 makes the dimension of the plates in Figure 6.23 the same as the physical dimension of a plate. See `help(levelplot)` for a description of the other arguments.

A drawback of using colour to encode magnitude is that a single outlier can compress the colour scale so that many values are mapped to a few colours. Most plates would have all dark squares with one prominent white outlier. Several solutions are available, including transforming the data by taking the square root of the counts. An alternative option is used below for Plate_5 only, to save space, but the same process should be applied to all plates. Instead of using a range of colours, only two are used, and they depend on whether a cell count value is above or below the median cell count for that plate. In the code below the median cell count for Plate_5 is calculated and then subtracted from each well; the result is stored in `cent.count`. Next, the `ifelse()` function assigns a value of $+1$ if the well is above zero (that is, above the median), and -1 otherwise (below the median). The result is stored in `above.below` and the first few lines for `plate5` are shown.

```
> # select only plate five
> plate5 <- subset(cellcount, plate=="Plate_5")
>
> # subtract the median
> plate5$cent.count <- plate5$cell.count - median(plate5$cell.count)
>
```

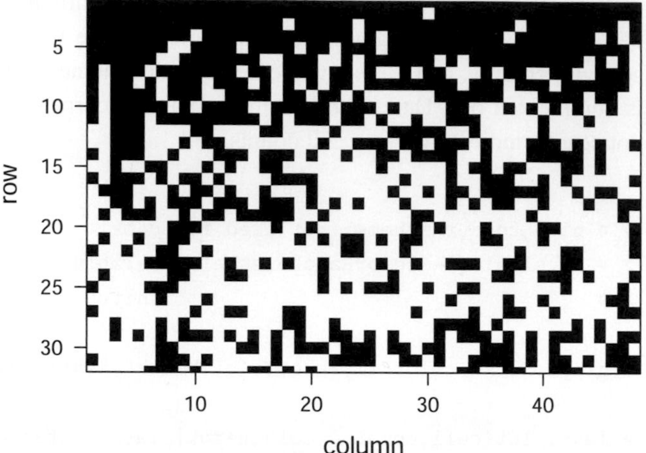

Fig. 6.24 Spatial effects for wells above (white) or below (black) the median. The first few rows tend to be black, indicating a spatial effect.

```
> # +1 if well is above plates median, -1 otherwise
> plate5$above.below <- ifelse(plate5$cent.count > 0, 1, -1)
>
> head(plate5)
        plate row column cell.count cent.count above.below
6145 Plate_5   1      1         77       -326          -1
6146 Plate_5   1      2        136       -267          -1
6147 Plate_5   1      3         38       -365          -1
6148 Plate_5   1      4         81       -322          -1
6149 Plate_5   1      5        141       -262          -1
6150 Plate_5   1      6        126       -277          -1
```

The same `levelplot()` function is used but now the outcome variable is `above.below` instead of the raw cell counts (Figure 6.24). The graph is only black and white because all values are either −1 or +1. This robust method is not influenced by outliers and shows that most wells in the first few rows are below the plate median, indicating an edge-effect, and consistent with previous graphs (Figure 6.22). The code below has a line commented out that spatially smooths the black and white squares to make trends easier to see.

```
> levelplot(above.below ~ column*row, data=plate5,
+           main="", aspect=0.67, ylim=c(32,1), colorkey=FALSE,
+           #panel = panel.2dsmoother, args = list(span=0.1), n=200
+           col.regions=greycols(100))
```

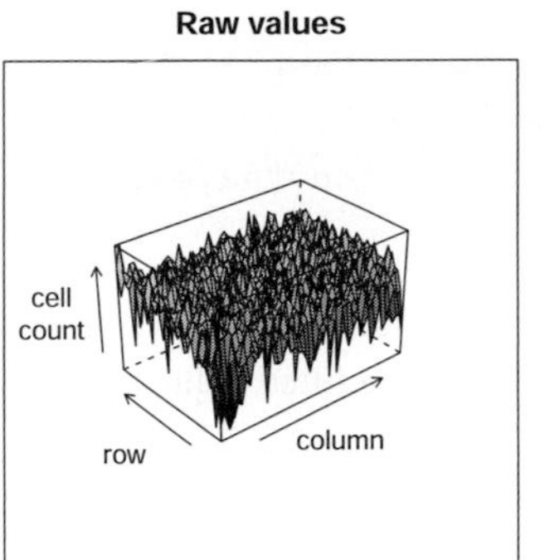

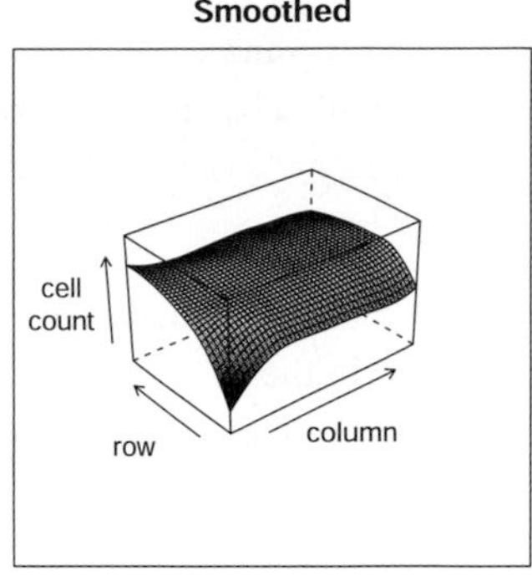

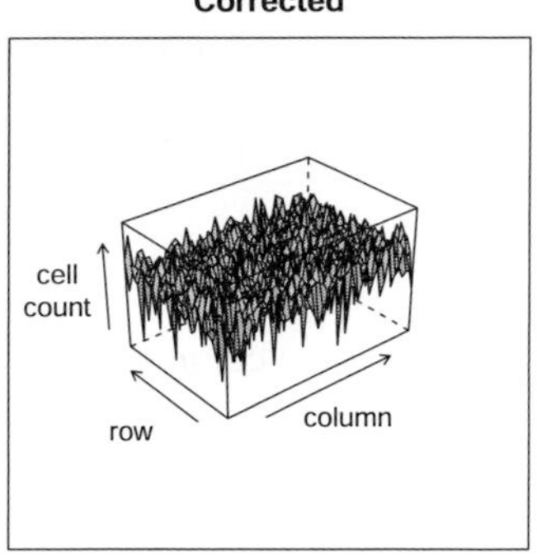

Fig. 6.25 Surface plots for spatial effects. The graphs show the raw cell count values for Plate 5, the smoothed values, and the corrected values.

The final plot is a surface plot, which represents cell counts by the height of the surface instead of by colour, although colouring the surface makes the differences starker. The raw cell counts are on the left in Figure 6.25, and the graph was made with the `wireframe()` function from the `lattice` package. The surface is lower towards the front, especially the front left corner. The code is below and resembles the `levelplot()` code; the new arguments are mainly to format the graph nicely.

```
> wireframe(cell.count ~ column*row, data=plate5, colorkey=FALSE,
+           scales=list(arrows=TRUE,distance=1.4), zlim=c(0,600),
+           drape=TRUE, col.regions=greycols(100), zoom=0.65,
+           zlab="cell\ncount", main="Raw values",  aspect=c(0.67,0.6))
```

The middle graph of Figure 6.25 shows a smoothed version of the cell counts. The trends in the data are easier to see when most of the well-to-well variation is removed. The code below uses the `loess()` function to fit a smoothed surface to the data and the results are stored in `sm1`. A `loess()` smoother was used behind the scenes to calculate the smoothed regression line in Figure 6.14 (p. 319). `cell.count` is the outcome and `column` and `row` are the predictor variables in the loess model. The `span` argument controls the amount of smoothing and is a value between 0 and 1; the higher the value the greater the smoothing. The `normalize` argument controls whether the predictor variables are normalised to a common scale, and it is set to `FALSE` because we do not want to normalise spatial coordinates. Setting `family="symmetric"` uses a robust method so that outliers have less influence. These data have no missing values, but it is good practice to set `na.action = "na.exclude"` which retains the NA values, if present. This ensures that when fitted values and residuals are calculated (see below) they have the same number of elements as the data. Without `na.exclude` the vector of fitted values and residuals will be shorter and will be misaligned with the vector of original data.

```
> sm1 <- loess(cell.count ~ column*row, data=plate5,
+              span=0.25, normalize = FALSE,
+              family="symmetric", na.action="na.exclude")
```

In the next chunk of code, the fitted values are extracted from `sm1` and stored in a new column called `smoothed` in the `plate5` data frame. The fitted values are the smoothed cell count data and are plotted in the middle graph of Figure 6.25. The code for the plot is not shown but it is identical to the graph for the raw data except for replacing `cell.count` with `smoothed`.

```
> # extract and save the smoothed values
> plate5$smoothed <- fitted(sm1)
```

The residuals are the distance of each well from the smoothed surface and can be extracted using the `resid()` function. The residuals are centred at zero because the wells above the smoothed surface have positive values and wells below the surface have negative values. The second line of code below adds the mean cell count to all wells to shift the values upwards and saves the result as `corrected.count`. This makes the corrected values comparable to the raw cell count values (`cell.count`), which can be seen in the summary below. Negative values are still present (the minimum value is −48.8), but this poses no analytical problems. The right graph in Figure 6.25 shows the corrected cell count values; note how the dip in the left front corner has been removed.

```
> # extract residuals
> plate5$resid <- resid(sm1)
>
> # add plate mean to shift the residuals to be positive
> plate5$corrected.count <- plate5$resid + mean(plate5$cell.count)
>
> summary(plate5[,c(4,5,8,9)])
   cell.count     cent.count          resid            corrected.count
 Min.   :  0   Min.   :-403.0   Min.   :-432.05   Min.   :-48.8
 1st Qu.:351   1st Qu.: -52.0   1st Qu.: -39.06   1st Qu.:344.2
 Median :403   Median :   0.0   Median :  -1.75   Median :381.5
 Mean   :383   Mean   : -19.7   Mean   : -15.44   Mean   :367.8
 3rd Qu.:443   3rd Qu.:  40.0   3rd Qu.:  31.54   3rd Qu.:414.8
 Max.   :602   Max.   : 199.0   Max.   : 147.63   Max.   :530.9
```

The corrected values are preprocessed data that could be used for downstream analyses instead of the raw cell counts. It is a good idea to check how well the preprocessing worked. The right graph of Figure 6.25 shows that the spatial trends have been removed. But were

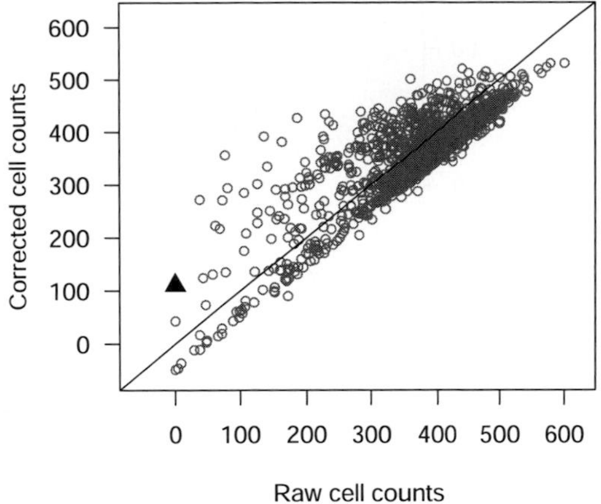

Fig. 6.26 Raw versus corrected cell counts. The black triangle indicates a point with a raw cell count of zero, but a corrected count of 110.

any artefacts introduced? Figure 6.26 plots the raw and corrected cell count data, which have a strong association, as expected. The data point highlighted with a black triangle has a raw cell count of zero, but a corrected count of 110 – cells have been generated from nowhere! Understanding these side effects of preprocessing is necessary for a sensible interpretation of the results. Wells with no cells should be removed, and possibly wells with few cells. This example used one of many methods to remove spatial effects, and the following references discuss other approaches [236, 249, 258, 414].

6.3.4 Individual profiles

This final section looks at repeated measure data and how mean and error bar plots hide interesting effects. The `locomotor` data from the `labstats` package are used and the data are from a real experiment. Rats were injected with either a compound or vehicle control at time = 0 and placed into an open field testing box. The outcome variable is the amount of locomotor activity in each 15 minute interval and a summary of the data is below.

```
> summary(locomotor)
      drug          animal           time             dist
 Control:138   Min.   : 1   Min.   :15.0   Min.   : 0.000
 Drug   :144   1st Qu.:12   1st Qu.:30.0   1st Qu.: 0.198
               Median :24   Median :52.5   Median : 0.538
               Mean   :24   Mean   :52.5   Mean   : 1.354
               3rd Qu.:36   3rd Qu.:75.0   3rd Qu.: 1.533
               Max.   :47   Max.   :90.0   Max.   :12.615
```

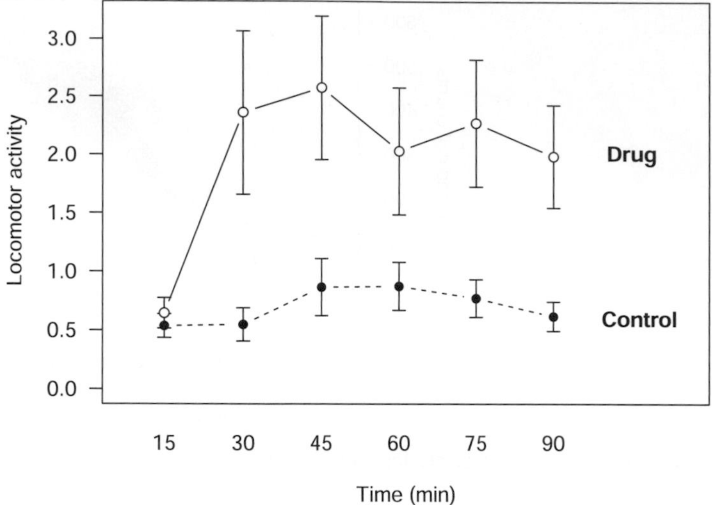

Fig. 6.27 Means and SEM. The data represent the total distance travelled by animals every 15 min. The two groups are similar at 15 min, and then the drug increases the distance travelled between 15 and 30 min, where it reaches its maximum effect and then remains stable until the last observation.

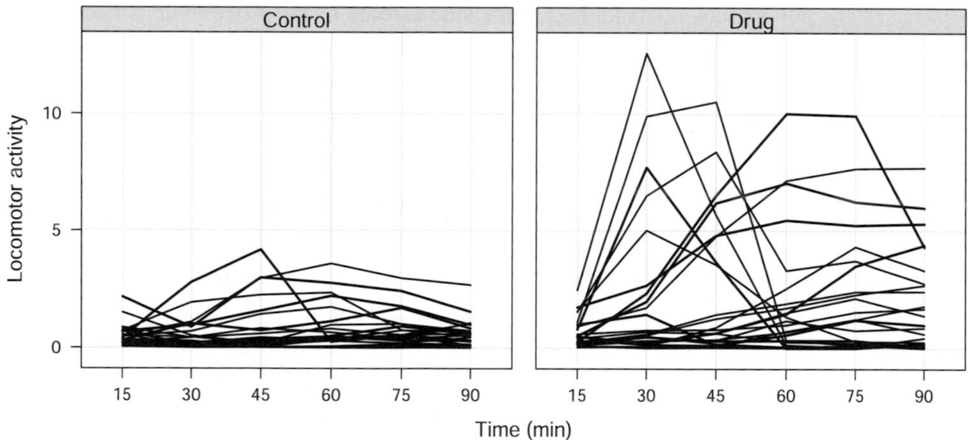

Fig. 6.28 Profile plot of each animal. No rat in the drug group follows the pattern of change in Figure 6.27.

The data are plotted in Figure 6.27 as a typical mean and SEM plot. The compound's effect could be described as follows: the two groups are similar 15 minutes after the injection, the compound increases activity and reaches its maximum effect by 30 minutes, and then remains stable until the last observation. The controls have low activity throughout, and the difference between the groups looks convincing.

⚠ The mean and SEM plot obscures an important fact – *no treated animal follows the trajectory of the group mean*. Figure 6.28 plots the profile for each animal across time with a line, and three patterns are visible. The compound has no effect on some animals (flat line), has a rapid effect on others, and a slower acting effect on the rest.

```
> xyplot(dist ~ factor(time)|drug, data=locomotor, group=animal,
+        type=c("g","l"), between=list(x=1), col="black", lty=1,
+        xlab="Time (min)", ylab="Locomotor activity",
+        strip=strip.custom(bg="lightgrey"),
+        scales=list(alternating=FALSE) )
```

A closer look at the rats in the drug group is warranted and the code below extracts these rats and saves their values in the `drug.only` data frame. Next, the data are converted into a wide format using the `unstack()` function and saved in the `drug.wide` data frame. The first few lines are shown and now each column is a time point and each row is a rat.

```
> # select only drug group
> drug.only <- locomotor[locomotor$drug=="Drug",]
>
> # convert data into wide format
> drug.wide <- unstack(drug.only, dist~time)
>
> # examine layout
> head(drug.wide)
    X15   X30   X45    X60   X75   X90
1 0.252 2.328 6.504 10.028 9.937 4.324
2 0.091 0.000 0.019  0.012 0.010 0.138
3 0.235 0.591 1.429  1.901 2.409 2.421
4 1.733 2.665 4.799  5.460 5.241 5.314
5 0.031 0.067 0.088  0.721 1.236 0.611
6 0.590 0.758 0.783  0.989 1.540 1.685
```

In the next step, the rats are clustered so that rats with similar profiles are placed in the same group. There are many (perhaps too many) clustering methods available and are not covered in this book. The clustering task view on CRAN lists the relevant R packages – over 100 of them.[14]

The k-means clustering algorithm is used, which works by minimising the sum of squares, a concept covered in Section 4.1.1 (p. 124).[15] This algorithm requires the user to specify the number of clusters, which is often unknown, but there appear to be three distinct profiles in Figure 6.28 and so the argument `centers=3` is specified in the `kmeans()` function in the code below. The k-means algorithm also requires starting values for the cluster centres and these are chosen randomly by the function (although user-defined values can be provided). The `set.seed()` function makes the results reproducible by setting

[14] `https://cran.r-project.org/web/views/Cluster.html`

[15] The data are partitioned into three clusters such that the sum of squares from each point to the cluster centres is minimised.

the random generator seed. Since the results might depend on the random values chosen, the `nstart` argument indicates that the clustering should be run 100 times with different starting values, and the best solution (smallest sum of squares) is saved. The final line of code prints the results.

```
> # perform clustering
> set.seed(1)
> km <- kmeans(drug.wide, centers=3, nstart=100)
>
> # show results
> km
K-means clustering with 3 clusters of sizes 4, 5, 15

Cluster means:
      X15    X30      X45      X60     X75     X90
1 0.85325 2.1715 5.563250 7.421250 7.27275 5.83450
2 1.49760 8.3480 6.360000 1.025200 0.83560 0.73240
3 0.30540 0.4164 0.519533 0.929867 1.42187 1.37927

Clustering vector:
 [1] 1 3 3 1 3 3 1 3 3 3 3 3 3 3 1 3 2 3 3 2 2 2 3 2

Within cluster sum of squares by cluster:
[1] 33.6392 97.4996 62.5906
 (between_SS / total_SS =  79.4 %)

Available components:

[1] "cluster"      "centers"      "totss"        "withinss"
[5] "tot.withinss" "betweenss"    "size"         "iter"
[9] "ifault"
```

The key output is the `Clustering vector`, a number indicating the cluster assignment for each rat. We want to integrate this information with the `drug.only` data so it can be used for plotting. The code below extracts the cluster information and repeats each value six times (one for each time point since `drug.only` is in the long format) and pastes the values to `"Drug Cluster"` to create a nice label. The `xyplot()` function is then used to plot the data, with each cluster plotted in a separate panel (Figure 6.29).

```
> # make the assigned cluster into a factor
> drug.only$clust <- as.factor(paste("Drug Cluster",
+                            rep(km$cluster, 6), sep=" "))
>
```

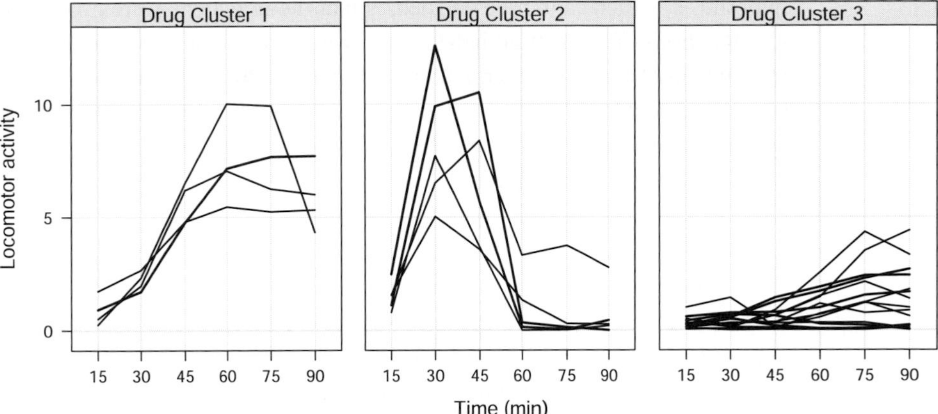

Fig. 6.29 Profile plot for each animal in the drug group. Some animals do not respond at all or have a small increase over time (cluster 3), some have a large early response but then drop back down to control levels (cluster 2), and some have a gradual increase that levels off (cluster 1).

```
> # make plot and conditon on cluster
> xyplot(dist ~ factor(time)|clust, group=animal, data=drug.only,
+         type=c("g","l"), between=list(x=1), col="black", lty=1,
+         xlab="Time (min)", ylab="Locomotor activity",
+         layout=c(3,1), scales=list(alternating=FALSE))
```

The rats in Cluster 3 look similar to the control animals (compare with Figure 6.28). The rats in Cluster 2 have a rapid onset but then drop down to low activity levels by 60 minutes, and rats in Cluster 1 have a gradual increase in activity that plateaus at around 60 minutes. Averaging over heterogeneous profiles gives the misleading average profile in the mean and SEM plot (Figure 6.27). Thus, the mean misrepresents the individuals.[16] Now it is clear why the error bars are bigger in the drug group (Figure 6.27); it is not because the data are 'more variable', but because the compound has different effects on different animals.

There are two explanations for these results. First, despite their genetic similarity and identical housing, interesting biological differences exist between the rats. These unplanned aspects of the experiment can often be the most informative and are the stuff that scientific discoveries are made of. Such anomalous results lead to further hypotheses, for example, about the compound's mechanism of action.

The second, and perhaps more likely, explanation is that uncontrolled technical factors are responsible. The obvious factors should be checked: do the clusters correspond to cages, the order of data collection, were multiple open field boxes used, and so on. One

[16] There is a distinction and debate in the statistics literature between the appropriateness of *marginal* or *population models*, which describe the relationship shown by the mean and SEM plots and *conditional models*, which model the individual profiles [226, 241].

hypothesis, which cannot be verified, is that the injections were given in different anatomical locations. They should have been given intraperitoneally, but some may have been in the intestine (non-responders), some intravascularly (fast responders), and some on target (slower responders). Whether the explanation is biological or technical, the experimental system is not under adequate control and is likely unsuitable for answering the research question that it was designed to.

* * *

To summarise, there are two key points of this chapter. First, before conducting a statistical analysis *look* at the data in many ways to (1) ensure the data pass quality control checks, (2) verify assumptions, (3) understand all the relationships and treatment, biological, and technical effects, and (4) understand how the preprocessing was done, or what preprocessing is required. Second, mean and SEM graphs can miss important relationships – look at the individual data points or profile plots for repeated measures designs. Create multiple graphs of the same data as some relationships are easy to see in one graph but not in another. Proceed to the statistical analysis only after you understand the data.

Further reading

Graphical methods: *The Visual Display of Quantitative Information* by Tufte [369] is a classic book, but it is more relevant to people making graphs for the general public. *Visualizing Data* and *The Elements of Graphing Data* by Cleveland are great books and relevant for scientists making graphs for other scientists [74, 75]. Good examples of displaying quantitative information in biology and medicine can be found in *A Picture is Worth a Thousand Tables: Graphics in Life Sciences* by Krause and O'Connell [196].

R implementation: *R Graphics* by Murrell is the most comprehensive book on graphing in R [288]. Sarkar describes the details of the `lattice` package in *Lattice: Multivariate Data Visualization with R* [343]. `ggplot2` is a popular graphing package (not used here) based on Wilkinson's *The Grammar of Graphics* [398], and Wickham [395] explains how to use `ggplot2`.

Appendix A Introduction to R

This chapter provides a basic introduction to R, focusing only on the features that are relevant for this book. Many topics are omitted and since there are many resources both online and in print, there is no need to duplicate them here. Quick-R is a great website that can be consulted in addition to this appendix to learn the basics.[1]

A.1 Installing R

R is available for Windows, Mac, and Linux operating systems and can be downloaded from the Comprehensive R Archive Network (CRAN).[2] For Windows and Mac users, download and install as you would any other program. For Linux users, packages are available for Debian, Redhat, SUSE, and Ubuntu. Ubuntu users can also install R from the synaptic package manager. Installation instructions are provided on the CRAN website. To run R, click the icon on the desktop or under a menu. Alternatively, R can be started on the Linux command line by typing R (capital).

In addition to the base installation there are over 7000 add-on packages contributed by R users. They provide additional functionality and can be installed by typing

```
> install.packages("package_name")
```

at the R command prompt. You will then be asked to specify a location, and choosing one close to you will result in a faster download. Once successfully downloaded and installed, the package will need to be loaded into the R session before it can be used by typing

```
> library(package_name)
```

Periodically running

```
> update.packages()
```

[1] http://www.statmethods.net/
[2] http://cran.r-project.org/

Table A.1 Packages that need to be installed.

Package	Details
`labstats`	Data sets for this book
`sciplot`	Mean and error bar plot
`plyr`	Data manipulation
`car`	Type II and III ANOVA tables
`phia`	*Post hoc* interaction analysis
`caret`	Preprocessing functions
`beeswarm`	Graphing package
`AlgDesign`	Optimal experimental design
`VIM`	Missing data
`beanplot`	Graphing package
`playwith`	Make graphics interactive
`latticeExtra`	Graphing package

will download newer versions of all of your installed packages. The packages listed in Table A.1 are used in this book but are not part of the base installation. You may wish to install them all at once with the following code

```
> install.packages(c("labstats", "sciplot", "plyr", "car", "phia",
+                    "caret", "beeswarm", "AlgDesign", "VIM",
+                    "beanplot", "playwith", "latticeExtra"))
```

A word of warning about packages: the quality and documentation can vary, and there is usually no guarantee that functions work as advertised. Packages submitted to CRAN by package developers must pass many checks before being accepted. These checks however do not test whether functions work properly. For example, a function called `reciprocal()` takes a number x and is supposed to return the number $1/x$, but it might return $2/x$ by accident. Package developers are responsible for ensuring that functions return the correct values. Do not let this warning put you off R. The basic functions and packages installed with R are extensively tested and the code is available for all to see, which means that bugs can be identified and quickly corrected. This is not true for commercial statistics software. Also, many packages are extensively tested.[3]

A.2 Writing and editing code

An R session starts with an uninspiring command prompt (>) that tells you R is ready to accept commands. R waits for you to give it instructions but it is almost impossible

[3] See the `testthat` package and the paper by Wickham for more on testing R code [396].

to figure out what to do without reading the documentation or following a book. One way to ease the transition from point-and-click statistics software is with the R Commander package (`Rcmdr`). Many graphical and statistical functions are available from menus, and a scripting window allows you to write your own scripts. When a function is selected from the menu the code is automatically added to the script window, which enables you to learn the R functions. `Rcmdr` can be downloaded and installed in the usual way (`install.packages("Rcmdr")`), and then type `Rcmdr` at the prompt to start the graphical user interface.

Most users eventually find that it is faster and easier to write R code directly instead of selecting options from a menu – provided the right tools are available. Although the base R installation contains a script window it is too rudimentary for serious use. RStudio[4] and Emacs[5] are two popular options that make writing code easier. They provide syntax highlighting, code completion, and smart indentation. R code can be run directly from the editor and it is easy to quickly move around a script file. RStudio is user-friendly, easier to learn, and is recommended if you are new to programming. The main drawback of RStudio is that it is only used for R, and so if you decide to learn another language then you have to find another editor.

Emacs is a highly extensible and customisable text editor that can be used for most computing languages. Emacs also does so much more that it has been (jokingly) called 'a great operating system, lacking only a decent editor'.[6] If you know how to program then you likely know about Emacs, and the Emacs Speaks Statistics (ESS)[7] add-on package provides the functionality for R and other statistics languages. Emacs is harder to learn, but once you do, you'll use it for everything.

A.3 Basic commands

R can be used as a simple calculator, for example two numbers can be added by typing

```
> 2 + 2
[1] 4
```

The `[1]` in the output is an index that numbers the elements of the output. The numbering is more useful when the output is long and breaks over multiple lines; some examples are seen later in this chapter.

It is often useful to store the result of a calculation, which can be done with the assignment operator (`<-`); for example

[4] https://www.rstudio.com/products/rstudio/
[5] https://www.gnu.org/software/emacs/
[6] https://en.wikipedia.org/wiki/Editor_war/
[7] http://ess.r-project.org/

```
> y <- 2 + 2
```

adds the two numbers and assigns the sum to a variable called y. The contents of y can be viewed by typing it on the command line.

```
> y
[1] 4
```

y can now be used in further operations:

```
> y + 3  # add 3 to y
[1] 7
>
> x <- 1 # make a new variable x
>
> x + y  # add the variables together
[1] 5
```

Everything after the hash (#) symbol in the above code is a comment and is not evaluated. Comments are useful for leaving notes to yourself or others to explain what the code does.

R contains all the basic maths operators and the most common ones are listed in Table A.2. If we want to calculate the square root of y the command is

```
> sqrt(y)
[1] 2
```

We created two variables above called x and y and they are examples of *objects*. An object can be the result of a calculation, a data set read into R, or functions that we make. Objects are temporarily stored in the *workspace*, which can be thought of as the top of your desk, and the objects are items on your desk, such as pens, paper, and a stapler. Many objects will be created during an analysis and the ls() function lists them in alphabetical order. The only objects in the workspace are x and y.

```
> ls()
[1] "x" "y"
```

To remove one or more objects enter them as arguments to the rm() function.

Table A.2 Basic mathematical operators and functions.

Function	Name
+	Addition
-	Subtraction
*	Multiplication
/	Division
^	Raising to a power
mean()	Mean
median()	Median
sd()	Standard deviation
var()	Variance
min()	Lowest value
max()	Highest
range()	Lowest and highest values
sum()	Sum of values
log()	Natural logarithm
exp()	*e* raised to a power
log10()	Log to the base 10
log2()	Log to the base 2
sqrt()	Square root
sin()	Sine
cos()	Cosine
round()	Round

```
> # do not run this code as x and y will be used later
> rm(x, y)
```

To clear the workspace and remove all objects use `rm(list=ls())`.[8] If you want to save all data sets, functions, and other objects in the workspace the `save.image()` function bundles and saves them into one large binary (not human readable) file with the '.RData' extension.

```
> save.image(file="all_objects.RData")
```

To read everything back into memory use the `load()` function.

```
> load("all_objects.RData")
```

[8] Yes, this is a strange and non-intuitive way of clearing a workspace. Just one of R's quirks.

When you are finished your R session use q() to quit. If you have not saved your workspace R will prompt you to save.

A.4 Obtaining help

All R functions provide help documentation and the format is standard across all packages. If you know the name of a function and want to learn more about it, use the help() function or preface the function name with a question mark.

```
> help("plot")
> ?plot          # is the same
```

The help.search() function searches all the documentation for a given term, including packages that are not loaded. The search can be restricted to the functions (file) name, title, or other fields using the field option. The code below searches for all functions that have the word plot in any field. The code is not evaluated because the output is long, but one representative line is shown. The output is formatted as the package name, two colons, the function name, and finally the title of the function. Below we see the barplot() function is from the graphics package and the title is 'Bar Plots'.

```
> help.search("plot")
>
> # graphics::barplot                    Bar Plots
```

When you remember only part of the function name you can use the apropos() function to find all functions containing the term. For example, suppose you cannot remember if the function is called barplot(), bar.plot(), or plotbars(). The code below returns functions matching the term plot, where the entry barplot can be seen. Since apropos() returns over 100 results, the head() function is used to limit the output to the first 10.

```
> head(apropos("plot"), 10)
 [1] "assocplot"        "barplot"          "barplot.default"
 [4] "biplot"           "boxplot"          "boxplot.default"
 [7] "boxplot.matrix"   "boxplot.stats"    "cdplot"
[10] "coplot"
```

Note that apropos() only searches functions in packages that are loaded, whereas help.search() searches packages that are installed but not loaded and therefore returns a much longer list. This means that your output will differ, depending on which packages you have loaded.

If you do not know how to do something in R, it is often easier to Google the question. It is unlikely that you are the first to have this problem and most likely someone will have answered it already.

A.5 Setting options

Each R session starts with over 50 predefined options that control how R looks and works. They can be viewed with the `options()` command, which returns a long list. To view the setting of a specific option give the name of the option after the dollar sign, for example

```
> options()$show.signif.stars
[1] TRUE
```

shows that the `show.signif.stars` option is set to `TRUE`. This option controls whether asterisks (*, **, and ***) are added to statistical summary tables to indicate levels of statistical significance. To change an option specify the new value within the `options()` function; for example, to exclude the stars set:

```
> options(show.signif.stars = FALSE) # set to FALSE
> options()$show.signif.stars  # check that it worked
[1] FALSE
```

Significance stars are now suppressed, and this setting is used throughout the book. To see the full list of options use `?options`.

A.6 Loading and saving data

Loading

Many R packages contain one or more data sets and they can be listed and loaded with the `data()` function. Several options are shown below, but the code is not run because the output is too long.

```
> data() # lists data sets in loaded packages
>
> data(package = .packages(all.available = TRUE)) # lists all data sets
```

```
>
> data(package="car") # lists all data sets for a given package
```

If the package has been loaded then the data set can be accessed with:

```
> library(car)          # load package
>
> data("ChickWeight")   # load data
>
> summary(ChickWeight) # summarise the data
     weight           Time             Chick        Diet
 Min.   : 35   Min.   : 0.0   13      : 12   1:220
 1st Qu.: 63   1st Qu.: 4.0   9       : 12   2:120
 Median :103   Median :10.0   20      : 12   3:120
 Mean   :122   Mean   :10.7   10      : 12   4:118
 3rd Qu.:164   3rd Qu.:16.0   17      : 12
 Max.   :373   Max.   :21.0   19      : 12
                              (Other):506
```

Most of the time you will want to load your own data, and the function used will depend on the data format. `read.table()` is the standard function to read tabular data and it has many options that provide flexibility. It is often easier however to use the `read.delim()` and `read.csv()` functions as they have many options predefined for tab and comma separated files, and usually only the file name needs to be specified, as shown in the code below.

```
> d1 <- read.delim("filename")  # read a tab-delimited file
> d2 <- read.csv("filename")    # read a comma separated values file
```

If you have data from another statistics program (e.g. SPSS, SAS, Stata, Minitab), the `foreign` package can read these files directly. The `xlsx` package reads files in Microsoft Excel format, but it is better to first save these files to a tab or comma delimited format and then read them using `read.delim()` or `read.csv()` as this will reduce the number of unanticipated consequences that come with reading in spreadsheet files.

Saving

Data frames and matrices can be written to tab or comma delimited plain-text files using the `write.table()` or `write.csv()` function. The 'object' is the data frame to be saved and a file name must be specified.

```
> write.table(object, filename="saved_data.txt", sep="\t", quote=FALSE,
+             row.names=FALSE)
> write.csv(object, filename="saved_data.csv")
```

By default `write.table()` separates variables with one space and the `sep` argument above changes this to a tab with the backslash `t`. By default quotation marks will be placed around character and factor variables, and setting `quote=FALSE` disables this option. Row names, which may contain useful information, are written to the file by default. But if the row names are just row numbers, then this option can be disabled by setting `row.names=FALSE`.

A.7 Objects, classes, and special values

Objects in R have a *class* that roughly tells you what the object is; for example, a matrix will have the class 'matrix' and data frames have the class 'data.frame'. Classes allow R functions to know how to operate on an object and the `class()` function returns an object's class. In the code below we see that y is 'numeric', the `festing` data set in the `labstats` package is a 'data.frame', and that variable `value` within the `festing` data frame is an integer and the variable `treatment` is a factor. The dollar sign (extraction operator) can be used to select a column within a data frame, as shown below.

```
> class(y)
[1] "numeric"
>
> library(labstats)
> class(festing)
[1] "data.frame"
>
> class(festing$value)       # class = integer
[1] "integer"
>
> class(festing$treatment) # class = factor
[1] "factor"
```

Classes work behind the scenes to provide appropriate output for a given type of input. For example, the `summary()` function knows to compute numeric summaries for integer variables such as `value` in the `festing` data set, and calculates the number of samples in each group for factors.

```
> summary(festing$value)
   Min. 1st Qu.  Median    Mean 3rd Qu.    Max.
    408     551     620     655     770    1000
>
> summary(festing$treatment)
Control      DS
      8       8
```

It is good practice to check the class of all variables in a data frame to ensure functions are doing what you think they are. The `sapply()` function below applies the function given in the second argument (`class`) to all columns in the data frame given in the first argument (`festing`). The output shows that the variable `batch` is an integer and thus the `summary()` function would calculate the mean, but batch numbers are arbitrary labels and the mean is not a useful summary. Statistical models also look at a predictor variable's class and will treat it differently in an analysis if it is numeric or categorical.

```
> sapply(festing, class)
   strain treatment     batch     value
 "factor"  "factor" "integer" "integer"
```

Classes can be changed by using functions beginning with `as.x`, where `x` is the name of the new class. So `as.factor()` in the code below changes `batch` into a factor. This new variable is saved back to the data frame as `fac.batch` and the last line of code verifies the class.

```
> festing$fac.batch <- as.factor(festing$batch) # convert to factor
>
> class(festing$fac.batch) # check class
[1] "factor"
```

In addition to the `as.x` set of functions the `is.x` functions test whether an object is of a given class, and they return `TRUE` or `FALSE` as appropriate.

```
> is.factor(festing$fac.batch) # is it a factor?
[1] TRUE
>
> is.integer(festing$fac.batch) # is it an integer?
[1] FALSE
```

To see all the `as.x` or `is.x` functions available type `as.` or `is.` at the command prompt and press the tab key twice. A list of word completions will then be displayed.

Looking at objects

Objects can be simple, like y, or they can be very complex, and we often need to understand all the parts of an object so we know where to find the relevant data. If the object is tabular, such as a data frame or matrix, the `View()` function (capital 'V') opens a window showing the values. The arrow, Page Up, Page Down, Home, and End keys can be used to move around in the table. Viewing tabular data in a new window is often more convenient than printing the object to the screen, especially when it is large.

One of the best functions for understanding objects is the `str()` function, which displays the object's structure. When it is used on the `festing` data set the first line of output shows that `festing` is a data frame and that there are 16 observations (rows) and 5 variables (columns). The output then lists the names of the five variables and for each variable shows their class, along with further class-specific information. For example, the first variable (`strain`) is a factor with four levels, and the first few factor levels are shown ('129/Ola' and 'A/J'). Complex objects can have lengthy output.

```
> str(festing) # look at structure
'data.frame': 16 obs. of  5 variables:
 $ strain   : Factor w/ 4 levels "129/Ola","A/J",..: 4 4 4 4 3 3 3 3 2 2 ...
 $ treatment: Factor w/ 2 levels "Control","DS": 1 1 2 2 1 1 2 2 1 1 ...
 $ batch    : int  1 2 1 2 1 2 1 2 1 2 ...
 $ value    : int  444 764 614 831 423 586 625 782 408 609 ...
 $ fac.batch: Factor w/ 2 levels "1","2": 1 2 1 2 1 2 1 2 1 2 ...
```

If you are only interested in obtaining some of the above information the functions below can extract them for data frames and matrices.

```
> dim(festing) # Dimensions (number of rows and columns)
[1] 16  5
>
> names(festing)  # Column names (use colnames() for a matrix)
[1] "strain"    "treatment" "batch"     "value"     "fac.batch"
>
> rownames(festing) # Row names
 [1] "1"  "2"  "3"  "4"  "5"  "6"  "7"  "8"  "9"  "10" "11" "12" "13" "14"
[15] "15" "16"
>
> head(festing) # Show the first few lines (rows)
  strain treatment batch value fac.batch
1    NIH   Control     1   444         1
2    NIH   Control     2   764         2
3    NIH        DS     1   614         1
4    NIH        DS     2   831         2
```

```
5 BALB/c   Control     1   423         1
6 BALB/c   Control     2   586         2
>
> tail(festing) # Show the last few lines (rows)
    strain treatment batch value fac.batch
11     A/J        DS     1   856         1
12     A/J        DS     2  1002         2
13 129/Ola   Control     1   447         1
14 129/Ola   Control     2   606         2
15 129/Ola        DS     1   719         1
16 129/Ola        DS     2   766         2
```

Special values

Numeric objects have several special values. The first is NA, which means 'not available' and is how missing values are represented in R. When reading in data from text files, NA will automatically be inserted where there are blanks, but it is better to explicitly include NA in the data file instead of having blanks. The code below creates an object called z that contains three numbers and a missing value. The c() function concatenates items separated by commas. Some functions by default will not calculate a value when there are missing values. For example, when calculating the average of z the mean() function returns NA instead of a number. To obtain values the na.rm ('NA remove') option must be set to TRUE.

```
> z <- c(3, 5, NA, 8)
> z
[1]  3  5 NA  8
>
> mean(z)
[1] NA
>
> mean(z, na.rm=TRUE)
[1] 5.33333
```

Another special value is NaN, which means 'not a number' and it can result from unusual calculations such as

```
> 0/0
[1] NaN
```

Table A.3 Logical operators.

Operator	Name
>	Greater than
>=	Greater than or equal to
<	Less than
<=	Less than or equal to
==	Equal
!=	Not equal

The final special values are `-Inf` and `Inf` which represent minus infinity and infinity. Instead of an error message R returns these values when dividing by zero. They can be used in further calculations such as adding a number to infinity, which is still infinity, without an error being generated.

```
> # division by zero
> 10/0
[1] Inf
>
> Inf + 1 # still infinity
[1] Inf
```

A.8 Conditional evaluation

Often you will want code to be run only when a condition is met, and in other situations you will want one piece of code to be run when a condition is met and another piece when the condition fails. The operators in Table A.3 are used to compare numbers or characters.

The code below shows how the comparison operators are used to compare items, and the output is always either `TRUE` or `FALSE`.

```
> # Is 5 greater than 3?
> 5 > 3
[1] TRUE
>
> # Are the words "hat" and "cat" equal (the same)?
> "hat" == "cat"
[1] FALSE
>
> # Are the words "hat" and "cat" unequal (different)?
> "hat" != "cat"
```

```
[1] TRUE
>
> # Is "hat" less than "cat" (is "hat" alphabetically before "cat")?
> "hat" <  "cat"
[1] FALSE
>
> # Does the word "cat" equal 5?
> "cat" == 5
[1] FALSE
>
> # Does the variable x equal the variable y?
> # Recall that we previously defined x=1 and y=4
> x == y
[1] FALSE
```

When combined with `if()`, the `else` and `ifelse()` functions can be used to test conditions and execute code based on whether a condition is true or false. The code below uses `if()` to test if five is greater than three. Since this is true, 'Bigger!' is printed to the screen. The second line of code tests if three is greater than five, and since this is false, nothing is printed.

```
> if (5 > 3) print("Bigger!")
[1] "Bigger!"
>
> if (3 > 5) print("Bigger!")
```

`if()` can be combined with `else` to string together a series of comparisons. The code below first tests if x is greater than y. If so, 'Bigger!' is printed. If not, then the code tests if x is less than y. If so, 'Smaller!' is printed, and if not, then 'The same!' is printed. Only one print statement is executed depending on which condition is met, but multiple lines of code between the braces '`{ }`' can be included.

```
> if (x > y) {
+
+    print("Bigger!")
+
+ } else if (x < y) {
+
+    print("Smaller!")
+
+ } else {
+
+    print("The same!")
```

```
+
+       }
[1] "Smaller!"
```

It is common to forget the braces '{ }' after if() and else, which can result in an error, or the code not evaluating as desired. Specifically, there should not be a new line between a right brace '}' and else to avoid a syntax error. For example, the code below will generate an error because the first line is read as a complete statement, and then else on the second is unconnected with if() above it. To let R know that the if() and else statements are connected, use the syntax like the above example, where the right brace '}' is on a new line and else is immediately after.

```
> # if (3 > 5) { print("Bigger!") }
> # else       { print("Smaller!") }
```

The ifelse() function is a more compact way of conditional evaluation if there is only one if-else statement. ifelse() takes three arguments separated by commas. The first is a test, the second is what should happen if the test is TRUE, and the third is what should happen if the test is false. The code below tests if x is equal to y. If so, 'Same' is saved to w, and if not, 'Different' is saved to w.

```
> # ifelse(condition, if TRUE, if FALSE)
> w <- ifelse(x == y, "Same", "Different") # Recall that x = 1, y =4
> w
[1] "Different"
```

A.9 Creating functions

One of the advantages of R over spreadsheet software is the possibility of collecting multiple computational steps into a single reusable function. For example, suppose we want to calculate the cube root of a number. There is no built-in function in R so we can make our own. Functions are created with the function() function and the name of the new function is created by assigning a function to it as in the example below. The arguments are the input that the function takes and are located between the brackets '( )'. The R code to be executed is placed between the braces '{ }'.

```
> function.name <- function(arguments){ code }
```

The code below creates a function called `cuberoot()` that takes only one argument. By default, the last line of code that is executed in the function is returned. Complex functions may generate values at multiple steps that need to be returned and they can be collected into a vector, data frame, matrix, or list and then returned using the `return()` function as the last line of code. An advantage of functions is that inputs can be checked to ensure they are of the correct type or that they meet other requirements such as being greater than zero. The code below checks the input to ensure that it is a number and if not, an error message is printed to the screen with the `stop()` function. This ensures that functions do not return nonsense if the input is not what it should be and also provides a helpful error message to the user, which is especially important when you share your code with others. It is also good practice to document what the function does, and this is indicated in the first line of the function code. Including comments within the function is also useful for both your future self and for others, as comments help users understand what the code is doing.

```
> cuberoot <- function(x){
+     ## calculates the cube root of a number
+
+     # check input
+     if (!is.numeric(x)) { stop("x must be a number!") }
+
+     # do calculation
+     output <- x^(1/3)
+
+     return(output)
+ }
>
> cuberoot(8)
[1] 2
>
> cuberoot("eight")
Error in cuberoot("eight"): x must be a number!
>
> cuberoot(-27)
[1] NaN
>
> cuberoot(0)
[1] 0
```

Once a function is created it is good practice to test that it returns correct values and manages unusual input appropriately. The code above correctly returns a value of two as the cube root of eight and an error message is printed when the input is text instead of a number. A negative number however returns `NaN`, but a cube root of a negative number exists. Thus the function does not return the desired result for negative inputs.[9] If we know the input should always be a positive number, the function can test and return an error when the input is negative. Alternatively, we can alter the code so that the function returns the correct result for a negative number. The code below modifies `cuberoot()` and returns a warning if the input is negative, but the function continues with the evaluation. This is done only to illustrate how to use the `warning()` function. The calculation line has been modified to handle negative numbers and the strategy is to remove the minus sign if the input is negative using `abs()`, calculate the cube root of the now always positive number, and then add the minus sign back to the result if the input is negative. The last step is done with the `sign()` function which returns a -1 if the input is negative and a $+1$ if the input is positive. The last line of code now returns the correct result and also issues a warning.

```
> cuberoot2 <- function(x){
+     ## calculates the cube root of a number
+
+     # check input
+     if (!is.numeric(x)) { stop("x must be a number!") }
+
+     # warn if input is less than zero
+     if (x < 0) warning("x is less than zero.")
+
+     # do calculation
+     output <- sign(x) * abs(x)^(1/3)
+
+     return(output)
+ }
>
> cuberoot2(-27)
Warning in cuberoot2(-27): x is less than zero.
[1] -3
```

A.10 Subsetting and indexing

We often need to select elements of a vector or a few rows or columns from a data frame or matrix. There are several ways to do this in R. One way is to index the elements that you want using square brackets. The vector `z` that we created before is shown below and the

[9] This occurs because there are three roots: one is a real number (the desired value) and the other two are complex numbers.

code shows how to use indices to select elements. In R, the indexing starts at one (in some languages it starts at zero) and the simplest way to index is to provide the index number or numbers for the elements that you want. So `z[1]` selects the first element in the vector `z`, which is 3.

```
> z
[1]  3  5 NA  8
>
> z[1]               # first element
[1] 3
>
> z[c(1, 4)]         # first and last element
[1] 3 8
```

A range of items can be selected using the sequence operator (`:`), which returns integers in increments of one using the following syntax: `from:to`. Thus, to get the numbers from 3 to 9 we use

```
> 3:9                # all integers from 3 to 9
[1] 3 4 5 6 7 8 9
```

The sequence operator can be used with brackets to select a range of elements.

```
> z[1:3]             # first three items (range)
[1]  3  5 NA
```

Any function or operation that returns a number can be used to subset. For example, the last element of `z` can be selected by using `length()` to count the number of elements in `z`, which is 4.

```
> z[length(z)]       # last item
[1] 8
```

Negative index numbers *exclude* items, so if we wanted to remove the third item use

```
> z[-3]              # all but the third item
[1] 3 5 8
```

In the example below the `is.na()` function tests whether each item in `z` is a missing value. It returns a vector of `TRUE` and `FALSE` values with the same length as `z`. `TRUE` and

FALSE values can also be used to filter or subset results. TRUE values are selected and FALSE values are excluded.

```
> # is the item missing?
> is.na(z)
[1] FALSE FALSE  TRUE FALSE
>
> # is the item NOT missing? = is the item present?
> !is.na(z)
[1]  TRUE  TRUE FALSE  TRUE
>
> z[!is.na(z)]     # exclude NAs
[1] 3 5 8
```

Similarly, any conditional expression that returns TRUE and FALSE values can be used for subsetting. For example, if we wanted only the items of z that are greater than four use

```
> z[z > 4]
[1]  5 NA  8
```

Matrices and data frames have two dimensions and all of the above methods can be used but there are now two indices, one for the rows and one for the columns. In R the format is always [row.index, column.index]. If an index is not provided for one dimension, R assumes that all elements should be retained. Several ways of subsetting the festing data frame are shown below.

```
> festing[1, 2]  # item in first row, second column
[1] Control
Levels: Control DS
>
> festing[3, ]   # all of third row
  strain treatment batch value fac.batch
3    NIH        DS     1   614         1
>
> festing[, 4]   # all of fourth column
 [1]  444  764  614  831  423  586  625  782  408  609  856 1002  447  606
[15]  719  766
>
> festing[1:4, c(1,3)] # rows 1-4, column 1 and 3
  strain batch
1    NIH     1
2    NIH     2
```

```
3    NIH    1
4    NIH    2
```

Columns from data frames can be selected with the extraction operator ($), and also by using brackets and providing the name of the column in quotes. The code below shows both ways of extracting the `strain` column. The extraction operator does not work for matrices and the brackets must be used.

```
> festing$strain
 [1] NIH      NIH      NIH      NIH      BALB/c   BALB/c   BALB/c   BALB/c
 [9] A/J      A/J      A/J      A/J      129/Ola  129/Ola  129/Ola  129/Ola
Levels: 129/Ola A/J BALB/c NIH
>
> festing[, "strain"]
 [1] NIH      NIH      NIH      NIH      BALB/c   BALB/c   BALB/c   BALB/c
 [9] A/J      A/J      A/J      A/J      129/Ola  129/Ola  129/Ola  129/Ola
Levels: 129/Ola A/J BALB/c NIH
```

With large data frames, often a subset of rows and columns that meet specific criteria need to be extracted for an analysis. The methods above can be used but providing an index of numbers has two drawbacks. First, if the data changes – for example, if the rows have been sorted – then the indexing may be incorrect. Second, numbers provide no information about what is selected. The methods below make the selection criteria more apparent. The first method tests whether the mouse strain is NIH using the double equals sign (==). If strain equals 'NIH' then a value of `TRUE` is returned, otherwise a value of `FALSE`. In the first line of code below brackets are used like the earlier examples to perform the subsetting. The second method uses the `subset()` function. The `subset` argument in the `subset()` function selects rows and the `select` argument selects columns. In the last line of code below the variable `batch` is removed using a minus sign.

```
> # select only NIH mice
> festing[festing$strain=="NIH", ]
  strain treatment batch value fac.batch
1    NIH   Control     1   444         1
2    NIH   Control     2   764         2
3    NIH        DS     1   614         1
4    NIH        DS     2   831         2
>
> # alternate method
> subset(festing, subset=strain=="NIH")
  strain treatment batch value fac.batch
1    NIH   Control     1   444         1
```

```
2     NIH   Control     2   764          2
3     NIH        DS     1   614          1
4     NIH        DS     2   831          2
>
> # also exclude the column "batch"
> subset(festing, subset=strain=="NIH", select=-batch)
  strain treatment value fac.batch
1     NIH   Control   444          1
2     NIH   Control   764          2
3     NIH        DS   614          1
4     NIH        DS   831          2
```

A.11 Looping and applying

In many programming languages, if you want to apply a function or calculation to all elements in a vector or matrix you have to explicitly loop over each element and perform the calculation. The variable `z` was created previously and is shown again below. Suppose that we want to multiply each element of `z` by two. First, we create a variable called `z.new` to store the results of our calculations. `z.new` is a vector of `NA` values that is as long as `z`. The `rep()` function replicates the first argument as many times as indicated in the second argument. Creating a variable to store results is called *preallocation* and is computationally efficient because R allocates memory once for the variable `z.new` when it is created, and then writes the output to the allocated position. If `z.new` is created with only one element it needs to be allocated more memory each time a new number is added to the vector, which is inefficient.

```
> z
[1]  3  5 NA  8
>
> # preallocate vector
> z.new <- rep(NA, length(z))
>
> z.new
[1] NA NA NA NA
>
> # This is inefficient computationally
> # z.new <- NA
```

In the code below a `for()` loop iterates through the numbers 1 to 4 (the number of elements in `z` calculated with `length()`). The letter `i` is used as an index but any letter or word can be substituted; i is just a convention. For the first iteration i equals 1. So the first line of code within the loop takes the first element of z, multiplies it by 2, and stores it as the first element of z.new. Note the use of the square brackets to subset z and z.new. The last line of code in the loop prints the iteration number followed by z and z.new to illustrate how the loop works but is unnecessary when using a loop. The final line of code then prints z.new.

```
> for (i in 1:length(z) ){
+      # multiply by two and save in z.new
+      z.new[i] <- z[i] * 2
+
+      # print iteration number
+      print(c("i"=i, "z"=z[i], "z.new"=z.new[i]))
+      }
     i      z z.new
     1      3     6
     i      z z.new
     2      5    10
     i      z z.new
     3     NA    NA
     i      z z.new
     4      8    16
>
> z.new
[1]  6 10 NA 16
```

There is an even faster way to multiply all elements of a vector by a number – just multiply the vector by the number as in the code below. The looping method above was only used to show how to use a for() loop but should be avoided as it requires more code and is computationally less efficient. Section 5.2.4 (p. 211) uses a more realistic example of a for() loop.

```
> z * 2
[1]  6 10 NA 16
```

In general, looping in R is slow, even when using preallocation. Fortunately, R has a family of apply functions that are both more efficient and require less code. They include apply(), lapply(), sapply(), and tapply().[10] To show how these methods are used we first create a matrix using cbind() to bind z and z.new and call it z.all. If we want

[10] Visser *et al.* discuss methods for speeding up computations in R [381].

to perform an operation on all elements of the matrix, say adding one to all the elements, then this can be done as before by adding one to the matrix.

```
> # combined into matrix
> z.all <- cbind(z, z.new)
>
> z.all
      z z.new
[1,]  3     6
[2,]  5    10
[3,] NA    NA
[4,]  8    16
>
> # add one to all elements
> z.all + 1
      z z.new
[1,]  4     7
[2,]  6    11
[3,] NA    NA
[4,]  9    17
```

Sometimes however we want to apply a function by row or column and below we show how to do this with apply(). The apply() function takes three arguments: a matrix or data frame, a number indicating whether the function should be applied across rows (1) or across columns (2), and the function to be applied. The example below shows how to calculate the sum of values across rows and how to find the maximum value in each column.

```
> # sum the values across rows
> apply(z.all, 1, sum)
[1]  9 15 NA 24
>
> # calculate the max value in each column
> apply(z.all, 2, max, na.rm=TRUE)
    z z.new
    8    16
```

sum() and max() are built-in functions but we can use functions that we have defined (Section A.9, p. 355). Also note that R has built-in functions for common calculations such as rowMeans(), colMeans(), rowSums(), and colSums().

The tapply() function applies a function to groups or subsets of a variable and is therefore useful for calculating summary statistics for experimental groups. tapply() takes three arguments: the first is the variable on which the calculation will be performed, the second is the grouping variable, and the third is the function to be applied. Thus, in the first line of code below the mean of the variable `value` is calculated for each treatment group. Multiple grouping variables can be entered by providing them as a list and is shown in the second line of code. The `with()` function passes the `festing` data to `tapply()`.

```
> # calculate mean for each treatment group
> with(festing, tapply(value, treatment, mean))
Control      DS
535.875 774.375
>
> # calculate SD for each treatment group by strain
> with(festing, tapply(value, list(strain, treatment), sd))
         Control      DS
129/Ola  112.430  33.234
A/J      142.128 103.238
BALB/c   115.258 111.016
NIH      226.274 153.442
```

A.12 Graphing data

R comes installed with two graphics systems: traditional (based on the `graphics` package) and grid (based on the `grid` package) [288]. High-level graphing functions will use one of these two systems to produce a plot and the distinction is mostly important when setting graphing options and when adding further information to a plot – you need to know which of the two systems produced the graph. Whole graphing packages have been developed that are based on one of these systems. For example, two packages used in this book are `sciplot`, based on traditional graphics, and `lattice`, based on `grid`. Many user contributed packages also have graphing functions and they will use one of these two systems.

Traditional graphics

Most graphing functions – both traditional and `grid` – use the formula method to specify the variables on the x- and y-axes using the following format

```
> y.var ~ x.var
```

where the variable to be plotted on the y-axis is to the left of the tilde (~) and the variable on the x-axis is on the right. For the `festing` data, we can plot the outcome by the treatment

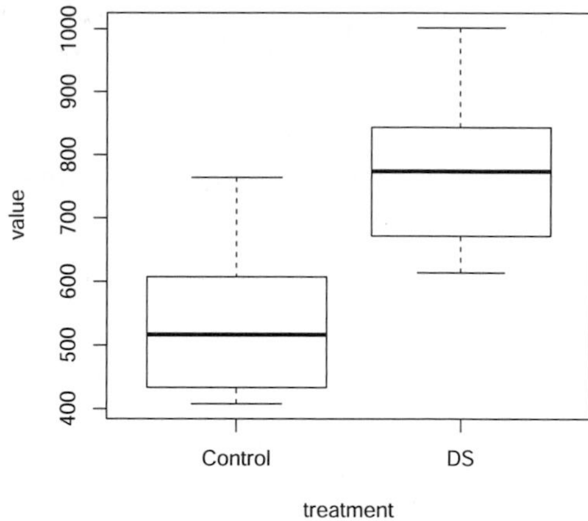

Fig. A.1 A basic traditional plot.

group with the following code (Figure A.1). Plotting functions will open a new window unless one is already open, and this window is called a *device*. A boxplot is generated because `treatment` is a factor, and if it was a numeric variable the individual points would have been plotted.

```
> plot(value ~ treatment, data=festing)
```

The graph can be improved and there are many options that can be changed. Some options are specific to the plotting function and some are general graphical parameters. To list all the graphical parameters and the default settings type `par()`. A long list will be generated and it is unclear what most options do, but they are described in the documentation (type `help(par)`).[11] The three most common options used in this book are `las`, which controls the orientation of the axis labels, `mfrow`, which controls the number of graphs on a page, and `mar`, which controls the amount of white space around a graph (the margin).

In Figure A.2A, we show an improved version of the graph. Setting `las=1` in the `par()` function changes the y-axis numbers to be parallel to the x-axis, making them easier to read. The range of the y-axis is set to 0 and 1100 with `ylim`, a title is added with `main`, a more informative y-axis label is added with `ylab`, and the x-axis label is suppressed by setting `xlab` to an empty string (nothing between the quotation marks). The boxes are shaded to make them stand out and their width is decreased using `boxwex`. Finally, a horizontal line (assume it is the limit of detection) at 100 is added to the plot with the `abline()` function and `lty` (line type) is set to 2, which makes a dashed line.

[11] Also see Paul Murrell's website associated with the *R Graphics* book [288] (`https://www.stat.auckland.ac.nz/~paul/RGraphics/rgraphics.html`).

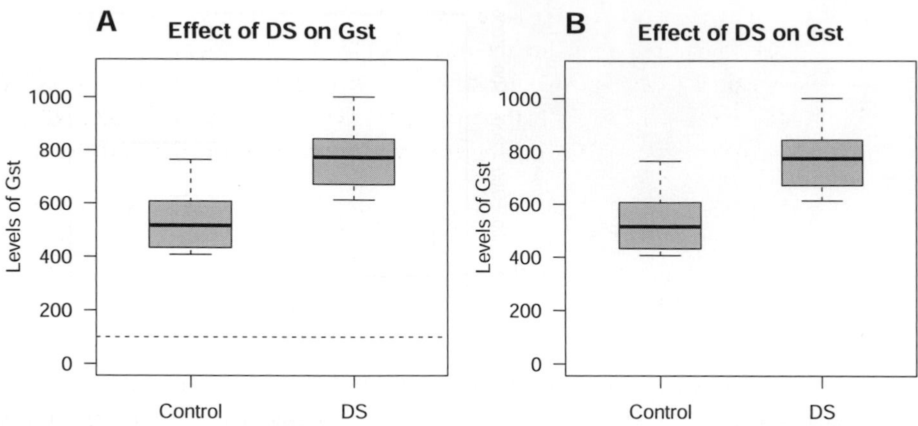

Fig. A.2 An improved graph by changing the global graphical parameters with `par()` and the local plotting options (A). The same plot generated in a different way (B).

```
> par(mfrow=c(1,2),                # plot two graphs in a 1 by 2 grid
+     mar=c(4,4,2.5,1),            # decrease the margin size
+     las=1)                       # rotate y-axis text; default is las=0
>
> plot(value ~ treatment, data=festing, ylim=c(0, 1100),
+      ylab="Levels of Gst", xlab="", col="darkgrey",
+      main="Effect of DS on Gst", boxwex=0.5)
> abline(h=100, lty=2)
> mtext("A", side=3, line=1, font=2, cex=1.5, adj=0)
>
> # alternate way of passing data and specifying variables
> with(festing, {
+          plot(x=treatment, y=value, ylim=c(0, 1100),
+               ylab="Levels of Gst", xlab="", col="darkgrey",
+               main="Effect of DS on Gst", boxwex=0.5)
+ })
> mtext("B", side=3, line=1, font=2, cex=1.5, adj=0)
```

Figure A.2B shows an alternative way to generate the same graph. First, some graphing functions do not have a `data` argument and so it is not possible to pass them data. The solution is to use the `with()` function, followed by the data frame, a comma, and then the plotting commands. Second, some functions cannot use the formula method for specifying variables and they need to be explicitly defined with the `x` and `y` arguments. Some plotting functions, like above, can use both methods. The code also shows how to use the `mtext()` function to add panel labels.

There are two ways to save graphs. The first is to make one or more plots like above, then save them to a file using the dev.copy2pdf() function. Recall that the plotting window is called a device, and therefore the function copies (i.e. saves) everything in the graph (device) to a PDF file. In the code below the file is called 'nice_plot.pdf'. Next, dev.off() closes the device. Without this last step the save is incomplete and the file cannot be viewed.

```
> plot(...)
> dev.copy2pdf("nice_plot.pdf")
> dev.off()
```

The second method is to first open a file of the desired type, write the graph to the file, and then close the device. The code below opens a PDF file and the functions png(), tiff(), jpeg(), and svg() work in the same way. Since the plot is saved directly to the file it cannot be viewed on the screen. The pdf() and other functions have several options that control the output and the code below shows how to set the height and width of the figure (the default units are inches).

```
> pdf("nice_plot.pdf", height=5, width=5)
> plot(...)
> dev.off()
```

Chapter 6 on Exploratory Data Analysis shows many graphs and some of the main plotting functions in the graphics package are the following:

```
> plot()
> boxplot()
> barplot()
> pairs()
> interaction.plot()
> plot.design()
> dotchart()
> contour()
> coplot()
```

Grid graphics

You rarely need to interact with the grid graphics system directly and will use a package that is built on top of it. This book uses the lattice package [343] but ggplot2 is a popular alternative [395].

The plotting functions in the lattice package are very flexible, and flexibility usually comes with greater complexity. Most functions from the lattice package use the

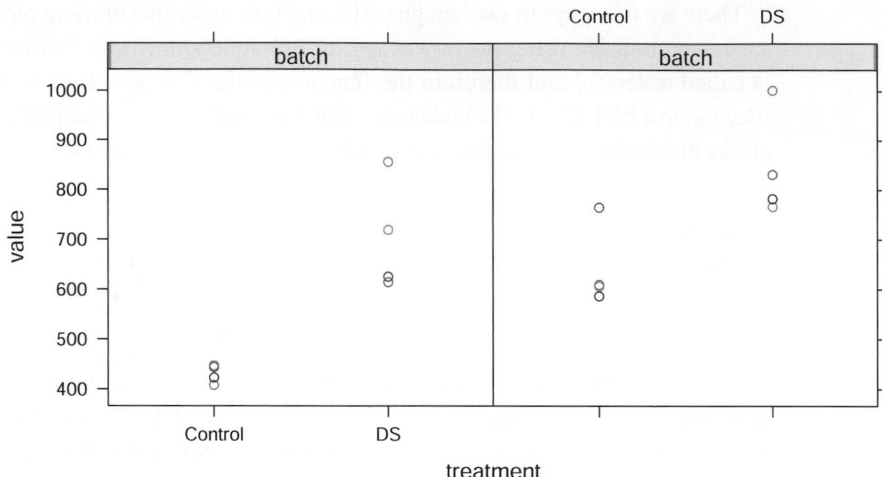

Fig. A.3 A basic plot using the `xyplot()` function from the `lattice` package.

formula method and the code below uses the `xyplot()` function to plot the `festing` data (Figure A.3). The outcome `value` and `treatment` are specified as before and there are two new features compared with the `plot()` function. After `treatment` there is a vertical bar (`|`) and the variable `batch`. The vertical bar is the conditioning operator and it indicates that the data should be plotted in a separate panel for each batch. The `groups` argument indicates that the data points should be distinguished by strain, and by default different colours are used, so the groups are not visible in Figure A.3.

```
> library(lattice)
>
> xyplot(value ~ treatment|batch, data=festing,
+        groups=strain)
```

Once again this basic graph can be improved in many ways by changing the global graphical parameters and the options for `xyplot()`. To view the global parameters use `trellis.par.get()`, which returns an even longer and harder to understand list than the list produced by `par()`. The book by Sarkar, the author of the `lattice` package, is the best place to start understanding what all of the options do, as well as the features not covered here [343].

In the code below the `trellis.par.set()` function sets three global parameters. The first is `superpose.symbol`, which controls the plotting symbols. They are all set to black and `pch` indicates the type of symbol, which is indicated with a number. The second is `superpose.line` which controls the lines. They are also set to black and `lty` controls the line type. These modifications make the strains distinguishable by symbol and line type instead of colour. Finally, `axis.components` controls the tick marks around the edge of the panels. Figure A.3 has ticks on the top and right edge of the panels and they are

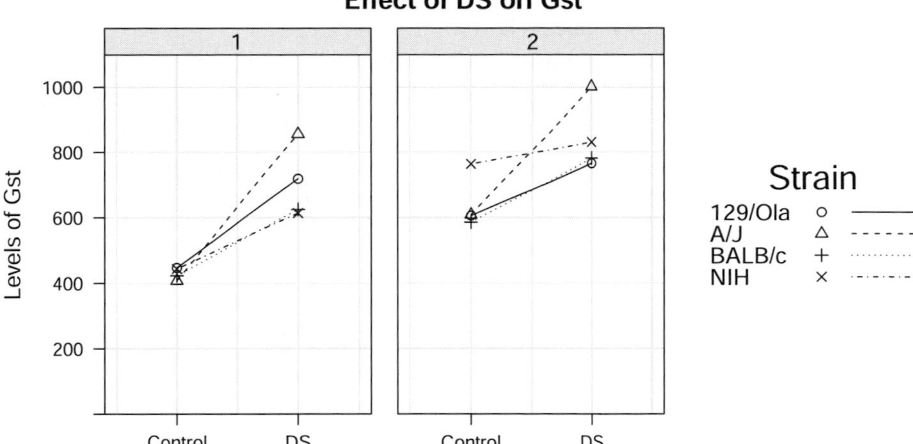

Fig. A.4 An improved graph by changing the global graphical parameters with `trellis.par.set()` and the local plotting options.

suppressed in Figure A.4 by setting `right=list(tck=0)` and `top=list(tck=0)`. This is just an aesthetic alteration that is used occasionally in the book but the code may not be shown to save space.

```
> trellis.par.set(superpose.symbol=list(col="black", pch=1:4),
+                 superpose.line=list(col="black", lty=1:4),
+                 axis.components=list(right=list(tck=0),
+                                      top=list(tck=0)))
>
> xyplot(value ~ treatment|factor(batch), data=festing,
+        groups=strain, type=c("g","p","l"), ylim=c(0, 1100),
+        xlab="", ylab="Levels of Gst", main="Effect of DS on Gst",
+        scales=list(alternating=FALSE), between=list(x=1),
+        auto.key=list(columns=1, lines=TRUE,
+            title="Strain", space="right"))
```

Another problem with Figure A.3 is that both panels are called 'batch', because in the `festing` data batch is a numeric variable. The panels are distinguished with a small strip of colour that cannot be seen, and so the code for Figure A.4 makes batch a factor with the `factor()` function. Now the factor labels are printed at the top of each panel (Figure A.4).

The `type` argument indicates that (1) a faint grid ("g") of lines should be drawn (which may be hard to see in print), (2) points should be drawn ("p"), and (3) lines should be drawn ("l"). The `scales` argument indicates that the axis ticks and numbers should not alternate (they are always on the left and bottom of a panel). The `between` argument indicates that a one unit gap should be introduced on the x-axis, which creates the space between the two panels. Finally, the `auto.key` argument provides all the information to create the legend on the right of Figure A.4.

Using `trellis.par.set()` before each graph generates a lot of code and clutter and it is often better to specify these details once and then use them where needed. The code below saves all of the graphical details as a list in an object called `par.set`. Then any function can use them with the `par.settings` argument. This is especially useful if you want all graphs in a paper or thesis to have the same theme; the options need only be specified once.

```
> par.set <- list(superpose.symbol=list(col="black", pch=1:4),
+                 superpose.line=list(col="black", lty=1:4),
+                 axis.components=list(right=list(tck=0),
+                                      top=list(tck=0)))
>
> xyplot(..., par.settings=par.set)
```

There is only one difference from traditional graphics when you want to save the output to a file: the plotting function must be wrapped with `print()`. Think of it as *printing* the plot to the file, and then closing the file with `dev.off()`. This step is easy to forget and results in blank files.

```
> pdf("nice_plot.pdf")
> print(
+     xyplot(...)
+ )
> dev.off()
```

Chapter 6 on Exploratory Data Analysis shows other graphs and some of the main plotting functions in the `lattice` package are the following:

```
> xyplot()
> dotplot()
> barchart()
> levelplot()
> splom()
> contourplot()
> densityplot()
> qqmath()
> wireframe()
```

Table A.4 Common distributions in R.

R function	Distribution
beta	Beta
binom	Binomial
chisq	Chi-squared
f	*F*
lnorm	Log-normal
nbinom	Negative binomial
norm	Normal (Gaussian)
pois	Poisson
t	Student's *t*
unif	Uniform

A.13 Distributions

There are many distributions available in R and the most common ones are listed in Table A.4. There are four functions associated with each of these distributions which have a single letter prefix added to the distribution name. For example, the prefix `r` generates random values from the named distribution, and so `rnorm()` generates random numbers from a normal distribution. The code below generates five random values from a normal distribution with a mean of 10 and a standard deviation of two and Figure A.5A shows 100 samples generated from this distribution. Random number generation is useful for power analyses and sample size calculations (Section 5.2.5, p. 212). The random numbers are not truly random but pseudo-random; given an initial seed number they are generated by a deterministic algorithm but serve well enough to be used as random. Unless specified, the seed is taken from the computer's clock. To make your results reproducible (and to match the results in this book) it is a good idea to set the seed for the random number generator using `set.seed()`.

```
> set.seed(1)
> rnorm(n=5, mean=10, sd=2)
[1]  8.74709 10.36729  8.32874 13.19056 10.65902
```

The second function associated with distributions calculates areas under the curve (AUC), which are *p*-values, and has the prefix `p`. It can be used to answer questions such as what is the probability of obtaining a value less than 12 from a normal distribution with a mean of 10 and a standard deviation of two?[12] Figure A.5B shows a normal distribution

[12] These questions are standard in introductory statistics classes, usually phrased as 'What is the probability that a randomly selected person will be greater than 180 cm tall if sampled from a population with a mean of 165 cm and a standard deviation of 15 cm?'

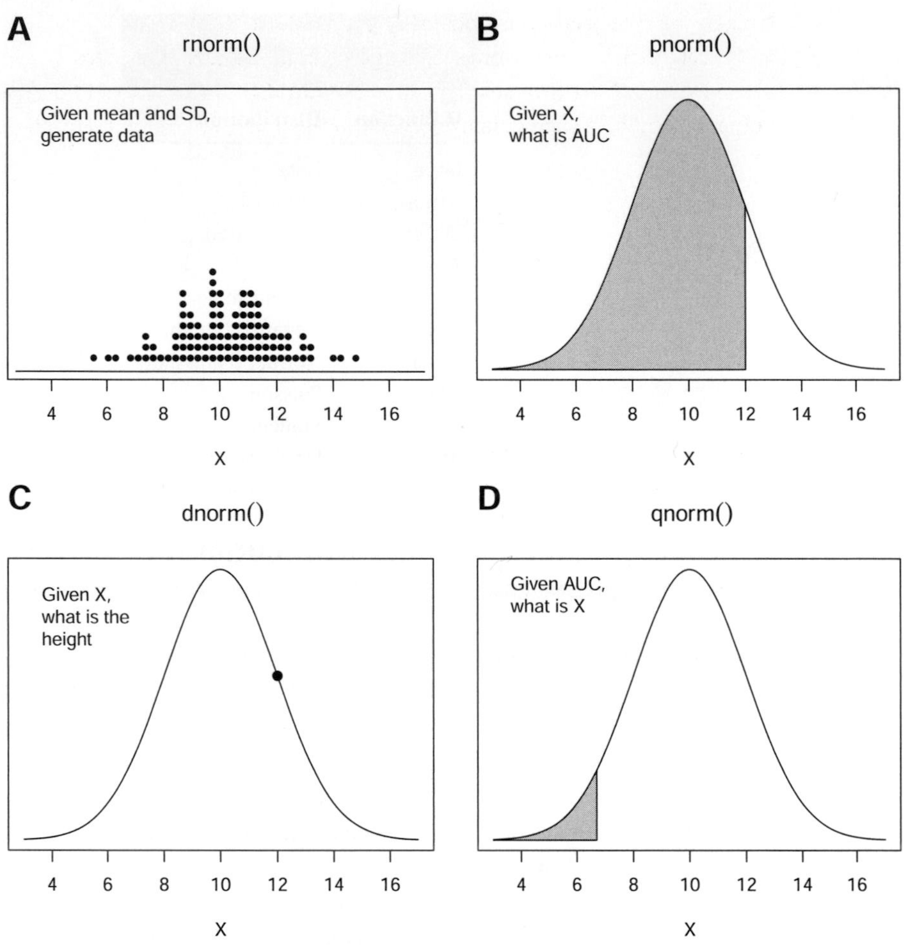

Fig. A.5 Functions associated with distributions in R. All four normal distributions have a mean of 10 and a SD of 2. `rnorm()` generates random data (A) and the other functions answer different but related questions. `pnorm()` is the distribution function (B), `dnorm()` is the density function (C), and `qnorm()` is the quantile function (D).

with a mean = 10 and SD = 2, and the code below shows how to use `pnorm()` to calculate the grey part of the curve (below 12). The default for `pnorm()` is to calculate the area under the curve *to the left of your specified value*. The default setting therefore provides the correct answer because the shaded region is to the left of 12. The code below shows that the shaded regions is approximately 84%.

```
> pnorm(12, mean=10, sd=2) # from -Inf to 12
[1] 0.841345
```

Suppose, however, that the question asked for the area under the curve *above* 12. This can be calculated in two ways. First, since the total area under the curve in Figure A.5B equals one (the area of a probability distribution always equals one), we can subtract the value calculated above from one to get the area under the curve to the right of 12. The second method is to specify `lower.tail=FALSE` in the `pnorm()` function (it is `TRUE` by default), which then calculates the area in the upper tail. Both methods are shown below.

```
> 1 - pnorm(12, mean=10, sd=2) # total area equals 1
[1] 0.158655
>
> pnorm(12, mean=10, sd=2, lower.tail=FALSE) # from 12 to Inf
[1] 0.158655
```

The distribution functions starting with p are not only for answering elementary homework problems but can also check reported p-values in publications. Suppose we read in a paper that there was a significant difference between groups using a two-tailed independent samples t-test and the results reported as ($t_{(10)} = 2.1, p < 0.05$). Since there is a one-to-one mapping between a t-statistic and df (indicated in the subscript) and a p-value, the reported information enables us to check the results. The code below uses the `pt()` function which is for the t-distribution. If there was no difference between the means of the groups then the t-statistic would equal zero. Since the value is positive in this example, we need to calculate the area under the curve to the right of 2.1 and therefore specify `lower.tail=FALSE` (if the t-statistic was negative, then we would calculate the AUC to the left of -2.1 and the default `lower.tail=FALSE` would be appropriate). The value of the t-statistic (2.1) and df (10) are also entered and everything is multiplied by two because it is a two-tailed test.

```
> pt(2.1, df=10, lower.tail=FALSE) * 2
[1] 0.0620772
```

The calculated p-value is not less than 0.05 as indicated in the above statement. But before we accuse the authors of fudging the numbers, consider that the t-statistic may have been rounded to one decimal and the unrounded value was slightly higher. The code below checks this assumption by using a value of 2.149999 for the t-statistic. If it was higher, then it would have been rounded to 2.2 instead of 2.1. The calculated p-value is still above 0.05 and is inconsistent with their reported results.

```
> pt(2.149999, df=10, lower.tail=FALSE) * 2
[1] 0.0570646
```

Suppose instead that the authors used a one-tailed test instead of a two-tailed test (despite stating that a two-tailed test was used). The calculation is below and the corresponding p-value is now below 0.05.

Table A.5 Common statistical models in R. `fac` = categorical predictor, `x` = continuous predictor, and `block` = categorical blocking variable.

Model	Notes
`y ~ 1`	Overall mean (intercept only)
`y ~ fac`	One factor with two or more levels (one-way ANOVA)
`y ~ fac1 + fac2`	Two crossed factors with no interaction effect (two-way ANOVA)
`y ~ fac1 * fac2`	Two crossed treatments with interaction effect (two-way ANOVA)
`y ~ fac + block`	One factor with blocking and either no or true replication
`y ~ fac + Error(subject)`	One factor with pseudoreplication and subject as a fixed factor (multiple observations per subject)
`y ~ fac + random=~1|subject`	One factor with pseudoreplication and subject as a random factor (`lme` notation)
`y ~ fac1 + fac2 + Error(subject)`	Split-unit design. Use unique identifiers to indicate nesting structure (see Section 4.3.4, p. 157)
`y ~ x`	One continuous predictor (regression)
`y ~ x1 + x2`	Two continuous predictors (multiple regression)
`y ~ x + fac`	One continuous and one categorical predictor (ANCOVA)
`y ~ x + I(x^2)`	Quadratic effect for x

```
> pt(2.1, df=10, lower.tail=FALSE)
[1] 0.0310386
```

The reason for the discrepancy is unclear and it could be the result of a rounding error, transcription error, incorrectly stating the type of test used (one- versus two-tailed), or fraudulent behaviour. Several studies have used this approach to examine the congruence between p-values and reported statistics in publications and the mismatch is approximately 10% [18, 37, 125, 198]. When peer-reviewing a paper it might be useful to check the reported results and the `pf()` and `pchisq()` functions can check ANOVA and chi-square results, respectively. Multiplication by two is unnecessary since both F and chi-square statistics are one-tailed.

The third function associated with distributions uses `d` as a prefix and calculates the height of the distribution for a given value (Figure A.5C). The final function uses `q` as a prefix and calculates the value of the variable given an area under the curve (Figure A.5D). As neither are used in the book they are not discussed further.

A.14 Fitting models

Whole books are devoted to fitting models in R and here we only cover one function, `aov()`, which stands for Analysis Of Variance. Despite the name, it can also be used for t-tests, analysis of covariance, and multiple regression. A related function is `lm()`, which stands for Linear Model, and the two functions are largely interchangeable. The main difference is that `aov()` has an extra `Error()` argument. The output is presented differently for `aov()` and `lm()`, but using `summary.lm()` on an `aov` model will give `lm`-like output and using `summary.aov()` on a `lm` model will give `aov`-like output, so it usually does not matter which function is used.

All models in R use the formula method for specifying the outcome (y) and predictor variables (x). Table A.5 lists several common models. The `festing` data set from the `labstats` package is used for illustration and the first few lines of the data frame are shown below. `value` is the outcome variable and is placed to the left of the tilde ($\sim$) and `treatment` is the only predictor variable for the first model. `data=festing` indicates the data frame where the outcome and predictor variables are located and the results are saved to an object called `mod1`. Summarising the model with `summary()` displays an ANOVA table and the sole p-value in the output is for the effect of treatment ($p = 0.002$). Interpreting ANOVA tables is described in Section 4.1 (p. 124).

```
> # first few lines of the data
> head(festing)
  strain treatment batch value fac.batch
1    NIH   Control     1   444         1
2    NIH   Control     2   764         2
3    NIH        DS     1   614         1
4    NIH        DS     2   831         2
5 BALB/c   Control     1   423         1
6 BALB/c   Control     2   586         2
>
> # fit model with one predictor variable
> mod1 <- aov(value ~ treatment, data=festing)
>
> summary(mod1)
            Df Sum Sq Mean Sq F value Pr(>F)
treatment    1 227529  227529    14.3  0.002
Residuals   14 223161   15940
```

After a model is fitted to the data, the suitability of the model needs to be established before we interpret the results. Diagnostic graphs are a good way to determine the suitability of a model and are easily generated by using `plot()`. Figure A.6 shows the diagnostic

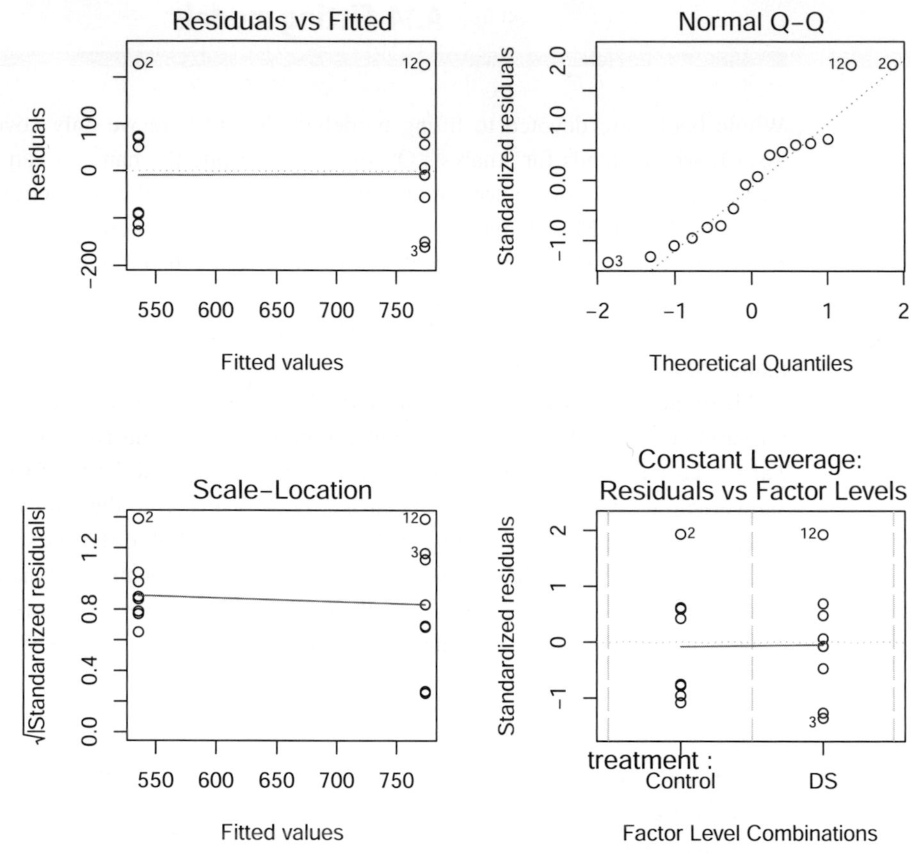

Fig. A.6 Diagnostic plots. These graphs help with assessing the normality and homogeneity of variance assumptions by looking at the model residuals.

graphs for `mod1`. By default four graphs are created and therefore we first use the `mfrow` option to arrange the graphs in a two-by-two grid.

```
> par(mfrow=c(2,2))
> plot(mod1)
```

The top left graph of Figure A.6 (Residuals vs Fitted) plots the residuals on the y-axis, which represent the variation in the outcome that is 'left over' after taking into account predictor variables. With this data set, the residuals are the distances of each point from their respective group means and they have the same units as the measured outcome variable. Residuals are discussed in Section 4.1.1 (p. 124) and are the vertical lines in Figure 4.1C (p. 125). The x-axis plots the fitted or predicted values, which are the model's best estimate for each sample. For models with only categorical predictors, the fitted values are the group means, and this explains why the points are either at approximately 540 or 775. If the predictor was continuous then the points would be scattered along the x-axis (see Figure 4.23, p. 190 for an example). Thus, this graph plots what the model predicts and what it has failed to predict, and there should be no relationships or patterns present. A common pattern is points that are more spread out in the vertical direction when going from left to right, giving a fan or wedge shape with the wide end on the right. Such a pattern indicates that the variance is increasing with the mean and thus violates the homogeneity of variance assumption. In Figure A.6, the points have a similar spread for both groups, indicating that the variances are similar. With such a simple design we can assess the variances by plotting the raw data. But residuals versus fitted plots become more useful with more complex designs, especially when they include continuous predictors.

The bottom left graph (Scale–Location) plot resembles the previous one except the residuals are first standardised to have a standard deviation of one, then the absolute value is taken (minus signs are removed so all values are positive), and finally the square root is calculated. Despite these extra calculations the graph tells the same story, but instead of looking for a wedge pattern we can look at the slope of the line. If the variance is greater at larger fitted values the line will slope upwards to the right. In this case it is flat, confirming our previous conclusion that the variances are equal between groups.

The top right graph (Normal Q–Q) plots the standardised residuals on the y-axis and the theoretical values for the residuals if they were from a normal distribution on the x-axis. This graph is useful for checking that the residuals are normally distributed – another assumption of linear models. Section 6.3.1 (p. 307) discusses how to interpret Q–Q plots for the assumption of normality.

The final graph on the bottom right is useful for understanding if any samples are influential or have undue weight. Influential observations are less likely in designs with only categorical variables because the values of the predictors are restricted to a few values, and therefore this graph is not very informative. An example of an influential observation is the point on the far right in Figure 6.1D (p. 273).

The code below shows how to include multiple crossed predictor variables in a model.[13] The predictors are included on the right side of the tilde and can be separated by either a plus (+) sign or asterisk (∗). A plus sign indicates that the main but not the interaction effects should be included in the model, and the output from mod2 includes the results for the main effects of strain and treatment.

```
> # main effects only
> mod2 <- aov(value ~ strain + treatment, data=festing)
> summary(mod2)
            Df Sum Sq Mean Sq F value Pr(>F)
strain       3  28613    9538    0.54 0.6651
treatment    1 227529  227529   12.86 0.0043
Residuals   11 194548   17686
```

An asterisk indicates that the interaction effect between the two variables should also be included in the model and is shown in the code below. An alternative way of including an

[13] See Section 2.7 (p. 66) for the difference between crossed and nested factors.

interaction is to use plus signs and then include the interaction effect as an additional term in the model, where the two variables that interact are joined by a colon.

```
> # main and interaction effects
> mod3 <- aov(value ~ strain * treatment, data=festing)
>
> # alternative specification
> mod3b <- aov(value ~ strain + treatment + strain:treatment,
+              data=festing)
>
> summary(mod3)
                 Df Sum Sq Mean Sq F value Pr(>F)
strain            3  28613    9538    0.53 0.6764
treatment         1 227529  227529   12.56 0.0076
strain:treatment  3  49590   16530    0.91 0.4771
Residuals         8 144957   18120
```

The code below includes batch as a third variable and the model has a main effect of batch, strain, and treatment, and the strain by treatment interaction. The `festing` data have the same number of observations in each group, but this will often not be the case. With unbalanced data the order that the variables are entered in the model matters – a different ordering will give different results. This is discussed in Section 4.1.1 (p. 128). The code below also shows how to use the `Anova` function from the `car` package. The results are identical to those produced by `summary()`, but this will not be the case for unbalanced data.

```
> mod4 <- aov(value ~ batch + strain * treatment, data=festing)
> summary(mod4)
                 Df Sum Sq Mean Sq F value  Pr(>F)
batch             1 124256  124256   42.02 0.00034
strain            3  28613    9538    3.23 0.09144
treatment         1 227529  227529   76.94   5e-05
strain:treatment  3  49591   16530    5.59 0.02832
Residuals         7  20701    2957
>
> # hierarchical sum of squares
> car::Anova(mod4)
Anova Table (Type II tests)

Response: value
                 Sum Sq Df F value   Pr(>F)
batch            124256  1  42.017  0.00034
strain            28613  3   3.225  0.09144
```

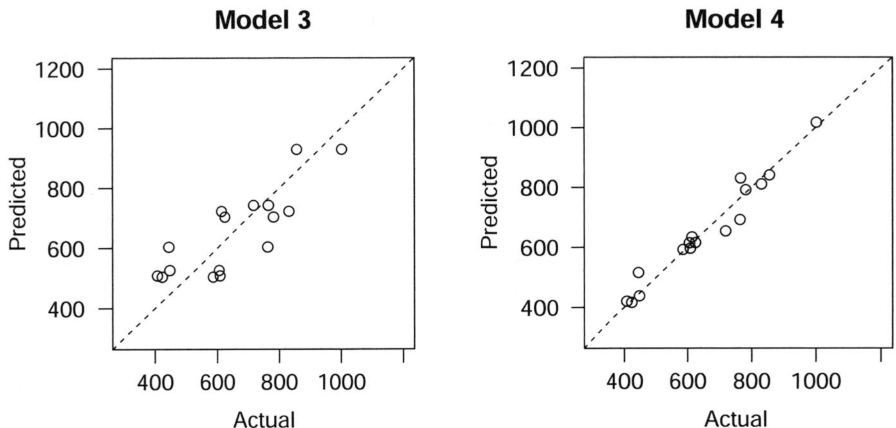

Fig. A.7 Prediction plot. The actual data values (*x*-axis) are plotted against the values predicted from the model (*y*-axis) for two different models. Note how the predictions are better (closer to the diagonal line) when batch is included as a variable in the model (right graph).

```
treatment            227529  1  76.939 5.04e-05
strain:treatment      49591  3   5.590  0.02832
Residuals             20701  7
```

Figure A.7 shows a final diagnostic plot that allows you to assess if the model predicts the data well. It plots the values of the measured outcome on the x-axis and the predicted values on the y-axis. If the model predicts the data perfectly the points will fall on the diagonal line. The predicted values are the same as the fitted values in Figure A.6 and can be calculated from a model using either the `predict()` or `fitted()`. The difference between the two functions is that `fitted()` extracts the values from the model while `predict()` uses the observed values of the predictor to predict the outcome. The advantage of `predict()` is that it can predict the outcome for new values of the predictor. For example, if the model has a continuous predictor variable then `predict()` can extrapolate or interpolate values for the outcome. Predict can also calculate confidence and prediction intervals (see the help menu for details).

```
> # calculated predicted values for mod3 and mod4
> pred.mod3 <- predict(mod3)      # same as fitted(mod3)
> pred.mod4 <- predict(mod4)      # same as fitted(mod4)
>
> par(mfrow=c(1,2),
+     las=1)
>
> plot(pred.mod3 ~ festing$value, ylab="Predicted", xlab="Actual",
+       xlim=c(300, 1200), ylim=c(300, 1200), main="Model 3")
> abline(0, 1, lty=2)
```

```
>
> plot(pred.mod4 ~ festing$value, ylab="Predicted", xlab="Actual",
+       xlim=c(300, 1200), ylim=c(300, 1200), main="Model 4")
> abline(0, 1, lty=2)
```

Figure A.7 plots actual versus predicted values for two models. Model 3 (`mod3`) was simpler and did not include batch, whereas Model 4 (`mod4`) did. The points are more tightly clustered around the diagonal line for Model 4, indicating a better fit. These graphs can also be used to check that predictions are equally good for all values. For example, most of the points may be equally scattered on either side of the diagonal line but at higher values the points may all be below the line. This indicates that the model (the diagonal line) over-predicts the actual values. This may be a problem if accuracy for higher values is more important than for low values and indicates that the model needs to be improved.

Appendix B Glossary

Page references indicate where the entry is discussed in greater detail and words in bold indicate terms defined elsewhere in the glossary.

Aliased effects Occur when some main or interaction effects cannot be estimated because they are **confounded**. Aliasing is done on purpose to simplify the design of the experiment. [p. 91]

Alpha (α) See **Critical value**.

Alternative hypothesis (H_1) Is the hypothesis that an association between variables is present or that an effect exists. It can be a general statement that the **null hypothesis** is not true, or it can be more specific and state the direction of the association or effect.

Analysis of covariance (ANCOVA) Is a **statistical model** with at least one **categorical** and one **continuous predictor variable** and a continuous **outcome**.

Analysis of variance (ANOVA) Is a **statistical model** with one or more categorical **predictor variables** and a continuous **outcome**.

Ancillary variable An **outcome** variable that is unrelated to the hypothesis or research question but is measured to provide more information about the subjects or the experimental system. Such variables are useful for quality control checks.

Argument Is an input into an R function. For example, if a function takes a number and returns the square root, the number is an argument to the square-root function.

Autocorrelation Is the 'self-correlation' of a vector across time or space.

Bias Is the difference between a measured or calculated value and the true value.

Biological effects Are variations that arise from intrinsic differences between biological samples or sample material. Examples include the sex or age of the subjects. [p. 52]

Biological unit Is the entity about which we would like to make an inference, test a hypothesis, estimate some property, or draw a conclusion in an experiment. This may or may not be the same as the **experimental unit**. [p. 95]

Blinding Occurs when either the experimenter, the subject, or both are unaware of the treatment conditions while the experiment is being conducted. Blinding can remove some sources of **bias**. In animal research only the experimenter is blinded. [p. 62]

Blocking factor Is a **predictor variable** included in the analysis because it is part of the experimental design, usually because there are restrictions on complete randomisation. [p. 60]

Carry-over Is the persistence of an effect applied at an earlier time period to a later time period; for example, in N-of-1 designs.

Categorical variable Is a variable that has **discrete** levels that can be either ordered such as low/medium/high or unordered such as male/female or healthy/diseased.

Cell Is an entry in a table, usually defined as the intersection of a row and column. For example, in a spreadsheet the cell B3 is the entry for the second row and third column.

Censored An observation is censored when it is known only up to a boundary value but not beyond. For example, many biochemical measurements have an upper and/or lower limit of detection. It may only be known that a sample is below the lower limit of detection but not its exact value. Thus, there is only partial information about the value of the sample. Censoring differs from **truncation**.

Citation bias The tendency for certain results to be cited over others, especially those that are statistically significant or support the hypothesis of the researcher.

Coefficient In mathematics, a coefficient is a number that is multiplied by another variable quantity in an expression. For example, in the term $3x$, 3 is the coefficient. In statistics, coefficients are usually **parameters** in a statistical model and the terms are often used interchangeably.

Coefficient of determination (R^2) Describes the proportion of variance in an outcome variable that is accounted for, or explained by, a **statistical model**. It is often used to compare models or to describe how well a model fits the data. However, it does not take model complexity into account.

Coefficient of variation (CV) Is defined as the **standard deviation** divided by the mean. It is a measure of variability in the data relative to the mean and is commonly used to quantify the variability amongst **experimental units** or **observational units**. A lower value is preferable as it indicates that measurements are precise. [p. 197]

Confidence interval (CI) Is an interval estimate of a **parameter** used in frequentist statistics. A 95% confidence interval tells us that in repeated experiments the true value of the parameter will lie within the upper and lower bound in 95% of those experiments. It does not tell us the probability of the parameter lying within a certain region (a common misinterpretation). [p. 43]

Confounding Occurs when two or more effects cannot be separately estimated. This is a problem when one effect is the experimental effect of interest and the other is a technical or biological effect. [p. 78]

Continuous variable Is a variable that can *theoretically* take any value within a range. However, due to the imprecision in the measurements, often only discrete values are obtained. For example, the body weight of a rat can be any value (between some lower and upper limit) but the scale may only record values to the nearest tenth of a gram. Body weight is still considered continuous however.

Covariate A generic term for a (usually continuous) **predictor variable** in a **statistical model**.

Critical value Is the number that defines the cut-off for statistical significance; the calculated p-value must be lower than this value to be considered significant. It is denoted by α and is set before the data are analysed; in practice it is almost always 0.05. α is set by the experimenter while a p-value is calculated from the data – these two concepts tend to be confused.

Data frame Is a table of data with columns as variables. Data in a column must be of the same type (e.g. all numbers) but column types can differ, such as one column of numbers and another of text. It is the main data structure used by R's analysis and graphing functions.

Degrees of freedom (df) A value calculated from the total number of samples minus the number of estimated parameters. [p. 132]

Dependent variable See **outcome variable**.

Design space It is the set of all possible values that predictor values can take in designed experiments.

Discrete variable Is a variable that can (theoretically) only take a finite number of values. An example is count data, which can be 0, 1, 2, ... If the number of values is large, the variable may be treated as **continuous** in an analysis.

Editor See **text editor**.

Effect size Is a single number that quantifies the size or strength of an effect. Examples include the difference between the means of two groups or the correlation between two variables. Effect sizes are often standardised; for example, by dividing the difference between two means by the within-group variance. This can make it easier to compare effects from different experiments or outcome variables but eliminates the units in which the data were measured and is therefore less intuitive. Many standardised effect sizes have been developed. [p. 204]

Efficiency Is a measure of the precision of an experimental design or statistical test. Two designs can be compared to obtain the relative efficiency. [p. 223]

End-aligned design Staggers the time of application of treatments and ends the experiment for all the subjects at the same time in experiments that have the duration of a treatment as an experimental factor. Compare with a **front-aligned design**. [p. 76]

Error Is the variation in the outcome that cannot be explained or attributed to the treatment, biological, or technical effects, or any combination of interactions. It is similar but not equivalent to the **residuals**. [p. 55]

Experimental error Is the natural biological variation from **experimental unit** to experimental unit, even after taking into account the relevant **biological effects** such as differences between sexes, ages, genotypes, and so on. It is the error used to test for treatment effects. [p. 55]

Experimental unit (EU) The smallest piece of experimental material that is randomly and independently assigned to a different treatment condition. Examples include a person, animal, litter, cage or holding pen, fish tank, culture dish, well, or a plot of land. The EU is also called the unit of allocation or unit of randomisation and it represents the unit to be replicated to increase the sample size (N). This may or may not correspond to the **biological unit** of interest. [p. 96]

Experimentwise error rate Is the probability of at least one **false positive** result across a set of statistical tests. Also see **per-comparison error rate** and **familywise error rate**. [p. 135]

Extreme value Is a value that is even further away from the bulk of data than an **outlier**.

Factor A categorical **predictor variable** which may be under the control of the experimenter (treatment), a property of the sample (sex), or a property of the experimental set-up (microtitre plate).

Factor levels Are the categories that a **factor** can take. For example, a factor called 'Treatment' might have 'Control', 'Drug A', and 'Drug B' as levels. A factor with only one level means that the variable has been held constant throughout the experiment; for example, if the factor 'Sex' has only the level 'Male'.

Factor-level combination Is the combination of all factor levels in experiments with multiple **factors**. For example, if an experiment has one factor called 'Sex' with levels 'Male' and 'Female' and another factor called 'Genotype' with levels 'WT' and 'KO', the factor level combinations are 'Male/WT', 'Male/KO', 'Female/WT', and 'Female/KO'.

False negative Concluding that no effect or relationship is present when one actually exists (also called a Type II error).

False positive Concluding that an effect or relationship exists when in fact there is none (also called a Type I error).

Familywise error rate Is the probability of at least one **false positive** result across a set or family of related statistical tests. Also see **per-comparison error rate**. [p. 135]

Fixed effect Relates the levels of a factor to the mean of an outcome variable. Compare with a **random effect**. [p. 65]

Front-aligned design Treatments are applied to all subjects at the same time at the start of the experiment, and then they are followed for different lengths of time in experiments that have the duration of a treatment as an experimental factor. Compare with **End-aligned design**. [p. 76]

Function In mathematics, it is a mapping between a set of inputs and a set of outputs (e.g. take each input and square it). In R, it is a set of instructions to perform a task (e.g. make a graph, save a file, or square a number).

Generalisability The degree to which conclusions from an experiment are applicable to the wider world. For example, do the conclusions apply to other experimental units, other similar treatments, other organisms, and so on.

Generalised linear model Is a **statistical model** used to analyse outcome variables that are counts, proportions, binary, or skewed (e.g. log-normal).

H_0 See **null hypothesis**.

H_1 See **alternative hypothesis**.

Hidden multiplicities All of the informal visual comparisons made and patterns examined that are not statistically tested. Usually only the most extreme or striking comparisons are then tested, without taking into account all of the other comparisons made. Such a procedure is highly likely to produce false positive results. [p. 135]

Index Is a number that refers to a location in a **vector**, **matrix**, or **data frame**. The vector `c("A","B","C")` has three elements where the index number 1 refers to `"A"`, 2 refers to `"B"`, and so on. Indices can be used to select a subset of elements, rows, or columns. [p. 357]

Independence In probability theory, two events, outcomes, or distributions are independent when knowledge of one tells us nothing about the other. A statistical analysis assumes that the **errors** are independent, and violations of this assumption can occur when there is **pseudoreplication**.

Independent variable See **Predictor variable**.

Interaction effect Occurs when the effect of one predictor variable depends on the value of another variable. [p. 68]

Latent variable Is a variable that is not directly measured, such as cognitive functioning or psychological and emotional states. These are inferred from tests, observations, or clinical assessments, but not directly measured like a person's height or weight. [p. 12]

Leverage Measures how far a sample is from the others based on the **predictor variables** and not the **outcome variables**. A sample with high leverage may be influential in an analysis.

Linear model Is a **statistical model** that describes how the **predictor variables** are related to the **outcome variables**. The 'linear' part describes how the *parameters* are related and does not refer to straight lines or linear relationships. Most of the standard statistical tests (e.g. *t*-test, ANOVA, ANCOVA, regression) are examples of linear models.

Main effect Is the effect of one predictor variable averaged over the others in an experiment with multiple predictors. Compare with an **interaction effect** and a **simple effect**.

Matrix In R, it is a data table where all elements must be of the same type, usually numeric. Compare with a **data frame**.

Measurement error Is variation in measurements because of the inability to perfectly measure the outcome. [p. 55]

Median Is the middlemost number in an ordered set of numbers. If there is no middle number because the set is even, then the median is the mean of the two middle numbers.

Meta-analysis Is a statistical method of combining the results from multiple studies.

Mixed-effects model A **statistical model** that contains both **fixed** and **random effects**.

Negative control Is an experimental condition that is known to induce no effect. It is sometimes called the 'all but *X*' condition, where *X* is the treatment or experimental intervention of interest. The negative control group should be as similar as possible to the treated groups, except that *X* is absent. [p. 74]

Nonparametric Refers to statistical methods that do not rely on a probability distribution to model the data.

Nuisance variable A term for a **predictor variable** that is of no scientific interest but may affect the outcome. It is usually a **technical** factor.

Null hypothesis (H_0) Is the hypothesis that there is no association between variables or no difference between groups. The data are used to reject the null hypothesis and to conclude that the **alternative hypothesis** is true.

Observational unit The biological entity on which measurements are made. It is also called the sampling or measurement unit. It may or may not correspond to the **experimental unit** or **biological unit**. [p. 99]

Omnibus test Is an overall test of a hypothesis, usually in an ANOVA; for example, testing if the means of several groups are equal. The overall F-statistic and p-value is an omnibus test of the equality of group means.

One-tailed test A statistical test in which the **null hypothesis** can only be rejected in one direction. For example, if we hypothesise that the mean of group X is greater than the mean of group Y, then a one-tailed test can only return a significant result in the hypothesised direction. If the mean of group X is much *less than* the mean of group Y, the test will never be significant. The trade-off is that a one-tailed test has greater power to detect an effect in the hypothesised direction compared with a **two-tailed test**.

Orthogonal In **statistical models**, two **predictor variables** are orthogonal if they are uncorrelated. [p. 128]

Outcome variable Is the variable that is measured and that you want to make an inference about. It is also called the response, criterion, or dependent variable and often denoted as Y. It is the variable to the left of the tilde ($\sim$) in R formulae.

Outlier Is defined as a data point that is far from the bulk of the other data points. Outliers in the raw data are not necessarily a problem because they may have little influence on the parameter estimates, and they may be accounted for by variables in the statistical model. Of greater concern are **residual** outliers.

Overfitting Occurs when a statistical model considers noise in the data as part of the signal. This can occur when the model has too many parameters relative to the number of observations or includes many irrelevant **predictor variables**. Such models usually have poor predictive performance on new data.

Parameter In the context of a probabilistic model, a parameter is a number that defines a particular distribution from a large family of possible distributions. For example, we often talk of a 'normal distribution', but there are infinitely many normal distributions having different means (μ) and variances (σ). The parameters $\mu = 1$ and $\sigma = 2.5$ specify one particular distribution, and often the purpose of an analysis is to estimate or determine the parameters given some data. **Statistical models** have parameters with unknown values and the data are used to obtain estimates for them. For example, in this equation for a straight line $y = \beta_0 + \beta_1 \times x$, β_0 and β_1 are the parameters which describe the intercept and slope for the variables y and x. β_0 and β_1 are also called **coefficients**.

Per-comparison error rate Is the probability of a **false positive** result when a single statistical test is conducted (is usually set by the researcher to 0.05). Compare with the **familywise** and **experimentwise error rate**. [p. 135]

Placebo effect Occurs when a treatment exhibits a response because the recipient believes that it will be effective. Withholding information about the treatment received (**blinding**) is the main method of controlling for it.

Population Is a complete set of items that we wish to make an inference about; for example, all people with a disease. It is usually not possible to observe all items and therefore a subset of the total population is usually taken – that is, a **sample**.

Positive control Are treatments or experimental interventions that are known to induce the effect that one is interested in detecting. [p. 74]

***Post hoc* test** Is a statistical test or analysis that is not specified before the data were collected and is often used when an interesting pattern is detected. This can lead to more **false positive** results. Many *post hoc* tests are available that try to control the number of false positives, with varying degrees of success. [p. 135]

Power Is the ability of a statistical test to detect true effects. More formally, it is the probability of rejecting the null hypothesis when it is false. If the power of a test is 0.8, there is an 80% chance of obtaining a significant result. [p. 206]

Predictor variable Is a variable that the experimenter manipulates (e.g. treatment condition) or is a property of the samples (e.g. sex). It is also called the explanatory or independent variable and is often denoted as X. It is the variable to the right of the tilde ($\sim$) in R formulae.

Pseudoreplication Occurs when the **experimental unit** is incorrectly defined in an analysis, usually because the sample size is incorrectly thought to be the number of **biological units** or **observational units**, instead of the number of experimental units. In such cases the number of experimental units is typically less than the number of biological or observational units, leading to an inflated sample size, p-values that are inappropriately small, and confidence intervals that are artificially precise. [p. 94]

Publication bias The tendency for certain results to be published over others, usually those with a p-value < 0.05 or that support the hypothesis of the researcher. This distorts the literature because not all information is available to assess treatment or experimental effects.

***p*-value** Is the probability of results equal to or more extreme than those obtained, given that the null hypothesis is true ($P(\text{Data}|H_0)$). [p. 38]

Quadratic From the Latin for 'square'. It refers to squaring a number or **variable**, usually a **term** in a statistical model. For example, $y = \beta_0 + \beta_1 x + \beta_2 x^2$ is a quadratic equation because of the x^2.

Quantile Is a generic term for divisions of the data into ordered subsets by taking cut-points at regular intervals. The quantiles are the values of the data that define the boundaries of the subsets. For example, if the data are divided into 100 subsets (also called percentiles) the 50th quantile is the value of the data point that cuts the distribution in half, such that 50% of the data is below (this is equivalent to the **median**).

R^2 See **coefficient of determination**.

Random effect Relates the levels of a factor to the variance of an outcome variable. Compare with a **fixed effect**. [p. 65]

Randomisation Is the process of using chance to group or order samples. The most common use is to allocate *experimental units* to treatment groups by a random process such as flipping a coin. This ensures that, on average, the groups will be equal on observed and unobserved characteristics. [p. 59]

Repeated measures Refers to an experiment where multiple measurements are taken on the same experimental units. Also called a longitudinal design. [p. 181]

Replication True or genuine replication consists of the application of an experimental intervention (or combinations of interventions) to multiple **experimental units**. [p. 94]

Residual Is the difference between the value of an outcome variable and the value predicted from a model. It is similar but not equivalent to the experimental **error**. For standard statistical models, the residuals should be normally distributed.

Residual sum of squares Is the variability remaining in the data that cannot be explained by the predictor variables in a **statistical model**. The equation is $\sum(x_i - \hat{x}_i)^2$, where x_i are the individual data points, and $\hat{x}_i$ are the predicted values from a statistical model.

Robust Refers to statistical methods or estimators that are not influenced by outliers or parametric assumptions. For example, the median is a robust estimate of the middle of a distribution because a single outlier will have little or no influence, unlike the mean.

Sample A set of items taken from a larger collection of items (the **population**).

Sample space Is the set of values that a variable can theoretically take. For example, the sample space for tossing a coin is {heads, tails}, whereas the sample space for the weight of a rat is all values greater than zero. Frequentist inference depends critically on the sample space being correctly defined.

Sampling error Occurs because a value calculated from a sample, such as the mean, will rarely be equal to the true population value (which is usually unknown). Increasing the sample size will decrease sampling error. [p. 55]

Simple effect Is the effect of one predictor variable at a fixed level of another predictor in an experiment with multiple predictors. Compare with a **main effect** and an **interaction effect**. [p. 155]

Skewness Is a measure of the asymmetry of a distribution. A distribution with negative skew has a long tail to the left and a distribution with a positive skew has a long tail to the right.

Standard deviation Is a measure of the variability of the data; the larger the standard deviation the further the data points are from the mean. It is the square root of the **variance**.

Standard error Is a measure of the precision of an estimate and is calculated by dividing the **standard deviation** by the square root of the sample size. Thus, as the sample size increases the standard error decreases, but the standard deviation remains the same.

Statistic Is any number calculated from a **sample** and common examples include the mean and variance as well as **test statistics** such as the t-statistic and F-statistic which are used for making inferences.

Statistical model Is a mathematical description of how **predictor variables** are related to the **outcome variables**.

Subsample Is the same as a **pseudoreplicate** in that it does not contribute to the sample size. It usually results from multiple observations on the same samples. [p. 94]

Sums of squares (SS) Is a measure of the variability in the data. It is the sum of squared deviations (distances) from the mean of the data. The equation is $\sum(x_i - \bar{x})^2$, where x_i are the individual data points, and $\bar{x}$ is the mean. The further the individual data points are from the mean, the larger the SS. The deviations from the mean are squared so that the negative values do not cancel out the positive values in the summation. [p. 124]

Technical effects Are the aspects of the experimental system which can influence the outcome and are usually not of direct interest. Examples include batches, cage effects, plate effects, trends over time, and experimenter effects. [p. 53]

Term In a mathematical or statistical equation a term is a number, parameter, variable, constant, or a combination of these multiplied together. Equations usually have multiple terms and are separated by + or − signs. For example, in the equation $y = \beta_0 + \beta_1 x + \beta_2 x^2$, the terms are β_0, $\beta_1 x$, and $\beta_2 x^2$.

Test statistic Is a single number calculated from the data used to test a hypothesis. The t- and F-statistic are the most common and a large test statistic corresponds to a small p-value.

Text editor Is software to write and edit plain text files. Microsoft's Notepad is an example, although it is not ideal for writing code. Editors used for writing code have features such as syntax highlighting, code completion, and smart indentation to make life easier. Text editors differ from word processors (e.g. Microsoft Word), which are unsuitable for writing code.

Two-tailed test A statistical test in which the **null hypothesis** can be rejected in either direction; for example, if the mean of group X is either much greater than or much less than the mean of group Y. Compare with a **one-tailed test**.

Treatment effect Is the effect due to the manipulations or interventions introduced by the experimenter. Drawing a conclusion about treatment effects is often the main reason for conducting an experiment. [p. 53]

Treatment error Is the inability to apply a treatment to all **experimental units** in exactly the same way. [p. 55]

Truncation An observation is truncated if values outside of a certain range are completely omitted, and it is unknown how many such values have been omitted. For example, suppose an automated image analysis uses a minimum value for cell size to consider an object a cell. Cells that are below this value will not be included in the analysis and thus the estimate of cell size can be biased. This is distinct from **censoring**, where the number of samples that reached the boundary are known.

Type I error See **false positive**.

Type II error See **false negative**.

Variable Is a generic term used to denote an **outcome** that is measured, a property of the sample material, a characteristic of the experimental system, or an attribute manipulated by the experimenter. Making inferences about relationships between variables is of primary interest in science and statistics.

Variance Is a measure of the spread of a set of numbers. It is the **sum of squares** divided by one less than the number of observations, $SS/n - 1$, or

$$\frac{\sum (x_i - \bar{x})^2}{(n-1)}.$$

Vector In R, it is a sequence of data elements of the same type. For example, `c(1, 3, 5, 6)` is a vector of numbers.

References

[1] (1988). When to believe the unbelievable. *Nature* 333(6176): 787.

[2] (2012). Must try harder. *Nature* 483(7391): 509.

[3] (2013). Announcement: reducing our irreproducibility. *Nature* 496: 398.

[4] Adler ID, Bootman J, Favor J, Hook G, Schriever-Schwemmer G, Welzl G, Whorton E, Yoshimura I, Hayashi M (1998). Recommendations for statistical designs of in vivo mutagenicity tests with regard to subsequent statistical analysis. *Mutat Res* 417(1): 19–30.

[5] Alberts B, Cicerone RJ, Fienberg SE, Kamb A, McNutt M, Nerem RM, Schekman R, Shiffrin R, Stodden V, Suresh S, Zuber MT, Pope BK, Jamieson KH (2015). Scientific integrity. Self-correction in science at work. *Science* 348(6242): 1420–1422.

[6] Aldrich J (1995). Correlations genuine and spurious in Pearson and Yule. *Statistical Science* 10(4): 364–376.

[7] Alexander GM, Erwin KL, Byers N, Deitch JS, Augelli BJ, Blankenhorn EP, Heiman-Patterson TD (2004). Effect of transgene copy number on survival in the G93A SOD1 transgenic mouse model of ALS. *Brain Res Mol Brain Res* 130(1–2): 7–15.

[8] Allison T, Cicchetti DV (1976). Sleep in mammals: ecological and constitutional correlates. *Science* 194(4266): 732–734.

[9] Altman DG, Bland JM (1997). Statistics notes. Units of analysis. *BMJ* 314(7098): 1874.

[10] Anglemyer AT, Krauth D, Bero L (2015). Industry sponsorship and publication bias among animal studies evaluating the effects of statins on atherosclerosis and bone outcomes: a meta-analysis. *BMC Med Res Methodol* 15(1): 12.

[11] Anscombe FJ (1973). Graphs in statistical analysis. *Am Stat* 27(1): 17–21.

[12] Austin PC, Brunner LJ (2004). Inflation of the type I error rate when a continuous confounding variable is categorized in logistic regression analyses. *Stat Med* 23(7): 1159–1178.

[13] Baddeley A, Vedel Jensen EB (2005). *Stereology for Statisticians*. Boca Raton, FL: CRC Press.

[14] Baggerly KA, Coombes KR (2009). Deriving chemosensitivity from cell lines: forensic bioinformatics and reproducible research in high-throughput biology. *Ann Appl Stat* 3(4): 1233–1830.

[15] Baggerly KA, Coombes KR, Neeley ES (2008). Run batch effects potentially compromise the usefulness of genomic signatures for ovarian cancer. *J Clin Oncol* 26(7): 1186–1187.

[16] Baggerly KA, Morris JS, Coombes KR (2004). Reproducibility of SELDI-TOF protein patterns in serum: comparing datasets from different experiments. *Bioinformatics* 20(5): 777–785.

[17] Bakker M, van Dijk A, Wicherts JM (2012). The rules of the game called psychological science. *Perspect Psychol Sci* 7(6): 543–554.

[18] Bakker M, Wicherts JM (2011). The (mis)reporting of statistical results in psychology journals. *Behav Res Methods* 43(3): 666–678.

[19] Bakker M, Wicherts JM (2014). Outlier removal and the relation with reporting errors and quality of psychological research. *PLoS One* 9(7): e103360.

[20] Bara M, Joffe AR (2014). The methodological quality of animal research in critical care: the public face of science. *Ann Intensive Care* 4: 26.

[21] Barber TX (1976). *Pitfalls in Human Research: Ten Pivotal Points*. New York, NY: Pergamon.

[22] Barnwell-Menard JL, Li Q, Cohen AA (2015). Effects of categorization method, regression type, and variable distribution on the inflation of Type-I error rate when categorizing a confounding variable. *Stat Med* 34(6): 936–949.

[23] Bate S, Karp NA (2014). A common control group: optimising the experiment design to maximise sensitivity. *PLoS One* 9(12): e114872.

[24] Bates DM, Watts DG (1988). *Nonlinear Regression Analysis and Its Applications*. Hoboken, NJ: Wiley.

[25] Bebarta V, Luyten D, Heard K (2003). Emergency medicine animal research: does use of randomization and blinding affect the results? *Acad Emerg Med* 10(6): 684–687.

[26] Bechard A, Meagher R, Mason G (2011). Environmental enrichment reduces the likelihood of alopecia in adult C57BL/6J mice. *J Am Assoc Lab Anim Sci* 50(2): 171–174.

[27] Beery AK, Zucker I (2011). Sex bias in neuroscience and biomedical research. *Neurosci Biobehav Rev* 35(3): 565–572.

[28] Begley CG (2013). Six red flags for suspect work. *Nature* 497(7450): 433–434.

[29] Begley CG, Ellis LM (2012). Drug development: raise standards for preclinical cancer research. *Nature* 483(7391): 531–533.

[30] Begley CG, Ioannidis JPA (2015). Reproducibility in science: improving the standard for basic and preclinical research. *Circ Res* 116(1): 116–126.

[31] Bello S, Krogsboll LT, Gruber J, Zhao ZJ, Fischer D, Hrobjartsson A (2014). Lack of blinding of outcome assessors in animal model experiments implies risk of observer bias. *J Clin Epidemiol* 67(9): 973–983.

[32] Benatar M (2007). Lost in translation: treatment trials in the SOD1 mouse and in human ALS. *Neurobiol Dis* 26(1): 1–13.

[33] Bennette C, Vickers A (2012). Against quantiles: categorization of continuous variables in epidemiologic research, and its discontents. *BMC Med Res Methodol* 12: 21.

[34] Benveniste J (1988). Benveniste on *Nature* investigation. *Science* 241(4869): 1028.

[35] Benveniste J (1988). Benveniste on the Benveniste affair. *Nature* 335(6193): 759.

[36] Berger MPF, Wong WK (2009). *An Introduction to Optimal Designs for Social and Biomedical Research*. Chichester, UK: Wiley.

[37] Berle D, Starcevic V (2007). Inconsistencies between reported test statistics and p-values in two psychiatry journals. *Int J Methods Psychiatr Res* 16(4): 202–207.

[38] Berrington de Gonzalez A, Cox DR (2007). Interpretation of interaction: a review. *Ann Appl Stat* 1(2): 371–385.

[39] Berry D (2012). Multiplicities in cancer research: ubiquitous and necessary evils. *J Natl Cancer Inst* 104(15): 1124–1132.

[40] Berry DA (2007). The difficult and ubiquitous problems of multiplicities. *Pharm Stat* 6(3): 155–160.

[41] Berry SM, Carlin BP, Peter Muller JJL (2010). *Bayesian Adaptive Methods for Clinical Trials*. Boca Raton, FL: CRC Press.

[42] Bissell M (2013). Reproducibility: the risks of the replication drive. *Nature* 503(7476): 333–334.

[43] Bland JM, Altman DG (1995). Comparing methods of measurement: why plotting difference against standard method is misleading. *Lancet* 346(8982): 1085–1087.

[44] Bland JM, Altman DG (2011). Comparisons against baseline within randomised groups are often used and can be highly misleading. *Trials* 12: 264.

[45] Bland JM, Altman DG (2011). Comparisons within randomised groups can be very misleading. *BMJ* 342: d561.

[46] Bland JM, Kerry SM (1997). Statistics notes. Trials randomised in clusters. *BMJ* 315(7108): 600.

[47] Bland JM, Kerry SM (1998). Statistics notes. Weighted comparison of means. *BMJ* 316(7125): 129.

[48] Bland M (2005). The *Horizon* homeopathic dilution experiment. *Significance* 2(3): 106–109.

[49] Blocker AW, Meng XL (2013). The potential and perils of preprocessing: building new foundations. *Bernoulli* 19(4): 1176–1211.

[50] Blume JD (2002). Likelihood methods for measuring statistical evidence. *Stat Med* 21(17): 2563–2599.

[51] Bolstad WM (2007). *Introduction to Bayesian Statistics*. Hoboken, NJ: Wiley.

[52] Bonate PL (2011). *Pharmacokinetic–Pharmacodynamic Modeling and Simulation*. New York, NY: Springer, 2nd edn.

[53] Borenstein M, Hedges LV, Higgins JPT, Rothstein HR (2009). *Introduction to Meta-Analysis*. Chichester, UK: Wiley.

[54] Box G (2006). *Improving Almost Anything: Ideas and Essays*. Hoboken, NJ.: Wiley.

[55] Box GEP, Cox DR (1964). An analysis of transformations (with Discussion). *J R Stat Soc B* 26: 211–252.

[56] Box GEP, Hunter JS, Hunter WG (2005). *Statistics for Experimenters: Design, Innovation, and Discovery*. Hoboken, NJ: Wiley, 2nd edn.

[57] Branham WS, Melvin CD, Han T, Desai VG, Moland CL, Scully AT, Fuscoe JC (2007). Elimination of laboratory ozone leads to a dramatic improvement in the reproducibility of microarray gene expression measurements. *BMC Biotechnol* 7: 8.

[58] Brembs B, Button K, Munafo M (2013). Deep impact: unintended consequences of journal rank. *Front Hum Neurosci* 7: 291.

[59] Breslow NE (2014). *Past, Present, and Future of Statistical Science*, chap. Lessons in biostatistics. Boca Raton, FL: CRC Press, 335–347.

[60] Bresnahan JF, Kitchell BB, Wildman MF (1983). Facial hair barbering in rats. *Lab Anim Sci* 33(3): 290–291.

[61] Brown JD (2014). *Linear Models in Matrix Form*. New York, NY: Springer.

[62] Brown RE, Wong AA (2007). The influence of visual ability on learning and memory performance in 13 strains of mice. *Learn Mem* 14(3): 134–144.

[63] Brudzynski SM (2013). Ethotransmission: communication of emotional states through ultrasonic vocalization in rats. *Curr Opin Neurobiol* 23(3): 310–317.

[64] Buja A, Cook D, Hofmann H, Lawrence M, Lee EK, Swayne DF, Wickham H (2009). Statistical inference for exploratory data analysis and model diagnostics. *Philos Transact A Math Phys Eng Sci* 367(1906): 4361–4383.

[65] Button KS, Ioannidis JPA, Mokrysz C, Nosek BA, Flint J, Robinson ESJ, Munafo MR (2013). Power failure: why small sample size undermines the reliability of neuroscience. *Nat Rev Neurosci* 14(5): 365–376.

[66] Casadevall A, Fang FC (2012). Reforming science: methodological and cultural reforms. *Infect Immun* 80(3): 891–896.

[67] Casella G (2008). *Statistical Design*. New York, NY: Springer.

[68] Chan AW, Hrobjartsson A, Haahr MT, Gotzsche PC, Altman DG (2004). Empirical evidence for selective reporting of outcomes in randomized trials: comparison of protocols to published articles. *JAMA* 291(20): 2457–2465.

[69] Chan AW, Krleza-Jeric K, Schmid I, Altman DG (2004). Outcome reporting bias in randomized trials funded by the Canadian Institutes of Health Research. *CMAJ* 171(7): 735–740.

[70] Chatfield C (1985). The initial examination of data. *J R Stat Soc* 148(3): 214–253.

[71] Chen H, Cohen P, Chen S (2007). Biased odds ratios from dichotomization of age. *Stat Med* 26(18): 3487–3497.

[72] Christensen R (2005). Testing Fisher, Neyman, Pearson, and Bayes. *Am Stat* 59(2): 121–126.

[73] Clayton JA, Collins FS (2014). Policy: NIH to balance sex in cell and animal studies. *Nature* 509(7500): 282–283.

[74] Cleveland WS (1993). *Visualizing Data*. Summit, NJ: Hobart Press.

[75] Cleveland WS (1994). *The Elements of Graphing Data*. Summit, NJ: Hobart Press, revised edn.

[76] Cohen J (1968). Multiple regression as a general data-analytic system. *Psychol Bull* 70(6): 426–443.

[77] Cohen J (1983). The cost of dichotomization. *Appl Psychol Meas* 7(3): 249–253.

[78] Cohen J (1988). *Statistical Power Analysis for the Behavioral Sciences*. Hillsdale, NJ: Lawrence Erlbaum Associates, 2nd edn.

[79] Cohen J (1994). The earth is round ($p < .05$). *Am Psychol* 49(12): 997–1003.

[80] Collins FS, Tabak LA (2014). Policy: NIH plans to enhance reproducibility. *Nature* 505(7485): 612–613.

[81] Colquhoun D (1971). *Lectures on Biostatistics: An Introduction to Statistics with Applications in Biology and Medicine*. Oxford, UK: Clarendon Press.

[82] Cordell HJ (2002). Epistasis: what it means, what it doesn't mean, and statistical methods to detect it in humans. *Hum Mol Genet* 11(20): 2463–2468.

[83] Couzin-Frankel J (2013). The power of negative thinking. *Science* 342(6154): 68–69.

[84] Couzin-Frankel J (2013). When mice mislead. *Science* 342(6161): 922–923, 925.

[85] Crawley MJ (2002). *Statistical Computing: An Introduction to Data Analysis Using S-Plus*. Chichester, UK: Wiley.

[86] Crawley MJ (2007). *The R Book*. Chichester, UK: Wiley.

[87] Crossley NA, Sena E, Goehler J, Horn J, van der Worp B, Bath PMW, Macleod M, Dirnagl U (2008). Empirical evidence of bias in the design of experimental stroke studies: a metaepidemiologic approach. *Stroke* 39(3): 929–934.

[88] Cumming G (2012). *Understanding the New Statistics: Effect Sizes, Confidence Intervals, and Meta-Analysis*. New York, NY: Routledge.

[89] Cumming G, Fidler F, Vaux DL (2007). Error bars in experimental biology. *J Cell Biol* 177(1): 7–11.

[90] D'Alonzo KT (2004). The Johnson–Neyman procedure as an alternative to ANCOVA. *West J Nurs Res* 26(7): 804–812.

[91] Davenas E, Beauvais F, Amara J, Oberbaum M, Robinzon B, Miadonna A, Tedeschi A, Pomeranz B, Fortner P, Belon P, Sainte-Laudy J, Poitevin B, Benveniste J (1988). Human basophil degranulation triggered by very dilute antiserum against IgE. *Nature* 333(6176): 816–818.

[92] de Winter JC, Dodou D (2015). A surge of p-values between 0.041 and 0.049 in recent decades (but negative results are increasing rapidly too). *PeerJ* 3: e733.

[93] Dempster AP (1998). Logicist statistics. I. Models and modeling. *Stat Sci* 13(3): 248–276.

[94] Dennis B (2004). Statistics and the scientific method, in ecology. In ML Tapper, SR Lele, eds, *The Nature of Scientific Evidence: Statistical, Philosophical, and Empirical Considerations*. Chicago, IL: University of Chicago Press, 327–378.

[95] Dienes Z (2011). Bayesian versus orthodox statistics: which side are you on? *Perspectives on Psychological Science* 6(3): 274–290.

[96] Diggle PJ (2003). *Statistical Analysis of Spatial Point Patterns*. London: Hodder Arnold, 2nd edn.

[97] Dirnagl U (2006). Bench to bedside: the quest for quality in experimental stroke research. *J Cereb Blood Flow Metab* 26(12): 1465–1478.

[98] Djulbegovic B, Kumar A, Glasziou P, Miladinovic B, Chalmers I (2013). Medical research: trial unpredictability yields predictable therapy gains. *Nature* 500(7463): 395–396.

[99] Donner A, Klar N (2004). Pitfalls of and controversies in cluster randomization trials. *Am J Public Health* 94(3): 416–422.

[100] Dopico XC, Evangelou M, Ferreira RC, Guo H, Pekalski ML, Smyth DJ, Cooper N, Burren OS, Fulford AJ, Hennig BJ, Prentice AM, Ziegler AG, Bonifacio E, Wallace C, Todd JA (2015). Widespread seasonal gene expression reveals annual differences in human immunity and physiology. *Nat Commun* 6: 7000.

[101] Drăghici S (2012). *Statistics and Data Analysis for Microarrays Using R and Bioconductor*. Boca Raton, FL: CRC Press, 2nd edn.

[102] Dunlap WP, Dietz J, Cortina JM (1997). The spurious correlation of ratios that have common variables: a Monte Carlo examination of Pearson's formula. *J Gen Psychol* 124(4): 182–193.

[103] Dunn HL (1929). Application of statistical methods in physiology. *Physiol Rev* 9(2): 275–398.

[104] Dwan K, Altman DG, Arnaiz JA, Bloom J, Chan AW, Cronin E, Decullier E, Easterbrook PJ, Elm EV, Gamble C, Ghersi D, Ioannidis JPA, Simes J, Williamson PR (2008). Systematic review of the empirical evidence of study publication bias and outcome reporting bias. *PLoS One* 3(8): e3081.

[105] Dwan K, Gamble C, Williamson PR, Kirkham JJ, Group RB (2013). Systematic review of the empirical evidence of study publication bias and outcome reporting bias: an updated review. *PLoS One* 8(7): e66844.

[106] Fanelli D (2009). How many scientists fabricate and falsify research? A systematic review and meta-analysis of survey data. *PLoS One* 4(5): e5738.

[107] Fanelli D (2012). Negative results are disappearing from most disciplines and countries. *Scientometrics* 90(3): 891–904.

[108] Fanelli D (2013). Positive results receive more citations, but only in some disciplines. *Scientometrics* 94(2): 701–709.

[109] Faraway JJ (2006). *Extending the Linear Model with R: Generalized Linear, Mixed Effects and Nonparametric Regression Models*. Boca Raton, FL: Chapman & Hall/CRC Press.

[110] Fare TL, Coffey EM, Dai H, He YD, Kessler DA, Kilian KA, Koch JE, LeProust E, Marton MJ, Meyer MR, Stoughton RB, Tokiwa GY, Wang Y (2003). Effects of atmospheric ozone on microarray data quality. *Anal Chem* 75(17): 4672–4675.

[111] Fedorov V, Mannino F, Zhang R (2009). Consequences of dichotomization. *Pharm Stat* 8(1): 50–61.

[112] Fedorov VV, Leonov SL (2014). *Optimal Design for Nonlinear Response Models*. Boca Raton, FL: Chapman & Hall/CRC Press.

[113] Feise RJ (2002). Do multiple outcome measures require p-value adjustment? *BMC Med Res Methodol* 2: 8.

[114] Festing MFW (2003). Principles: the need for better experimental design. *Trends Pharmacol Sci* 24(7): 341–345.

[115] Festing MFW (2014). Randomized block experimental designs can increase the power and reproducibility of laboratory animal experiments. *ILAR J* 55(3): 472–476.

[116] Fiedler K (2011). Voodoo correlations are everywhere: not only in neuroscience. *Perspect Psychol Sci* 6(2): 163–171.

[117] Fields RD (2014). NIH policy: mandate goes too far. *Nature* 509(7505): 340.

[118] Filardo G, Hamilton C, Hamman B, Ng HKT, Grayburn P (2007). Categorizing BMI may lead to biased results in studies investigating in-hospital mortality after isolated CABG. *J Clin Epidemiol* 60(11): 1132–1139.

[119] Firebaugh G, Gibbs JP (1985). User's guide to ratio variables. *Am Sociol Rev* 50(5): 713–722.

[120] Fisher RA (1947). The analysis of covariance method for the relation between a part and the whole. *Biometrics* 3(2): 65–68.

[121] Fisher RA (1971). *The Design of Experiments*. New York, NY: Hafner Publishing Company, 8th edn.

[122] Franco A, Malhotra N, Simonovits G (2014). Social science. Publication bias in the social sciences: unlocking the file drawer. *Science* 345(6203): 1502–1505.

[123] Freedman LP, Inglese J (2014). The increasing urgency for standards in basic biologic research. *Cancer Res* 74(15): 4024–4029.

[124] Freeman R, Weinstein E, Marincola E, Rosenbaum J, Solomon F (2001). Careers. Competition and careers in biosciences. *Science* 294(5550): 2293–2294.

[125] Garcia-Berthou E, Alcaraz C (2004). Incongruence between test statistics and P values in medical papers. *BMC Med Res Methodol* 4: 13.

[126] Garner JP (2014). The significance of meaning: why do over 90 neuroscience results fail to translate to humans, and what can we do to fix it? *ILAR J* 55(3): 438–456.

[127] Gautier L, Moller M, Friis-Hansen L, Knudsen S (2004). Alternative mapping of probes to genes for Affymetrix chips. *BMC Bioinformatics* 5: 111.

[128] Gelman A, Carlin J (2014). Beyond power calculations: assessing Type S (Sign) and Type M (Magnitude) errors. *Perspec Psychol Sci* 9(6): 641–651.

[129] Gelman A, Hill J (2007). *Data Analysis Using Regression and Multilevel/Hierarchical Models*. Cambridge, UK: Cambridge University Press.

[130] Gelman A, Loken E (2014). The AAA tranche of subprime science. *Chance* 27(1): 51–56.

[131] Gelman A, O'Rourke K (2014). Discussion: difficulties in making inferences about scientific truth from distributions of published *p*-values. *Biostatistics* 15(1): 18–23; discussion 39–45.

[132] Gelman A, Stern H (2006). The difference between 'significant' and 'not significant' is not itself statistically significant. *Am Stat* 60(4): 328–331.

[133] Gigerenzer G (2004). Mindless statistics. *J Socio-Econ* 33(5): 587–606.

[134] Giner-Sorolla R (2012). Science or art? How aesthetic standards grease the way through the publication bottleneck but undermine science. *Perspect Psychol Sci* 7(6): 562–571.

[135] Glass DJ (2007). *Experimental Design for Biologists*. Cold Spring Harbor, NY: Cold Spring Harbor Laboratory Press.

[136] Goodman S (2008). A dirty dozen: twelve *p*-value misconceptions. *Semin Hematol* 45(3): 135–140.

[137] Goodman SN (1999). Toward evidence-based medical statistics. 1: the P value fallacy. *Ann Intern Med* 130(12): 995–1004.

[138] Goodman SN, Berlin JA (1994). The use of predicted confidence intervals when planning experiments and the misuse of power when interpreting results. *Ann Intern Med* 121(3): 200–206.

[139] Goodman SN, Royall R (1988). Evidence and scientific research. *Am J Public Health* 78(12): 1568–1574.

[140] Grace JB (2006). *Structural Equation Modeling and Natural Systems*. Cambridge, UK: Cambridge University Press.

[141] Greenberg SA (2009). How citation distortions create unfounded authority: analysis of a citation network. *BMJ* 339: b2680.

[142] Greenberg SA (2011). Understanding belief using citation networks. *J Eval Clin Pract* 17(2): 389–393.

[143] Greenwald AG (1975). Consequences of prejudice against the null hypothesis. *Psychol Bull* 82(1): 1–20.

[144] Grieve AP (2015). How to test hypotheses if you must. *Pharm Stat* 14(2): 139–150.

[145] Gueorguieva R, Krystal JH (2004). Move over ANOVA: progress in analyzing repeated-measures data and its reflection in papers published in the Archives of General Psychiatry. *Arch Gen Psychiatry* 61(3): 310–317.

[146] Guo Y, Logan HL, Glueck DH, Muller KE (2013). Selecting a sample size for studies with repeated measures. *BMC Med Res Methodol* 13: 100.

[147] Harper KN, Peters BA, Gamble MV (2013). Batch effects and pathway analysis: two potential perils in cancer studies involving DNA methylation array analysis. *Cancer Epidemiol Biomarkers Prev* 22(6): 1052–1060.

[148] Haseman JK, Hogan MD (1975). Selection of the experimental unit in teratology studies. *Teratology* 12(2): 165–171.

[149] Healy MJR (1984). Prospects for the future: where has statistics failed? *J R Stat Soc* 147(2): 368–374.

[150] Hector A, von Felten S, Schmid B (2010). Analysis of variance with unbalanced data: an update for ecology & evolution. *J Anim Ecol* 79(2): 308–316.

[151] Hilbe JM (2011). *Negative Binomial Regression*. Cambridge, UK: Cambridge University Press, 2nd edn.

[152] Hilbe JM (2014). *Modeling Count Data*. Cambridge, UK: Cambridge University Press.

[153] Hinkelmann K, Kempthorne O (2008). *Design and Analysis of Experiments, Volume 1: Introduction to Experimental Design*. Hoboken, NJ: Wiley, 2nd edn.

[154] Hirst JA, Howick J, Aronson JK, Roberts N, Perera R, Koshiaris C, Heneghan C (2014). The need for randomization in animal trials: an overview of systematic reviews. *PLoS One* 9(6): e98856.

[155] Hoekstra R, Morey RD, Rouder JN, Wagenmakers EJ (2014). Robust misinterpretation of confidence intervals. *Psychon Bull Rev* 21(5): 1157–1164.

[156] Hoenig J, Heisey D (2001). The abuse of power: the pervasive fallacy of power calculations for data analysis. *Am Stat* 55(1): 19–24.

[157] Holland T, Holland C (2011). Unbiased histological examinations in toxicological experiments (or, the informed leading the blinded examination). *Toxicol Pathol* 39(4): 711–714.

[158] Holman L, Head ML, Lanfear R, Jennions MD (2015). Evidence of experimental bias in the life sciences: why we need blind data recording. *PLoS Biol* 13(7): e1002190.

[159] Holson RR, Pearce B (1992). Principles and pitfalls in the analysis of prenatal treatment effects in multiparous species. *Neurotoxicol Teratol* 14(3): 221–228.

[160] Hooijmans CR, Rovers MM, de Vries RBM, Leenaars M, Ritskes-Hoitinga M, Langendam MW (2014). SYRCLE's risk of bias tool for animal studies. *BMC Med Res Methodol* 14: 43.

[161] Horwitz RI, Abell JE, Christian JB, Wivel AE (2014). Right answers, wrong questions in clinical research. *Sci Transl Med* 6(221): 221fs5.

[162] Hu J, Coombes KR, Morris JS, Baggerly KA (2005). The importance of experimental design in proteomic mass spectrometry experiments: some cautionary tales. *Brief Funct Genomic Proteomic* 3(4): 322–331.

[163] Hubbard R, Bayarri MJ (2003). Confusion over measures of evidence (p's) versus errors (α's) in classical statistical testing. *Am Stat* 57(3): 171–178.

[164] Hughes CW (1979). Outcome of early experience studies as affected by between-litter variance. *J Nutr* 109(4): 642–645.

[165] Hurlbert SH (1984). Pseudoreplication and the design of ecological field experiments. *Ecol Monogr* 54(2): 187–211.

[166] Imbens GW, Rubin DB (2015). *Causal Inference for Statistics, Social, and Biomedical Sciences: An Introduction*. Cambridge, UK: Cambridge University Press.

[167] International Conference on Harmonisation (1993). Detection of toxicity to reproduction for medicinal products and toxicity to male fertility. *S5(R2)*.

[168] Ioannidis JPA (2005). Why most published research findings are false. *PLoS Med* 2(8): e124.

[169] Ioannidis JPA (2008). Why most discovered true associations are inflated. *Epidemiology* 19(5): 640–648.

[170] Ioannidis JPA (2012). Scientific inbreeding and same-team replication: type D personality as an example. *J Psychosom Res* 73(6): 408–410.

[171] Ioannidis JPA (2012). Why science is not necessarily self-correcting. *Perspect Psychol Sci* 7(6): 645–654.

[172] Ioannidis JPA (2014). How to make more published research true. *PLoS Med* 11(10): e1001747.

[173] Ioannidis JPA, Allison DB, Ball CA, Coulibaly I, Cui X, Culhane AC, Falchi M, Furlanello C, Game L, Jurman G, Mangion J, Mehta T, Nitzberg M, Page GP, Petretto E, van Noort V (2009). Repeatability of published microarray gene expression analyses. *Nat Genet* 41(2): 149–155.

[174] Irwin J, McClelland G (2003). Negative consequences of dichotomizing continuous predictor variables. *J Mark Res* 40: 366–371.

[175] Jaynes ET (2003). *Probability Theory: The Logic of Science*. Cambridge, UK: Cambridge University Press.

[176] Jergas H, Baethge C (2014). Quotation accuracy in medical journal articles: a systematic review and meta-analysis. *PeerJ* 3: e1364.

[177] John LK, Loewenstein G, Prelec D (2012). Measuring the prevalence of questionable research practices with incentives for truth telling. *Psychol Sci* 23(5): 524–532.

[178] Jones LV (1955). Statistical theory and research design. *Annu Rev Psychol* 6: 405–430.

[179] Jonker RM, Guenther A, Engqvist L, Schmoll T (2013). Does systematic variation improve the reproducibility of animal experiments? *Nat Methods* 10(5): 373.

[180] Kagan M, Lindman H (1980). The proper experimental unit, once again. *J Res Sci Teach* 17(4): 351–358.

[181] Kalueff AV, Minasyan A, Keisala T, Shah ZH, Tuohimaa P (2006). Hair barbering in mice: implications for neurobehavioural research. *Behav Processes* 71(1): 8–15.

[182] Kelley K, Maxwell SE, Rausch JR (2003). Obtaining power or obtaining precision. Delineating methods of sample-size planning. *Eval Health Prof* 26(3): 258–287.

[183] Kelner KL (2013). Playing our part. *Sci Transl Med* 5: 190ed7.

[184] Kenny PW, Montanari CA (2013). Inflation of correlation in the pursuit of drug-likeness. *J Comput Aided Mol Des* 27(1): 1–13.

[185] Kerr NL (1998). HARKing: hypothesizing after the results are known. *Pers Soc Psychol Rev* 2(3): 196–217.

[186] Kerry SM, Bland JM (1998). Analysis of a trial randomised in clusters. *BMJ* 316(7124): 54.

[187] Kerry SM, Bland JM (1998). The intracluster correlation coefficient in cluster randomisation. *BMJ* 316(7142): 1455.

[188] Kerry SM, Bland JM (1998). Sample size in cluster randomisation. *BMJ* 316(7130): 549.

[189] Kilkenny C, Parsons N, Kadyszewski E, Festing MFW, Cuthill IC, Fry D, Hutton J, Altman DG (2009). Survey of the quality of experimental design, statistical analysis and reporting of research using animals. *PLoS One* 4(11): e7824.

[190] Kimmelman J, Mogil JS, Dirnagl U (2014). Distinguishing between exploratory and confirmatory preclinical research will improve translation. *PLoS Biol* 12(5): e1001863.

[191] Kleikers PW, Hooijmans C, Gob E, Langhauser F, Rewell SS, Radermacher K, Ritskes-Hoitinga M, Howells DW, Kleinschnitz C, Schmidt HHW (2015). A combined pre-clinical meta-analysis and randomized confirmatory trial approach to improve data validity for therapeutic target validation. *Sci Rep* 5: 13428.

[192] Klein G (2014). *Seeing What Others Don't*. London, UK: Nicholas Brealey Publishing.

[193] Kline RB (2004). *Beyond Significance Testing: Reforming Data Analysis Methods in Behavioral Research*. Washington, DC: APA.

[194] Klotz IM (1980). The N-Ray affair. *Sci Am* 242(5): 168–175.

[195] Kono H, Rock KL (2008). How dying cells alert the immune system to danger. *Nat Rev Immunol* 8(4): 279–289.

[196] Krause A, O'Connell M (Eds.) (2012). *A Picture is Worth a Thousand Tables: Graphics in Life Sciences*. New York, NY: Springer.

[197] Krauth D, Anglemyer A, Philipps R, Bero L (2014). Nonindustry-sponsored preclinical studies on statins yield greater efficacy estimates than industry-sponsored studies: a meta-analysis. *PLoS Biol* 12(1): e1001770.

[198] Krawczyk M (2015). The search for significance: a few peculiarities in the distribution of *p* values in experimental psychology literature. *PLoS One* 10(6): e0127872.

[199] Kristensen M, Hansen T (2004). Statistical analyses of repeated measures in physiological research: a tutorial. *Adv Physiol Educ* 28(1–4): 2–14.

[200] Kronmal RA (1993). Spurious correlation and the fallacy of the ratio standard revisited. *J R Stat Soc* 156(3): 379–392.

[201] Kruschke JK (2010). What to believe: Bayesian methods for data analysis. *Trends Cogn Sci* 14(7): 293–300.

[202] Kruschke JK (2011). Bayesian assessment of null values via parameter estimation and model comparison. *Perspect Psychol Sci* 6(3): 299–312.

[203] Kruschke JK (2011). *Doing Bayesian Data Analysis: A Tutorial with R and BUGS*. New York, NY: Academic Press.

[204] Kruschke JK (2013). Bayesian estimation supersedes the *t* test. *J Exp Psychol Gen* 142(2): 573–603.

[205] Kuhn M, Johnson K (2013). *Applied Predictive Modeling*. New York, NY: Spinger.

[206] Kuhn TS (1996). *The Structure of Scientific Revolutions*. Chicago, IL: University of Chicago Press, 3rd edn.

[207] Kurien BT, Gross T, Scofield RH (2005). Barbering in mice: a model for trichotillomania. *BMJ* 331(7531): 1503–1505.

[208] Kuss O (2013). The danger of dichotomizing continuous variables: a visualization. *Teaching Statistics* 35(2): 78–79.

[209] Kyzas PA, Denaxa-Kyza D, Ioannidis JPA (2007). Almost all articles on cancer prognostic markers report statistically significant results. *Eur J Cancer* 43(17): 2559–2579.

[210] Laber K, Veatch LM, Lopez MF, Mulligan JK, Lathers DMR (2008). Effects of housing density on weight gain, immune function, behavior, and plasma corticosterone concentrations in BALB/c and C57BL/6 mice. *J Am Assoc Lab Anim Sci* 47(2): 16–23.

[211] Landsheer JA, van den Wittenboer G (2015). Unbalanced 2×2 factorial designs and the interaction effect: a troublesome combination. *PLoS One* 10(3): e0121412.

[212] Lauss M, Visne I, Kriegner A, Ringner M, Jonsson G, Hoglund M (2013). Monitoring of technical variation in quantitative high-throughput datasets. *Cancer Inform* 12: 193–201.

[213] Lawson J (2015). *Design and Analysis of Experiments with R*. Boca Raton, FL: CRC Press.

[214] Lazic SE (2008). Why we should use simpler models if the data allow this: relevance for ANOVA designs in experimental biology. *BMC Physiol* 8: 16.

[215] Lazic SE (2009). Statistical evaluation of methods for quantifying gene expression by autoradiography in histological sections. *BMC Neurosci* 10: 5.

[216] Lazic SE (2010). The problem of pseudoreplication in neuroscientific studies: is it affecting your analysis? *BMC Neurosci* 11(1): 5.

[217] Lazic SE (2010). Relating hippocampal neurogenesis to behavior: the dangers of ignoring confounding variables. *Neurobiol Aging* 31(12): 2169–2171.

[218] Lazic SE (2012). Using causal models to distinguish between neurogenesis-dependent and -independent effects on behaviour. *J R Soc Interface* 9(70): 907–917.

[219] Lazic SE (2013). Comment on 'Stress in puberty unmasks latent neuropathological consequences of prenatal immune activation in mice'. *Science* 340(6134): 811; discussion 811.

[220] Lazic SE (2015). Analytical strategies for the marble burying test: avoiding impossible predictions and invalid *p*-values. *BMC Res Notes* 8(1): 141.

[221] Lazic SE (2015). Ranking, selecting, and prioritising genes with desirability functions. *PeerJ* 3: e1444.

[222] Lazic SE, Essioux L (2013). Improving basic and translational science by accounting for litter-to-litter variation in animal models. *BMC Neurosci* 14(1): 37.

[223] Lazic SE, Fuss J, Gass P (2014). Quantifying the behavioural relevance of hippocampal neurogenesis. *PLoS One* 9(11): e113855.

[224] Lecoutre MP, Poitevineau J, Lecoutre B (2003). Even statisticians are not immune to misinterpretations of null hypothesis significance tests. *Int J Psychol* 38(1): 37–45.

[225] Lee MD, Wagenmakers EJ (2013). *Bayesian Cognitive Modeling: A Practical Course*. Cambridge, UK: Cambridge University Press.

[226] Lee Y, Nelder JA (2004). Conditional and marginal models: another view. *Stat Sci* 19(2): 219–238.

[227] Leek JT, Scharpf RB, Bravo HC, Simcha D, Langmead B, Johnson WE, Geman D, Baggerly K, Irizarry RA (2010). Tackling the widespread and critical impact of batch effects in high-throughput data. *Nat Rev Genet* 11(10): 733–739.

[228] Leggett NC, Thomas NA, Loetscher T, Nicholls MER (2013). The life of p: 'just significant' results are on the rise. *Q J Exp Psychol (Hove)* 66(12): 2303–2309.

[229] Lenth RV (2007). Statistical power calculations. *J Anim Sci* 85(13 Suppl): E24–E29.

[230] Levey WA, Manore MM, Vaughan LA, Carroll SS, VanHalderen L, Felicetta J (1995). Blood pressure responses of white men with hypertension to two low-sodium metabolic diets with different levels of dietary calcium. *J Am Diet Assoc* 95(11): 1280–1287.

[231] Levin JR, Serlin RC, Seaman MA (1994). A controlled, powerful multiple-comparison strategy for several situations. *Psychol Bull* 115(1): 153–159.

[232] Levine M, Ensom MH (2001). Post hoc power analysis: an idea whose time has passed? *Pharmacotherapy* 21(4): 405–409.

[233] Lew M (2007). Good statistical practice in pharmacology. Problem 1. *Br J Pharmacol* 152(3): 295–298.

[234] Lew M (2007). Good statistical practice in pharmacology. Problem 2. *Br J Pharmacol* 152(3): 299–303.

[235] Lew MJ (2008). On contemporaneous controls, unlikely outcomes, boxes and replacing the 'Student': good statistical practice in pharmacology, problem 3. *Br J Pharmacol* 155(6): 797–803.

[236] Liang Y, Woodle SA, Shibeko AM, Lee TK, Ovanesov MV (2013). Correction of microplate location effects improves performance of the thrombin generation test. *Thromb J* 11(1): 12.

[237] Lin LI (1989). A concordance correlation coefficient to evaluate reproducibility. *Biometrics* 45: 255–268.

[238] Lin LI (2000). A note on the concordance correlation coefficient. *Biometrics* 56: 324–325.

[239] Lindley D, Novick M (1981). The role of exchangeability in inference. *Ann Stat* 9(1): 45–58.

[240] Lindner MD (2007). Clinical attrition due to biased preclinical assessments of potential efficacy. *Pharmacol Ther* 115(1): 148–175.

[241] Lindsey JK, Lambert P (1998). On the appropriateness of marginal models for repeated measurements in clinical trials. *Stat Med* 17(4): 447–469.

[242] Listgarten J, Kadie C, Schadt EE, Heckerman D (2010). Correction for hidden confounders in the genetic analysis of gene expression. *Proc Natl Acad Sci USA* 107(38): 16465–16470.

[243] Liu H, Zeeberg BR, Qu G, Koru AG, Ferrucci A, Kahn A, Ryan MC, Nuhanovic A, Munson PJ, Reinhold WC, Kane DW, Weinstein JN (2007). AffyProbeMiner: a web resource for computing or retrieving accurately redefined Affymetrix probe sets. *Bioinformatics* 23(18): 2385–2390.

[244] Loftus GR (1978). On interpretation of interactions. *Mem Cognition* 6(3).

[245] Loftus GR (1996). Psychology will be a much better science when we change the way we analyze data. *Curr Dir Psychol* 5(6): 161–171.

[246] Lovell DP (1997). Issues in the experimental design and statistical analysis of in vitro mutagenicity tests. *Drug Inf J* 31: 345–356.

[247] Loven J, Orlando DA, Sigova AA, Lin CY, Rahl PB, Burge CB, Levens DL, Lee TI, Young RA (2012). Revisiting global gene expression analysis. *Cell* 151(3): 476–482.

[248] Lubin JH, Colt JS, Camann D, Davis S, Cerhan JR, Severson RK, Bernstein L, Hartge P (2004). Epidemiologic evaluation of measurement data in the presence of detection limits. *Environ Health Perspect* 112(17): 1691–1696.

[249] Lundholt BK, Scudder KM, Pagliaro L (2003). A simple technique for reducing edge effect in cell-based assays. *J Biomol Screen* 8(5): 566–570.

[250] MacCallum RC, Zhang S, Preacher KJ, Rucker DD (2002). On the practice of dichotomization of quantitative variables. *Psychol Methods* 7(1): 19–40.

[251] Macleod M (2011). Why animal research needs to improve. *Nature* 477(7366): 511.

[252] Macleod M (2014). Some salt with your statin, professor? *PLoS Biol* 12(1): e1001768.

[253] Macleod MR, Fisher M, O'Collins V, Sena ES, Dirnagl U, Bath PMW, Buchan A, van der Worp HB, Traystman R, Minematsu K, Donnan GA, Howells DW (2009). Good laboratory practice: preventing introduction of bias at the bench. *Stroke* 40(3): e50–e52.

[254] Macleod MR, O'Collins T, Howells DW, Donnan GA (2004). Pooling of animal experimental data reveals influence of study design and publication bias. *Stroke* 35(5): 1203–1208.

[255] Maddox J, Randi J, Stewart WW (1988). 'High-dilution' experiments a delusion. *Nature* 334(6180): 287–291.

[256] Maiväli U (2015). *Interpreting Biomedical Science: Experiment, Evidence, and Belief.* London, UK: Academic Press.

[257] Malik M (2002). The imprecision in heart rate correction may lead to artificial observations of drug induced QT interval changes. *Pacing Clin Electrophysiol* 25(2): 209–216.

[258] Malo N, Hanley JA, Cerquozzi S, Pelletier J, Nadon R (2006). Statistical practice in high-throughput screening data analysis. *Nat Biotechnol* 24(2): 167–175.

[259] Manning WG, Mullahy J (2001). Estimating log models: to transform or not to transform? *J Health Econ* 20(4): 461–494.

[260] Martinson BC, Anderson MS, de Vries R (2005). Scientists behaving badly. *Nature* 435(7043): 737–738.

[261] Masicampo EJ, Lalande DR (2012). A peculiar prevalence of *p* values just below .05. *Q J Exp Psychol (Hove)* 65(11): 2271–2279.

[262] Matthews JN, Altman DG (1996). Statistics notes. Interaction 2: compare effect sizes not P values. *BMJ* 313(7060): 808.

[263] Maurissen J (2010). Practical considerations on the design, execution and analysis of developmental neurotoxicity studies to be published in *Neurotoxicology and Teratology*. *Neurotoxicol Teratol* 32(2): 121–123.

[264] Maxwell S, Delaney H (1993). Bivariate median splits and spurious statistical significance. *Quant Methods Psychol* 113(1): 181–190.

[265] Maxwell SE (2004). The persistence of underpowered studies in psychological research: causes, consequences, and remedies. *Psychol Methods* 9(2): 147–163.

[266] Maxwell SE, Kelley K, Rausch JR (2008). Sample size planning for statistical power and accuracy in parameter estimation. *Annu Rev Psychol* 59: 537–563.

[267] Mayo DG (1996). *Error and the Growth of Experimental Knowledge*. Chicago, IL: Chicago University Press.

[268] McClelland GH (1997). Optimal design in psychological research. *Psyhological Methods* 2(1): 3–19.

[269] McElreath R (2016). *Statistical Rethinking: A Bayesian Course with Examples in R and Stan*. Boca Raton, FL: CRC Press.

[270] McNutt M (2014). Raising the bar. *Science* 345(6192): 9.

[271] McNutt M (2014). Reproducibility. *Science* 343(6168): 229.

[272] McPherson G (1989). The scientists' view of statistics: a neglected area. *J R Stat Soc* 152(Part 2): 221–240.

[273] McShane BB, Bockenholt U (2014). You cannot step into the same river twice: when power analyses are optimistic. *Perspect Psychol Sci* 9(6): 612–625.

[274] Mead R, Gilmour SG, Mead A (2012). *Statistical Principles for the Design of Experiments: Applications to Real Experiments*. Cambridge, UK: Cambridge University Press.

[275] Mehta MV, Gandal MJ, Siegel SJ (2011). mGluR5-antagonist mediated reversal of elevated stereotyped, repetitive behaviors in the VPA model of autism. *PLoS One* 6(10): e26077.

[276] Miclaus K, Wolfinger R, Vega S, Chierici M, Furlanello C, Lambert C, Hong H, Zhang L, Yin S, Goodsaid F (2010). Batch effects in the BRLMM genotype calling algorithm influence GWAS results for the Affymetrix 500K array. *Pharmacogenomics J* 10(4): 336–346.

[277] Miekisch W, Herbig J, Schubert JK (2012). Data interpretation in breath biomarker research: pitfalls and directions. *J Breath Res* 6(3): 036007.

[278] Mobley A, Linder SK, Braeuer R, Ellis LM, Zwelling L (2013). A survey on data reproducibility in cancer research provides insights into our limited ability to translate findings from the laboratory to the clinic. *PLoS One* 8(5): e63221.

[279] Moja L, Pecoraro V, Ciccolallo L, Dall'Olmo L, Virgili G, Garattini S (2014). Flaws in animal studies exploring statins and impact on meta-analysis. *Eur J Clin Invest* 44(6): 597–612.

[280] Morey RD, Hoekstra R, Rouder JN, Lee MD, Wagenmakers EJ (2016). The fallacy of placing confidence in confidence intervals. *Psychon Bull Rev* 23(1): 103–123.

[281] Morrison DA, Morris EC (2000). Pseudoreplication in experimental designs for the manipulation of seed germination treatments. *Austral Ecology* 25(3): 292–296.

[282] Motulsky HJ (2014). Common misconceptions about data analysis and statistics. *J Pharmacol Exp Ther* 351(1): 200–205.

[283] Mouton PR (2002). *Principles and Practices of Unbiased Stereology*. Baltimore, MD: Johns Hopkins University Press.

[284] Mudge JF, Baker LF, Edge CB, Houlahan JE (2012). Setting an optimal α that minimizes errors in null hypothesis significance tests. *PLoS One* 7(2): e32734.

[285] Mudge JF, Barrett TJ, Munkittrick KR, Houlahan JE (2012). Negative consequences of using $\alpha = 0.05$ for environmental monitoring decisions: a case study from a decade of Canada's Environmental Effects Monitoring Program. *Environ Sci Technol* 46(17): 9249–9255.

[286] Mudge JF, Penny FM, Houlahan JE (2012). Optimizing α for better statistical decisions: a case study involving the pace-of-life syndrome hypothesis: optimal α levels set to minimize Type I and II errors frequently result in different conclusions from those using $\alpha = 0.05$. *Bioessays* 34(12): 1045–1049.

[287] Mullard A (2011). Reliability of 'new drug target' claims called into question. *Nat Rev Drug Discov* 10(9): 643–644.

[288] Murrell P (2005). *R Graphics*. Boca Raton, FL: Chapman & Hall/CRC Press.

[289] Naggara O, Raymond J, Guilbert F, Roy D, Weill A, Altman DG (2011). Analysis by categorizing or dichotomizing continuous variables is inadvisable: an example from the natural history of unruptured aneurysms. *Am J Neuroradiol* 32(3): 437–440.

[290] Nelder JA (1999). From statistics to statistical science. *J R Stat Soc D* 48(2): 257–269.

[291] Nelder JA, Wedderburn RWM (1972). Generalized linear models. *J R Stat Soc* 135(3): 370–384.

[292] Nevalainen T (2014). Animal husbandry and experimental design. *ILAR J* 55(3): 392–398.

[293] Nicholson A, Malcolm RD, Russ PL, Cough K, Touma C, Palme R, Wiles MV (2009). The response of C57BL/6J and BALB/cJ mice to increased housing density. *J Am Assoc Lab Anim Sci* 48(6): 740–753.

[294] Nieuwenhuis S, Forstmann BU, Wagenmakers EJ (2011). Erroneous analyses of interactions in neuroscience: a problem of significance. *Nat Neurosci* 14(9): 1105–1107.

[295] Nuzzo R (2014). Scientific method: statistical errors. *Nature* 506(7487): 150–152.

[296] Nye MJ (1980). N-rays: an episode in the history and psychology of science. *Hist Stud Phys Sci* 11(1), 125–156.

[297] OECD (2007). *Guideline for the Testing of Chemicals: Developmental Neurotoxicity Study*. Paris: OECD, 1–26.

[298] O'Hara RB, Kotze DJ (2010). Do not log-transform count data. *Methods Ecol Evol* 1(2): 118–122.

[299] Olsen CH (2003). Review of the use of statistics in infection and immunity. *Infect Immun* 71(12): 6689–6692.

[300] Olson R (2015). *Houston, We Have a Narrative: Why Science Needs Story*. Chicago, IL: University of Chicago Press.

[301] Open Science Collaboration (2015). PSYCHOLOGY. Estimating the reproducibility of psychological science. *Science* 349(6251): aac4716.

[302] Owen SV, Froman RD (2005). Why carve up your continuous data? *Res Nurs Health* 28(6): 496–503.

[303] Parker HS, Leek JT (2012). The practical effect of batch on genomic prediction. *Stat Appl Genet Mol Biol* 11(3): Article 10.

[304] Paylor R (2009). Questioning standardization in science. *Nat Methods* 6(4): 253–254.

[305] Peers IS, Ceuppens PR, Harbron C (2012). In search of preclinical robustness. *Nat Rev Drug Discov* 11(10): 733–734.

[306] Perneger TV, Courvoisier DS (2010). Interpretation of evidence in data by untrained medical students: a scenario-based study. *BMC Med Res Methodol* 10: 78.

[307] Pfannkuch M, Wild CJ (2000). Statistical thinking and statistical practice: themes gleaned from professional statisticians. *Stat Sci* 15(2): 132–152.

[308] Philip M, Benatar M, Fisher M, Savitz SI (2009). Methodological quality of animal studies of neuroprotective agents currently in phase II/III acute ischemic stroke trials. *Stroke* 40(2): 577–581.

[309] Phillips PC (2008). Epistasis: the essential role of gene interactions in the structure and evolution of genetic systems. *Nat Rev Genet* 9(11): 855–867.

[310] Pinheiro JC, Bates DM (2000). *Mixed-Effects Models in S and S-Plus*. London: Springer.

[311] Pocock SJ (1977). Group sequential methods in the design and analysis of clinical trials. *Biometrika* 64(2): 191–199.

[312] Pohl RF (Ed.) (2004). *Cognitive Illusions: A Handbook on Fallacies and Biases in Thinking Judgement and Memory*. New York, NY: Psychology Press.

[313] Poitevineau J, Lecoutre B (2001). Interpretation of significance levels by psychological researchers: the .05 cliff effect may be overstated. *Psychon Bull Rev* 8(4): 847–850.

[314] Pollitzer E (2013). Biology: cell sex matters. *Nature* 500(7460): 23–24.

[315] Poste G (2011). Bring on the biomarkers. *Nature* 469(7329): 156–157.

[316] Pound P, Bracken MB (2014). Is animal research sufficiently evidence based to be a cornerstone of biomedical research? *BMJ* 348: g3387.

[317] Prendergast BJ, Onishi KG, Zucker I (2014). Female mice liberated for inclusion in neuroscience and biomedical research. *Neurosci Biobehav Rev* 40: 1–5.

[318] Prinz F, Schlange T, Asadullah K (2011). Believe it or not: how much can we rely on published data on potential drug targets? *Nat Rev Drug Discov* 10(9): 712.

[319] Prosser JI (2010). Replicate or lie. *Environ Microbiol* 12(7): 1806–1810.

[320] Quinn GP, Keough MJ (2002). *Experimental Design and Data Analysis for Biologists*. Cambridge, UK: Cambridge University Press.

[321] Ramirez CC, Fuentes-Contreras E, Rodriguez LC, Niemeyer HM (2000). Pseudoreplication and its frequency in olfactometric laboratory studies. *Journal of Chemical Ecology* 26(6): 1423–1431.

[322] Ransohoff DF, Gourlay ML (2010). Sources of bias in specimens for research about molecular markers for cancer. *J Clin Oncol* 28(4): 698–704.

[323] Richter SH, Garner JP, Auer C, Kunert J, Wuerbel H (2010). Systematic variation improves reproducibility of animal experiments. *Nat Methods* 7(3): 167–168.

[324] Richter SH, Garner JP, Wuerbel H (2009). Environmental standardization: cure or cause of poor reproducibility in animal experiments? *Nat Methods* 6(4): 257–261.

[325] Ridley J, Kolm N, Freckelton RP, Gage MJG (2007). An unexpected influence of widely used significance thresholds on the distribution of reported P-values. *J Evol Biol* 20(3): 1082–1089.

[326] Ritz C, Streibig JC (2008). *Nonlinear Regression with R*. New York, NY: Springer.

[327] Roberts I, Kwan I, Evans P, Haig S (2002). Does animal experimentation inform human healthcare? Observations from a systematic review of international animal experiments on fluid resuscitation. *BMJ* 324(7335): 474–476.

[328] Rodgers JL, Nicewander WA, Toothaker L (1984). Linearly independent, orthogonal, and uncorrelated variables. *Am Stat* 38(2): 133–134.

[329] Rooke EDM, Vesterinen HM, Sena ES, Egan KJ, Macleod MR (2011). Dopamine agonists in animal models of Parkinson's disease: a systematic review and meta-analysis. *Parkinsonism Relat Disord* 17(5): 313–320.

[330] Rosenbaum PR (2001). Replicating effects and biases. *Am Stat* 55(3): 223–227.

[331] Rosenthal R, Gaito J (1963). The interpretation of levels of significance by psychological researchers. *J Psychol* 55: 33–38.

[332] Rosenthal R, Gaito J (1964). Further evidence for the cliff effect in the interpretation of levels of significance. *Psychol Rep* 15: 570.

[333] Rothman KJ (1990). No adjustments are needed for multiple comparisons. *Epidemiology* 1(1): 43–46.

[334] Rouder JN (2014). Optional stopping: no problem for Bayesians. *Psychon Bull Rev* 21(2): 301–308.

[335] Royston P, Altman DG, Sauerbrei W (2006). Dichotomizing continuous predictors in multiple regression: a bad idea. *Stat Med* 25(1): 127–141.

[336] Rubin DB (1976). Inference and missing data. *Biometrika* 63(3): 581–592.

[337] Rubin DB (1980). Randomization analysis of experimental data: the Fisher randomization test. *J Am Stat Assoc* 75(371): 591–593.

[338] Sackett DL (1979). Bias in analytic research. *J Chronic Dis* 32(1–2): 51–63.

[339] Sanborn AN, Hills TT (2014). The frequentist implications of optional stopping on Bayesian hypothesis tests. *Psychon Bull Rev* 21(2): 283–300.

[340] Sanborn AN, Hills TT, Dougherty MR, Thomas RP, Yu EC, Sprenger AM (2014). Reply to Rouder (2014): good frequentist properties raise confidence. *Psychon Bull Rev* 21(2): 309–311.

[341] Sandercock P, Roberts I (2002). Systematic reviews of animal experiments. *Lancet* 360(9333): 586.

[342] Sarewitz D (2012). Beware the creeping cracks of bias. *Nature* 485(7397): 149.

[343] Sarkar D (2008). *Lattice: Multivariate Data Visualization with R*. New York, NY: Springer.

[344] Schnabel J (2008). Neuroscience: standard model. *Nature* 454(7205): 682–685.

[345] Schroeder A, Mueller O, Stocker S, Salowsky R, Leiber M, Gassmann M, Lightfoot S, Menzel W, Granzow M, Ragg T (2006). The RIN: an RNA integrity number for assigning integrity values to RNA measurements. *BMC Mol Biol* 7: 3.

[346] Scott S, Kranz JE, Cole J, Lincecum JM, Thompson K, Kelly N, Bostrom A, Theodoss J, Al-Nakhala BM, Vieira FG, Ramasubbu J, Heywood JA (2008). Design, power, and interpretation of studies in the standard murine model of ALS. *Amyotroph Lateral Scler* 9(1): 4–15.

[347] Searle SR, Casella G, McCulloch CE (1992). *Variance Components*. New York, NY: Wiley.

[348] Sena ES, van der Worp HB, Bath PMW, Howells DW, Macleod MR (2010). Publication bias in reports of animal stroke studies leads to major overstatement of efficacy. *PLoS Biol* 8(3): e1000344.

[349] Senn S (2001). Two cheers for P-values? *J Epidemiol Biostat* 6(2): 193–204; discussion 205–10.

[350] Senn S (2003). Disappointing dichotomies. *Pharm Stat* 2(4): 239–240.

[351] Senn S, Julious S (2009). Measurement in clinical trials: a neglected issue for statisticians? *Stat Med* 28(26): 3189–3209.

[352] Senn SJ (2002). Power is indeed irrelevant in interpreting completed studies. *BMJ* 325(7375): 1304.

[353] Sheiner LB (1997). Learning versus confirming in clinical drug development. *Clin Pharmacol Ther* 61(3): 275–291.

[354] Shipley B (2000). *Cause and Correlation in Biology: A User's Guide to Path Analysis, Structural Equations and Causal Inference*. Cambridge, UK: Cambridge University Press.

[355] Simmons JP, Nelson LD, Simonsohn U (2011). False-positive psychology: undisclosed flexibility in data collection and analysis allows presenting anything as significant. *Psychol Sci* 22(11): 1359–1366.

[356] Simpson EH (1951). The interpretation of interaction in contingency tables. *J R Stat Soc B* 13(2): 238–241.

[357] Smith AH, Bates MN (1992). Confidence limit analyses should replace power calculations in the interpretation of epidemiologic studies. *Epidemiology* 3(5): 449–452.

[358] Sorge RE, Martin LJ, Isbester KA, Sotocinal SG, Rosen S, Tuttle AH, Wieskopf JS, Acland EL, Dokova A, Kadoura B, Leger P, Mapplebeck JCS, McPhail M, Delaney A, Wigerblad G, Schumann AP, Quinn T, Frasnelli J, Svensson CI, Sternberg WF, Mogil JS (2014). Olfactory exposure to males, including men, causes stress and related analgesia in rodents. *Nat Methods* 11(6): 629–632.

[359] Spiegelhalter DJ, Abrams KR, Myles JP (2004). *Bayesian Approaches to Clinical Trials and Health-Care Evaluation*. Hoboken, NJ: Wiley.

[360] Stang A, Poole C, Kuss O (2010). The ongoing tyranny of statistical significance testing in biomedical research. *Eur J Epidemiol* 25(4): 225–230.

[361] Steward O, Popovich PG, Dietrich WD, Kleitman N (2012). Replication and reproducibility in spinal cord injury research. *Exp Neurol* 233(2): 597–605.

[362] Strasak AM, Zaman Q, Pfeiffer KP, Gobel G, Ulmer H (2007). Statistical errors in medical research: a review of common pitfalls. *Swiss Med Wkly* 137(3–4): 44–49.

[363] Streiner DL (2002). Breaking up is hard to do: the heartbreak of dichotomizing continuous data. *Can J Psychiatry* 47(3): 262–266.

[364] Sui Y, Wu Z (2007). Alternative statistical parameter for high-throughput screening assay quality assessment. *J Biomol Screen* 12(2): 229–234.

[365] Taylor J, Yu M (2002). Bias and efficiency loss due to categorizing an explanatory variable. *J Multivar Anal* 83(1): 248–263.

[366] ter Riet G, Korevaar DA, Leenaars M, Sterk PJ, Noorden CJFV, Bouter LM, Lutter R, Elferink RPO, Hooft L (2012). Publication bias in laboratory animal research: a survey on magnitude, drivers, consequences and potential solutions. *PLoS One* 7(9): e43404.

[367] Tetlock PE, Gardner D (2015). *Superforecasting: The Art and Science of Prediction*. London, UK: Random House.

[368] Tsilidis KK, Panagiotou OA, Sena ES, Aretouli E, Evangelou E, Howells DW, Salman RAS, Macleod MR, Ioannidis JPA (2013). Evaluation of excess significance bias in animal studies of neurological diseases. *PLoS Biol* 11(7): e1001609.

[369] Tufte ER (2001). *The Visual Display of Quantitative Information*. Cheshire, CT: Graphics Press, 2nd edn.

[370] Tukey JW (1969). Analyzing data: sanctification or detective work? *Am Psychol* 24(2): 83–91.

[371] van Belle G (2002). *Statistical Rules of Thumb*. New York, NY: Wiley.

[372] van Buuren S (2012). *Flexible Imputation of Missing Data*. Boca Raton, FL: CRC Press.

[373] Van Vleck LD, Henderson CR (1965). Statistics in the design and analysis of physiology experiments. *J Anim Sci* 24(2): 559–567.

[374] van Walraven C, Hart RG (2008). Leave 'em alone: why continuous variables should be analyzed as such. *Neuroepidemiology* 30(3): 138–139.

[375] Vandenbroeck P, Wouters L, Molenberghs G, Gestel JV, Bijnens L (2006). Teaching statistical thinking to life scientists: a case-based approach. *J Biopharm Stat* 16(1): 61–75.

[376] Vaux DL (2012). Research methods: know when your numbers are significant. *Nature* 492(7428): 180–181.

[377] Vaux DL, Fidler F, Cumming G (2012). Replicates and repeats: what is the difference and is it significant? A brief discussion of statistics and experimental design. *EMBO Rep* 13(4): 291–296.

[378] Vesterinen HM, Sena ES, French C, Williams A, Chandran S, Macleod MR (2010). Improving the translational hit of experimental treatments in multiple sclerosis. *Mult Scler* 16(9): 1044–1055.

[379] Vickers AJ (2001). The use of percentage change from baseline as an outcome in a controlled trial is statistically inefficient: a simulation study. *BMC Med Res Methodol* 1: 6.

[380] Vickers AJ (2003). How many repeated measures in repeated measures designs? Statistical issues for comparative trials. *BMC Med Res Methodol* 3: 22.

[381] Visser MD, McMahon SM, Merow C, Dixon PM, Record S, Jongejans E (2015). Speeding up ecological and evolutionary computations in R; essentials of high performance computing for biologists. *PLoS Comput Biol* 11(3): e1004140.

[382] Wagenmakers EJ, Krypotos AM, Criss AH, Iverson G (2012). On the interpretation of removable interactions: a survey of the field 33 years after Loftus. *Mem Cognit* 40(2): 145–160.

[383] Wagenmakers EJ, Wetzels R, Borsboom D, van der Maas HLJ, Kievit RA (2012). An agenda for purely confirmatory research. *Perspect Psychol Sci* 7(6): 632–638.

[384] Wainer H (2009). *Picturing the Uncertain World: How to Understand, Communicate, and Control Uncertainty through Graphical Display*. Princeton, NJ: Princeton University Press.

[385] Wainer H, Gessaroli M, Verdi M (2006). Finding what is not there through the unfortunate binning of results: the Mendel effect. *CHANCE* 19(1): 49–52.

[386] Wainwright PE (1998). Issues of design and analysis relating to the use of multiparous species in developmental nutritional studies. *J Nutr* 128(3): 661–663.

[387] Wainwright PE, Leatherdale ST, Dubin JA (2007). Advantages of mixed effects models over traditional ANOVA models in developmental studies: a worked example in a mouse model of fetal alcohol syndrome. *Dev Psychobiol* 49(7): 664–674.

[388] Wald A (1945). Sequential tests of statistical hypotheses. *Ann Math Stat* 16(2): 117–186.

[389] Warton DI, Hui FKC (2011). The arcsine is asinine: the analysis of proportions in ecology. *Ecology* 92(1): 3–10.

[390] Watts DJ (2011). *Everything is Obvious: How Common Sense Fails Us*. London, UK: Atlantic Books.

[391] Weinberg CR (2001). It's time to rehabilitate the P-value. *Epidemiology* 12(3): 288–290.

[392] West BT, Welch KB, Galecki AT (2015). *Linear Mixed Models: A Practical Guide Using Statistical Software*. Boca Raton, FL: Chapman & Hall/CRC Press, 2nd edn.

[393] White CR (2003). Allometric analysis beyond heterogeneous regression slopes: use of the Johnson–Neyman technique in comparative biology. *Physiol Biochem Zool* 76(1): 135–140.

[394] Wicherts JM, Bakker M, Molenaar D (2011). Willingness to share research data is related to the strength of the evidence and the quality of reporting of statistical results. *PLoS One* 6(11): e26828.

[395] Wickham H (2009). *ggplot2: Elegant Graphics for Data Analysis*. New York, NY: Springer.

[396] Wickham H (2011). testthat: get started with testing. *The R Journal* 3(1).

[397] Wild CJ, Pfannkuch M (1999). Statistical thinking in empirical enquiry. *Int Stat Rev* 67(3): 223–248.

[398] Wilkinson L (2005). *The Grammar of Graphics*. New York, NY: Springer, 2nd edn.
[399] Wolfinger RD (2013). Reanalysis of Richter *et al.* (2010) on reproducibility. *Nat Methods* 10(5): 373–374.
[400] Wong AA, Brown RE (2013). Prevention of vision loss protects against age-related impairment in learning and memory performance in DBA/2J mice. *Front Aging Neurosci* 5: 52.
[401] Wuerbel H, Richter SH, Garner JP (2013). Reply to: 'Reanalysis of Richter *et al.* (2010) on reproducibility'. *Nat Methods* 10(5): 374.
[402] Xie Y (2015). *Dynamic Documents with R and knitr*. Boca Raton, FL: Chapman & Hall/CRC Press, 2nd edn.
[403] Yang H, Harrington CA, Vartanian K, Coldren CD, Hall R, Churchill GA (2008). Randomization in laboratory procedure is key to obtaining reproducible microarray results. *PLoS One* 3(11): e3724.
[404] Yee D, Ho A (2015). Discreteness causes bias in percentage-based comparisons: a case study from educational testing. *Am Stat* 69(3): 174–181.
[405] Yildiz A, Hayirli A, Okumus Z, Kaynar O, Kisa F (2007). Physiological profile of juvenile rats: effects of cage size and cage density. *Lab Anim (NY)* 36(2): 28–38.
[406] Yin J, McLoughlin S, Jeffery IB, Glaviano A, Kennedy B, Higgins DG (2010). Integrating multiple genome annotation databases improves the interpretation of microarray gene expression data. *BMC Genomics* 11: 50.
[407] Young ME (2016). The problem with categorical thinking by psychologists. *Behav Processes* 123: 43–53.
[408] Young NS, Ioannidis JPA, Al-Ubaydli O (2008). Why current publication practices may distort science. *PLoS Med* 5(10): e201.
[409] Yu EC, Sprenger AM, Thomas RP, Dougherty MR (2014). When decision heuristics and science collide. *Psychon Bull Rev* 21(2): 268–282.
[410] Yu H, Wang F, Tu K, Xie L, Li YY, Li YX (2007). Transcript-level annotation of Affymetrix probesets improves the interpretation of gene expression data. *BMC Bioinformatics* 8: 194.
[411] Yule GU (1924). The function of statistical method in scientific investigation. Tech. rep., Industrial Fatigue Research Board, Med. Res. Council, Report 28, 1–14.
[412] Zhang J, Chung T, Oldenburg K (1999). A simple statistical parameter for use in evaluation and validation of high throughput screening assays. *J Biomol Screen* 4(2): 67–73.
[413] Zhang XD (2007). A pair of new statistical parameters for quality control in RNA interference high-throughput screening assays. *Genomics* 89(4): 552–561.
[414] Zimmermann H, Gerhard D, Dingermann T, Hothorn LA (2010). Statistical aspects of design and validation of microtitre-plate-based linear and non-linear parallel in vitro bioassays. *Biotechnol J* 5(1): 62–74.
[415] Zorrilla EP (1997). Multiparous species present problems (and possibilities) to developmentalists. *Dev Psychobiol* 30(2): 141–150.
[416] Zuur AF, Ieno EN, Walker NJ, Saveliev AA, Smith GM (2009). *Mixed Effects Models and Extensions in Ecology with R*. New York, NY: Springer.

Index